PROSTHETICS AND ASSISTIVE TECHNOLOGY IN ANCIENT GREECE AND ROME

This is the first comprehensive study of prosthetics and assistive technology in classical antiquity, integrating literary, documentary, archaeological, and bioarchaeological evidence to provide as full a picture as possible of their importance for the lived experience of people with disabilities at that time. The volume is not only a work of disability history but also one of medical, scientific, and technological history, and so will be of interest to members of multiple academic disciplines across multiple historical periods. The chapters cover extremity prostheses; facial prostheses; prosthetic hair; the design, commission, and manufacture of prostheses and assistive technology; and the role of caregivers in the lives of ancient people with impairments and disabilities. Lavishly illustrated, the study further contains informative tables that collate the aforementioned different types of evidence in an easily accessible way.

JANE DRAYCOTT is Lecturer in Ancient History at the University of Glasgow. Her research investigates science, technology, and medicine in the ancient world. She has published extensively on the history and archaeology of medicine, impairment, and disability in the ancient world, including the monographs *Roman Domestic Medical Practice in Central Italy from the Middle Republic to the Early Empire* (2019) and *Approaches to Healing in Roman Egypt* (2012), and the edited volumes *Prostheses in Antiquity* (2019) and *Bodies of Evidence: Ancient Anatomical Votives Past, Present and Future* (2017).

PROSTHETICS AND ASSISTIVE TECHNOLOGY IN ANCIENT GREECE AND ROME

JANE DRAYCOTT
University of Glasgow

CAMBRIDGE
UNIVERSITY PRESS

CAMBRIDGE
UNIVERSITY PRESS

University Printing House, Cambridge CB2 8BS, United Kingdom

One Liberty Plaza, 20th Floor, New York, NY 10006, USA

477 Williamstown Road, Port Melbourne, VIC 3207, Australia

314–321, 3rd Floor, Plot 3, Splendor Forum, Jasola District Centre, New Delhi – 110025, India

103 Penang Road,#05–06/07, Visioncrest Commercial, Singapore 238467

Cambridge University Press is part of the University of Cambridge.

It furthers the University's mission by disseminating knowledge in the pursuit of education, learning, and research at the highest international levels of excellence.

www.cambridge.org
Information on this title: www.cambridge.org/9781009168397
DOI: 10.1017/9781009168410

First published 2023

A catalogue record for this publication is available from the British Library.

ISBN 978-1-009-16839-7 Hardback

For Isabel Ruffell, with thanks.

Contents

List of Figures — *page* viii
List of Tables — x
Acknowledgements — xi
List of Abbreviations — xiii

Introduction — 1
1 Extremity Prostheses and Assistive Technology — 40
2 Facial Prostheses — 73
3 Hair Prostheses — 102
4 Design, Commission, and Manufacture of Prostheses — 124
5 Living Prostheses — 154
Conclusion — 169

References — 176
Index Locorum — 195
Index — 200

Figures

I.1	Page from Jacob de Voragine's *The Golden Legend* manuscript.	*page* 3
I.2	Greek votive relief.	6
I.3	Anglesey Leg.	13
I.4	Naturally useful greave.	17
I.5	Gleed 3D greave.	18
I.6	Auldearn Antiques greave.	19
I.7	Medical corset belonging to Frida Kahlo.	20
I.8	Prosthetic leg belonging to Frida Kahlo.	21
I.9	Vine Arm designed by the Alternative Limb Project for Kelly Knox.	22
I.10	Snake Arm designed by the Alternative Limb Project for Jo-Jo Cranfield.	23
I.11	Floral Leg designed by the Alternative Limb Project for Kiera Roche.	24
I.12	Turfan Limb.	26
1.1	Terracotta figurine.	41
1.2	Roman bone saw.	46
1.3	Roman tourniquet.	48
1.4	Silver denarius, Rome, 116–115 BCE.	52
1.5	Longobard knife prosthesis.	60
1.6	Greville Chester Toe.	62
1.7	Cairo Toe.	62
1.8	Replica of the Capua Limb.	64
1.9	Red-figure chous, Attica, circa 440–430 BCE.	70
1.10	Detail from a Roman marble sarcophagus.	70
2.1	Graeco-Roman-Egyptian voodoo doll.	75
2.2	Graeco-Roman-Egyptian Mummy portrait.	78
2.3	Graeco-Roman dental forceps.	80
2.4	Scythian vase.	80

2.5 Etruscan dental appliance. 95
2.6 Etruscan dental appliance. 95
3.1 Corinthian *Pyxides*, circa fifth century BCE. 103
3.2 Terracotta ex votos. 107
3.3 Terracotta ex voto, Temple of Minerva Medica, Rome, third or second century BCE. 108
3.4 Gold aureus, Rome, 69 CE. 113
3.5 Roman wig, York, late-third to early-fifth century CE. 118
3.6 Roman hairpiece from Gurob in the Fayum, late first or early second century CE. 118
4.1 'Memento Mori' mosaic from the triclinium of the House/ Workshop I.5.2, Pompeii, 30 BCE–14 CE. 128
4.2 Italian statuette, third century or second century BCE. 131
4.3 Funerary monument of Xanthippos, circa 420 BCE. 136
4.4 Roman relief, second century CE. 138
4.5 Macedonian greaves, from the tomb of Philip II of Macedonia, Amphipolis. 140
4.6 Detail of the Thermae Boxer, Baths of Constantine, Rome, third–second century BCE. 141
4.7 Egyptian straw hat, circa 420–568 CE. 145
4.8 'Cupids as Goldsmiths' fresco from the House of the Vettii, Pompeii, 62–79 CE. 148
5.1 'Thetis bittet Hephaistos, für ihren Sohn Achilleus eine Rüstung zu schmieden' by Johann Heinrich Füssli. 155
5.2 Fresco from St Archangel Michael's Church, the Lesnovo Monastery, Macedonia, 1347 CE. 160
5.3 Section from the 'Forum Frieze' fresco from the atrium of the Praedia of Julia Felix, Pompeii, 62–79 CE. 161
6.1 Still from *Assassin's Creed Odyssey*. 170

Tables

I.1 All ancient literary references to prostheses found to date. *page* 32

I.2 Types of prostheses mentioned in ancient literature, and natures of prosthesis users. 33

I.3 Types of prostheses mentioned in ancient literature, and genders of prosthesis users. 33

I.4 Materials the prostheses mentioned in ancient literature are made from. 34

I.5 Archaeological and bioarchaeological evidence for ancient prostheses. 36

Acknowledgements

My research into ancient prostheses began in earnest in 2015, and I would like to thank the Wellcome Trust for funding the Prostheses in Antiquity conference (Wellcome Trust Small Grant 108557/Z/15/Z). I would also like to thank the Royal Society of Edinburgh for funding the Accessing the Lived Experience of Ancient Impairment and Disability through Prostheses (Artefacts and Replicas) research project (Arts and Humanities Small Research Grant 58730). Over the course of this research project, I spent time at the British Museum and the Science Museum in London, the World Museum in Liverpool, and the Surgeons' Hall Museum in Edinburgh, and was lucky enough to access items in their collections. I would like to thank all the curatorial staff who assisted me: Dr Hannah Pethen and Dr Julie Anderson, the Curators at the British Museum; Natasha Logan, the Collections Administrator and Access Coordinator at Blythe House; Dr Chrissy Partheni, the Curator of Antiquities at the World Museum; and Dr Louise Wilkie, the Assistant Curator at the Surgeons' Hall Museums. I would also like to thank Dr Jacky Finch for sharing her research into the experimental archaeological reconstruction of ancient Egyptian prosthetic toes with me and for allowing me access to the resultant replicas, and Dr Campbell Price, the Curator of Egypt and the Sudan at the Manchester Museum, for providing us with space to have our discussion.

I undertook the research and writing of the first draft of this manuscript over the course of the three years that I spent at the University of Glasgow as Lord Kelvin Adam Smith Postdoctoral Research Fellow in Classics (Ancient Science and Technology) between 2016 and 2019, and I gained valuable insights discussing the subject of impairment, disability, and assistive technology in classical antiquity from my colleagues, notably Professor Isabel Ruffell, and from the students who took the Impairment and Disability in the Ancient World, Ancient Technology in Context, and Ancient Medicine undergraduate and postgraduate courses I either convened or taught on during this time. I partially revised the manuscript during a Visiting Scholarship in the Department of History and Philosophy of Science at the University of Cambridge during the spring of 2019 and a Visiting Fellowship at the Institute of Classical Studies during the summer of 2019, and I completed the revisions in the spring and summer of 2021.

I would like to thank Dr Ellen Adams, Dr Emma-Jayne Graham, Dr Maria Gerolemou, Dr Jessica Hughes, Professor Christian Laes, Dr Alexia Petsalis-Diomidis, Professor Isabel Ruffell, Dr Debby Sneed, Dr Laurence Totelin, and Dr Katherine van Schaik for discussing my research with me at various points and events over the last six years.

Finally, I would like to thank Dr Virginia Campbell, Dr Debby Sneed, Dr Robert Cromarty, and Professor Christian Laes for reading various parts and drafts of this manuscript and offering feedback, and the Cambridge University Press anonymous reviewers for their suggestions on how to improve the manuscript.

Abbreviations

ANRW	*Aufstieg und Niedergang der römischen Welt* (1972–)
CIL	*Corpus Inscriptionum Latinarum* (1863–)
Crawford	*Roman Republican Coinage* (1974)
IG	*Inscriptiones Graecae* (1873–)
ILS	*Inscriptiones Latinae Selectae* (1892–1916)
LIMC	*Lexicon Iconographicum Mythologiae Classicae*
P.Giss.	*Griechische Papyri im Museum des oberhessischen Geschichtsvereins zu Giessen*, ed. O. Eger, E. Kornemann, and P. M. Meyer. Leipzig-Berlin 1910–12. Pt. I, nos. 1–35 (1910); Pt. II, nos. 36–57 (1910); Pt. III, nos. 58–126 (1912). [Rp. CG].
P.Giss.Apoll.	*Briefe des Apollonios-Archives aus der Sammlung Papyri Gissenses*, ed. M. Kortus. Giessen 1999. (Berichte und Arbeiten aus der Universitätsbibliothek und dem Universitätsarchiv Giessen 49.) Nos. 1–43.
RCV	*Roman Coins and Their Values* (1988)
RSC	*Roman Silver Coins* (1952–89)
W.Chr	L. Mitteis and U. Wilcken, *Grundzüge und Chrestomathie der Papyruskunde*, I Bd. *Historischer Teil*, II Hälfte *Chrestomathie*. Leipzig-Berlin 1912. Nos. 1–382. [MF 2.120–121 (with Grundzüge); Rp. GO].

Sources

Achilles Tatius, *Leucippe and Clitophon*	Ach. Tat.
Aelian, *Historical Miscellany*	Ael. *VH.*
Aelian, *On the Nature of Animals*	Ael. *NA.*

Agnellus of Ravenna, *Agnelli Liber Pontificalis Ecclesiae Ravennatis.*	
Ammianus Marcellinus, *Roman History*	Amm. Marc.
Andocides, *On the Mysteries.*	
Antiphilus of Byzantium, *Greek Anthology*	
Appian, *Civil War*	App. *B Civ.*
Appian, *Roman History: The Hannibalic War*	App. *Hann.*
Apuleius, *Metamorphoses*	Apul. *Met.*
Aristophanes, *Birds*	Arist. *Aves.*
Aristophanes, *Ecclesiazusae*	Arist. *Eccl.*
Aristophanes, *Frogs*	Arist. *Ran.*
Aristophanes, *Peace*	Arist. *Pax.*
Aristophanes, *Wasps*	Arist. *Sph.*
Aristophanes, *Women of the Thesmophoria*	Arist. *Thesm.*
Aristotle, *Categories*	Arist. *Cat.*
Aristotle, *Household Management*	Arist. [*Oec.*]
Aristotle, *Metaphysics*	Arist. *Metaph.*
Aristotle, *Nicomachean Ethics*	Arist. *Eth. Nic.*
Aristotle, *On Marvellous Things Heard.*	
Aristotle, *On the Generation of Animals*	Arist. *Gen. an.*
Aristotle, *On the History of Animals*	Arist. *Hist. an.*
Aristotle, *On the Parts of Animals*	Arist. *Part. an.*
Aristotle, *On the Soul*	Arist. *De an.*
Aristotle, *Politics*	Arist. *Pol.*
Aristotle, *Problems*	Arist. [*Pr.*]
Aristotle, *Rhetoric*	Arist. *Rhet.*
Arrian, *Anabasis of Alexander*	Arr. *Anab.*
Arrian, *Indica*	Arr. *Ind.*
Artemidorus, *The Interpretation of Dreams*	Artem. *On.*

Athenaeus, *Dinner Sophists*	Ath.
Augustine, *Letters*	August. *Ep.*
Augustus, *Res Gestae*	Aug. *RG.*
Avienus, *Fables*	
Babylonian Talmud	
Caelius Aurelianus, *Chronic Diseases*	
Caesar, *Civil Wars*	Caes. *BCiv.*
Caesar, *Gallic Wars*	Caes. *BGall.*
Caesar, *Spanish War*	Caes. *BHisp.*
Calpurnius Siculus, *Eclogues*	Calp. *Ecl.*
Cassius Dio, *Roman History*	Cass. Dio.
Cato the Elder, *On Agriculture*	Cato, *Agr.*
Celsus, *On Medicine*	Celsus, *Med.*
Charles Dickens, *Barnaby Rudge*	
Charles Dickens, *David Copperfield*	
Charles Dickens, *Our Mutual Friend*	
Charles Dickens, *The Old Curiosity Shop*	
Charles Dickens, *The Pickwick Papers*	
Cicero, *Against Piso*	Cic. *Pis.*
Cicero, *On Duties*	Cic. *Off.*
Cicero, *On the Laws*	Cic. *Leg.*
Cicero, *Philippics*	Cic. *Phil.*
Cicero, *Tusculan Disputations*	Cic. *Tusc.*
Cinesias, *Testimonia*	
Claudian, *On the Fourth Consulship of the Emperor Honorius*	Claud. *Cons. Hon.*
Clement of Alexandria, *The Instructor*	Clem. Al.
Cyprian, *Letters*	
Demosthenes, *Orations*	Dem.
Digest	*Dig.*
Dinarchus, *Against Demosthenes*	Din.
Dio Chrysostom, *Eighth Discourse: On Virtue*	Dio Chrys. *Or.*
Diodorus Siculus, *Library of History*	Diod. Sic.

Diogenes Laertius, *Anaxarchus*	Diog. Laert.
Diogenes Laertius, *Lives of the Eminent Philosophers*	Diog. Laert.
Dionysius of Halicarnassus, *Roman Antiquities*	Dion. Hal. *Ant. Rom.*
Dioscorides, *On Medical Materials*	Diosc.
Epidaurian Iamata	
Epiphanius, *Against Heresies*	Epiph. *Adv. haeres.*
Erycius, *Greek Anthology*	
Eugentius, *Mythologies*	
Euripides, *Hecuba*	Eur. *Hec.*
Euripides, *Phoenician Women*	Eur. *Phoen.*
Eutropius, *Brief History of Rome*	Eutr.
Florus, *Epitome*	Flor.
Frontinus, *Strategems*	Frontin. *Str.*
Galen, *An Outline of Empiricism*	Gal. *Subf. Emp.*
Galen, *Commentary on Hippocrates' On Joints*	Gal. *Hipp. Art.*
Galen, *Method of Medicine*	Gal. *MM*
Galen, *On Avoiding Distress*	Gal. *Ind.*
Galen, *On Passions and Errors of the Soul*	Gal. *Aff. Dig.*
Galen, *On the Composition of Medicines According to Place*	Gal. *Comp. Loc.*
Galen, *On the Natural Faculties*	Gal. *Nat. Fac.*
Gregory of Tours, *Libri de Virtutibus Sancti Martini Episcopi*	Gregory of Tours, *VM*
Hermesianax, *Fragments*	
Herodas, *Mimes*	Herod.
Herodotus, *Histories*	Hdt.
Hesiod, *Works and Days*	Hes. *Op.*

Hippocrates, *Instruments of Reduction*	Hippoc. *Mochl.*
Hippocrates, *On Fleshes*	Hippoc. *Carn.*
Hippocrates, *On Glands*	Hippoc. *Gland.*
Hippocrates, *On Joints*	Hippoc. *Art.*
Hippocrates, *On the Affections of Women*	Hippoc. *Mul.*
Hippocrates, *On the Nature of Women*	Hippoc. *Nat. mul.*
Hippocrates, *On the Nature of the Child*	Hippoc. *Nat. puer.*
Hippocrates, *On the Sacred Disease*	Hippoc. *Morb. sacr.*
Homer, *Iliad*	Hom. *Il.*
Homer, *Odyssey*	Hom. *Od.*
Horace, *Epodes*	Hor. *Epod.*
Horace, *Satires*	Hor. *Sat.*
Jacob de Voragine, *Legenda Aurea*/*The Golden Legend*	
John Damascene, *Baarlam and Ioasaph*	
Josephus, *Jewish Antiquities*	Joseph. *AJ*
Josephus, *Jewish War*	Joseph. *BJ*
Josephus, *Life of Josephus*	Joseph. *Vit.*
Juvenal, *Satires*	Juv.
Laws of the Twelve Tables	
Leonidas of Alexandria, *Greek Anthology*	
Leviticus	
Lev Rabbah	
Livy	
Livy, *Epitome*	Livy, *Epit.*
Lucan, *Pharsalia*	
Lucian, *Alexander the False Prophet*	Luc. *Alex.*
Lucian, *Apology for the Salaried Posts in Great Houses*	Luc. *De Merc. cond.*
Lucian, *Dialogues of the Courtesans*	Luc. *Dial. meret.*
Lucian, *Essays in Portraiture Defended*	Luc. *Imag.*
Lucian, *Friendship*	Luc. *Tox.*

Lucian, *Gout*	Luc. *Pod.*
Lucian, *Ignorant Book-Collector*	Luc. *Ind.*
Lucian, *Professor of Public Speaking*	Luc. *Rhet.*
Lucian, *The Dance*	Luc. *De Salt.*
Lucian, *The Dream*	Luc. *Somn.*
Lucian, *True Story*	Luc. *Ver. hist.*
Lucillius, *Greek Anthology*	
Luke	
Lycophron, *Alexandra*	Lycoph. *Alex.*
Lysias	Lys.
Macedonius, *Greek Anthology*	
Macrobius, *Saturnalia*	Macrob. *Sat.*
Mardonius the Consul, *Greek Anthology*	
Mark	
Martial, *Epigrams*	Mart.
Matthew	
Mekilta on Exodus	
Menander, *The Girl with Her Hair Cut Short*	Men. *Pk.*
Musonius Rufus, *Discourse 21 On Cutting the Hair*	Muson.
Myrinus, *Greek Anthology*	
Nonius, Scholiast to Lucian, *The Dependent Scholar*	Non.
Nonnus, *Dionysiaca*	Nonnus, *Dion.*
Oribasius, *Medical Collection*	
Ovid, *Amores*	Ov. *Am.*
Ovid, *Arts of Love*	Ov. *Ars am.*
Ovid, *Heroides*	Ov. *Her.*
Ovid, *Metamorphoses*	Ov. *Met.*
Palaephatus, *On Unbelievable Things*	
Palestinian Talmud	
P.Giss.	
Paul, *Corinthians*	
Paul of Aegina, *Medical Compendium*	
Pausanias, *Description of Greece*	Paus.

Persius, *Satires*	Pers.
Petronius, *Satyricon*	Petron. *Sat.*
Philippus or Isodorus, *Greek Anthology*	
Philo, *That the Worse Is Wont to Attack the Better*	
Philostratus, *Apollonios of Tyana*	Philostr. *VA*
Philostratus, *Lives of the Philosophers*	Philostr. *VS*
Philostratus the Elder, *Epistles*	Philostr. *Ep.*
Philostratus the Elder, *Imagines*	Philostr. *Imag.*
Pindar, *Olympian Odes*	Pind. *Ol.*
Plato the Younger, *Greek Anthology*	
Plautus, *Amphitryon*	Plaut. *Amph.*
Plautus, *A Three Coin Day*	Plaut. *Trin.*
Plautus, *Pot of Gold*	Plaut. *Aul.*
Plautus, *The Braggart Soldier*	Plaut. *Mil.*
Plautus, *The Persian*	Plaut. *Pers.*
Plautus, *The Rope*	Plaut. *Rud.*
Plautus, *Weevil*	Plaut. *Cur.*
Pliny the Elder, *Natural History*	Plin. *HN*
Pliny the Younger, *Letters*	Plin. *Ep.*
Plutarch, *A Letter of Condolence to Apollonios*	[Plut.] *Cons. Ad Apoll.*
Plutarch, *Caesar*	Plut. *Vit. Caes.*
Plutarch, *Camillus*	Plut. *Vit. Cam.*
Plutarch, *Eumenes*	Plut. *Vit. Eum.*
Plutarch, *Flaminius*	Plut. *Vit. Flam.*
Plutarch, *Galba*	Plut. *Vit. Galb.*
Plutarch, *Lysander*	Plut. *Vit. Lys.*
Plutarch, *Moralia*	Plut. *Mor.*
Plutarch, *Moralia: Lives of the Ten Orators: Antiphon*	

Plutarch, *Moralia: On Brotherly Love*	Plut. *Mor. De frat. amor.*
Plutarch, *Moralia: On Exile*	
Plutarch, *Moralia: The Dialogue on Love*	
Plutarch, *On Isis and Osiris*	Plut. *Mor. De Is. et Os.*
Plutarch, *Pericles*	Plut. *Vit. Per.*
Plutarch, *Pompey*	Plut. *Vit. Pomp.*
Plutarch, *Sertorius*	Plut. *Vit. Sert.*
Polybius, *Histories*	Polyb.
Porphyry, *Life of Pythagoras*	Porph. *Pyth.*
Procopius, *History of the Wars*	Procop.
Prudentius, *Crowns of Martyrdom*	Prudent.
Pseudo-Apollodorus, *Library*	Apollod. *Bibl.*
Pseudo-Hyginus, *Fables*	Hyg. *Fab.*
Quintilian, *Lesser Declamations*	Quint.
Quintilian, *The Orator's Education*	Quint. *Inst.*
Quintus Curtius, *History of Alexander.*	
Quintus Smyrnaeus, *The Fall of Troy*	Quint. Smyrn. *Rig Veda.*
Sallust, *Histories*	Sall. *Hist.*
Scribonius Largus, *Compositiones medicamentorum*	
Seneca the Elder, *Controversiae*	Sen. *Controv.*
Seneca the Younger, *Moral Epistles*	Sen. *Ep.*
Seneca the Younger, *Natural Questions*	Sen. *QNat.*
Seneca the Younger, *On Anger*	Sen. *Ira.*
Seneca the Younger, *Thyestes*	Sen. *Thy.*
Servius	Serv.
Sextus Empiricus, *Against the Professors*	Sext. Emp. *Math.*
Sophocles, *Oedipus at Colonus*	Soph. *OC*
Sophocles, *Philoctetes*	Soph. *Phil.*
Soranus, *Gynaecology*	Sor. *Gyn.*
Statius, *Silvae*	Stat. *Silv.*

Statius, *Thebaid*	Stat. *Theb.*
Strabo, *Geography*	Strabo, *Geog.*
	Suda.
Suetonius, *Augustus*	Suet. *Aug.*
Suetonius, *Caligula*	Suet. *Calig.*
Suetonius, *Claudius*	Suet. *Claud.*
Suetonius, *Domitian*	Suet. *Dom.*
Suetonius, *Galba*	Suet. *Galb.*
Suetonius, *Julius Caesar*	Suet. *Iul.*
Suetonius, *Nero*	Suet. *Ner.*
Suetonius, *Otho*	Suet. *Oth.*
Suetonius, *Tiberius*	Suet. *Tib.*
Tacitus, *Agricola*	Tac. *Agr.*
Tacitus, *Germania*	Tac. *Germ.*
Tacitus, *Histories*	Tac. *Hist.*
Talmud Sanhedrin	
Tertullian, *On the Apparel of Women*	Tert.
Theophanes the Confessor, *Chronicle*	
Theophrastus, *Enquiry into Plants*	Theophr. *Hist. pl.*
Tibullus, *Elegies*	Tib.
Tosephta, *Parah*	
Tractate Nedarim	
Valerius Maximus, *Memorable Deeds and Sayings*	Val. Max.
Varro, *On Agriculture*	Varro, *Rust.*
Virgil, *Georgics*	Verg. *G.*
Vitruvius, *On Architecture*	Vitr. *De arch.*
Xenophon, *Cyropaedia*	Xen. *Cyr.*
Xenophon, *Estate Management*	Xen. *Oec.*
Xenophon, *Hellenica*	Xen. *Hell.*
Xenophon, *Memorabilia*	Xen. *Mem.*

Introduction

> Pope Felix, a predecessor of Saint Gregory, built a noble church in Rome in honour of Saints Cosmas and Damian. In this church there was a man, a devoted servant of holy martyrs. One of the man's legs had been totally consumed by a cancer. While he was asleep, the two saints appeared to their devoted servant, bringing salves and surgical instruments. One of them said to the other: 'Where can we get flesh to fill in where we cut away the rotted leg?' The other said: 'Just today an Ethiopian was buried in the cemetery of Saint Peter in Chains. Go and take his leg, and we'll put it in place of the bad one.' So, he sped to the cemetery and brought back the Moor's leg, and the two saints cut off the sick man's leg and inserted the Moor's in its place, carefully anointing the wound. Finally, they took the amputated leg and attached it to the body of the dead Moor. The man woke up, felt no pain, put his hand to his leg, and detected no lesion. He held a candle to the leg and could see nothing wrong with it and began to wonder whether he was himself or someone else. Then he came to his senses, bounded joyfully from his bed, and told everyone what he had seen in his dreams and how he had been healed. They sent at once to the Moor's tomb and found that his leg had indeed been cut off and the aforesaid man's limb put in its place in the tomb.[1]

Over time, Cosmas and Damian, twin brothers reportedly martyred for their Christian faith in 297 CE, part of the persecutions during the reign of the

[1] Jacob de Voragine, *Legenda Aurea*/*The Golden Legend* 2.143.4 (trans. W. G. Ryan, with minor adjustments): *Felix papa attavus sancti Gregorii in honore sanctorum Cosmae et Damiani nobilem ecclesiam Romae construxit. In hac ecclesia quidam vir sanctis martiribus serviebat, cui cancer unum crus totum consumserat. Et ecce dormiente illo sancti Cosmas et Damianus devoto suo apparuerunt unguenta et ferramenta secum portantes; quorum unus alteri dixit: ubi carnes accipiemus, ut abscisca carne putrida locum vacuum repleamus? Tunc ait alter: in cimiterio sancti Petri ad vincula hodie Aethiops recens sepultus est, de illo autem affer, ut huic suppleamus. Et ecce ad cimiterium properavit et coxam Mauri attulit, praecidentesque coxam infirmi loco ejus coxam Mauri inseruerunt et plagam diligenter ungentes coxam infirmi ad corpus Mauri mortui detulerunt. Evigilans autem cum se sine dolore sensisset, manum ad coxam apposuit et nil laesionis invenit, apponensque candelam cum in crure nil mali videret, cogitabat, an non ipse, qui erat, sed alius alter isset. Rediens autem ad se prae gaudio de lectulo prosiliit et quid in somnis viderat et qualiter sanatus fuerat, omnibus enarravit. Qui conciti ad tumulum Mauri miserunt et coxam Mauri praecisam et coxam praedicti viri loco illius in tumulo positam repererunt.*

emperor Diocletian (283–303 CE), became venerated as the patron saints of medicine, surgery, pharmacy, and, perhaps somewhat surprisingly to a contemporary reader, organ transplantation.[2] The pair are said to have been born in the mid-third century CE at Aegae in the Roman province of Cicilia (modern-day Çukurova in Turkey) on the Bay of Alexandretta (modern-day Iskenderun), and to have studied medicine in Syria. Once they began practicing medicine, they became renowned for refusing to accept payment for their services. Their most famous healing episode, and the reason for their role as patron saints of organ transplantation, is known as the 'miracle of the black leg'.[3] This miracle involved the twins treating a white man suffering from a gangrenous wound in his leg by amputating the afflicted limb and replacing it with the limb of a deceased black man (in some versions described as an Ethiopian, in others a Moor).[4] Whatever the original motivation for telling the story in this way and making a concerted effort to differentiate between the patient and the donor on the grounds of race, it is clear that the 'miracle' would have been at once apparent to an individual hearing or reading this story, or seeing a visual representation of it.[5] The source for this episode, the writings of the archbishop of Genua Jacob de Voragine's *The Golden Legend*, dates to the late thirteenth century (a specific date between 1252 and 1260 has been proposed), so well after the lives and deaths of Cosmas and Damian and the establishment of their cult. The earliest known illustration of this episode is found in a late-thirteenth-century manuscript of de Voragine's work, and depicts Cosmas and Damian in the middle of the transplantation; they have removed the gangrenous white leg, which lies discarded to one side of the patient's bed, and are in the process of attaching the black leg.[6] However, it soon became a popular subject for medieval artists and numerous later depictions of the event survive.[7]

[2] On the association of the saints with organ transplantation, see Decker, 2016, pp. 51–4. See also Duffin, 2013.

[3] In medieval eyes, this is an example of 'incarnatyf' medicine, which not only made new flesh but also required this new flesh to bind with existing flesh or non-flesh through a process equated with knitting that was analogous with grafting or soldering; for discussion, see Walter, 2016.

[4] For Africans in classical antiquity, see Snowden, 1970, 1991. On racism in antiquity, see Isaac, 2004. On the racial implications of this version of the story, see Fracchia, 2013.

[5] An alternative version of the myth, found in Greek sources dating from the fifth century, describes Cosmas and Damian replacing a patient's gangrenous leg with the leg of a corpse, but it does not mention the ethnicity of the leg; for this, see Deubner, 1907. It is necessary for the legs to be exchanged so that upon the Day of Judgement and the Resurrection each man would be given back his own leg because of the importance of having a complete body; see Walter, 2016, p. 1354.

[6] Huntington Library manuscript HM 3027, folio 132r.

[7] Danilevicius, 1967; Zimmerman, 1998; Zimmerman et al., 2013.

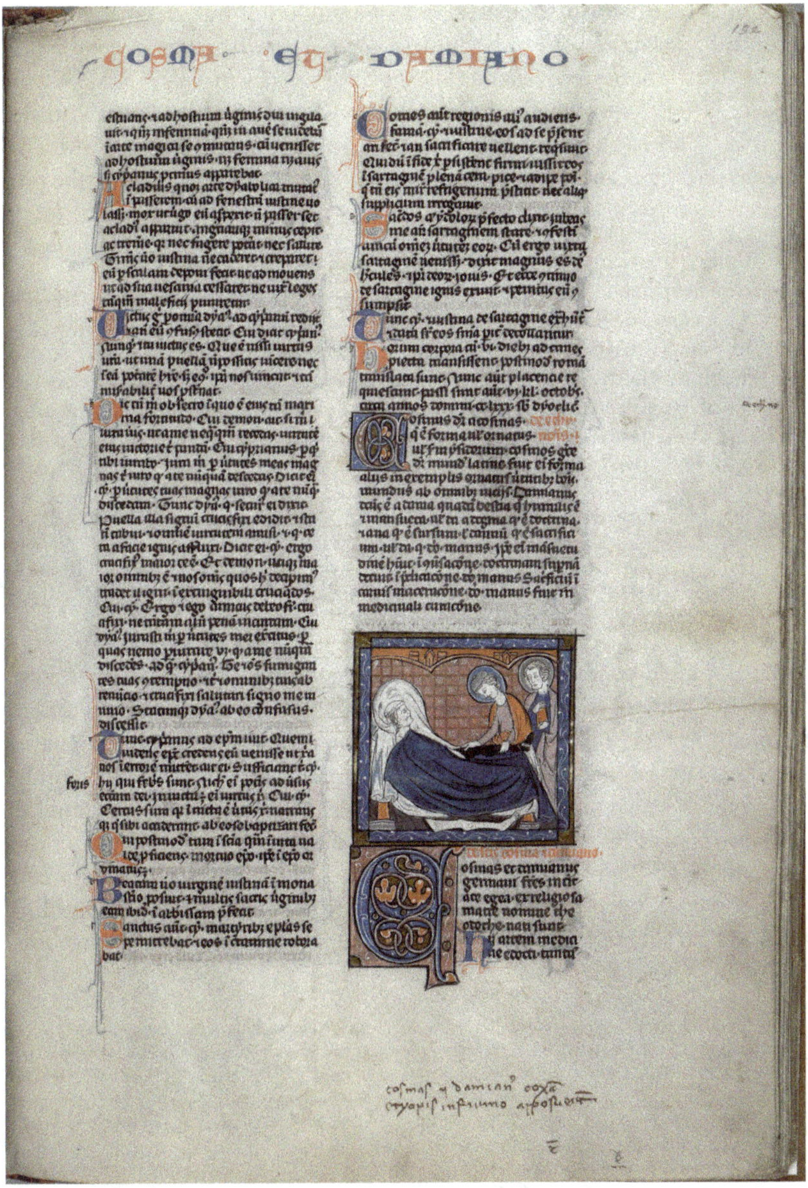

Figure I.1 Page from Jacob de Voragine's *The Golden Legend* manuscript. Huntington Library manuscript HM 3027, folio 132 r. Image courtesy of the Huntingdon Library, San Marino, California.

Cosmas and Damian are part of a long tradition of miraculous healing in which the restoration of lost body parts serves as a demonstration of divine power. Inscriptions recovered from the healing sanctuary of Asklepios at Epidauros and dating to the fourth century BCE claim that visitors to the sanctuary underwent incubation rituals, and during these rituals the god appeared to them and cured their ailments.[8] One man claimed that the god restored his missing eye:

> Once a man came as a supplicant to the god who was so blind in one eye that, while he still had the eyelids of that eye, there was nothing within them and they were completely empty. Some of the people in the sanctuary were laughing at his simple-mindedness in thinking that he could be made to see, having absolutely nothing, not even the beginnings of an eye, but only the socket. Then in his sleep, a vision appeared to him. It seemed the god boiled some drug, and then drew apart his eyelids and poured it in. When day came he departed with both eyes.[9]

Another, Heraieos of Mytilene, claimed that the god restored his lost hair:

> This man had no hair on his head, but plenty on his chin. Ashamed because he was laughed at by the others, he slept here. The god anointed his head with a drug and made it have hair.[10]

It was not just Asklepios, the Greek god of medicine, who was purported to restore lost body parts. Other examples include the goddess Minerva Medica reportedly restoring a woman named Tullia Superiana's lost hair at a sanctuary near Travo in the Trébbia valley in northern Italy during the Roman period.[11] Additionally, early Christianity was replete with tales of the restoration of lost body parts, with Jesus supposedly restoring the ear of a high priest's servant that was cut off by his disciple Peter in an attempt to prevent Jesus' arrest.[12]

There have been numerous attempts to rationalise ancient healing miracles.[13] If one felt inclined to do so, one could rationalise these stories

[8] The link between Cosmas and Damian and Asklepios is made explicit by Santing, 2013, p. 128.

[9] Epidaurian iamata A9 (trans. L. R. LiDonnici): Ἀνὴρ ἀφίκετο ποὶ τὸν θεὸν ἱκέτας ἀτερόπτιλλος οὕτως, ὥστε τὰ βλέφαρα μόνον ἔχειν, ἐνεῖμεν δ'ἐν αὐτοῖς μηθέν, ἀλλὰ κενεὰ ε[ἶ]μεν ὅλως. ἐ(γ)έ(λω)ν δή τινες τῶν ἐν τῶι ἱαρῶι τὰν εὐηθίαν αὐτοῦ, τὸ νομίζειν βλεψεῖσθαι ὅλως μηδεμίαν ὑπαρχὰν ἔχοντος ὀπτίλλου ἀλλ' ἢ χώραμ μόνον. ἐγκαθ[εύδο]ντι οὖν αὐτῶι ὄψις ἐφάνη· ἐδόκει τὸν θεὸν ἑψῆσαί τι φά[ρμακον, ἔπε]ιτα διαγαγόντα τὰ βλέφαρα ἐγχέαι εἰς αὐτά· ἁμέρ[ας δὲ γενομέν]ας βλέπων ἁμερ[ας δὲ γενομέν]ας βλέπων ἀμφοῖν ἐξῆλθε.

[10] Epidaurian iamata A 19 (trans. L. R. LiDonnici): Ἡραιεὺς Μυτιληναῖος. οὗτος οὐκ εἶχε ἐν τᾶι κεφαλᾶι τρίχας, ἐν δὲ τωῖ γενείωι παμπόλλας. αἰσχυνόμενος δὲ [ὡς] καταγελάμενος ὑπ[ὸ] τῶν ἄλλων ἐνεκάθευδε. τὸν δὲ ὁ θεὸς χρίσας φαρμάκωι τὰν κεφαλὰν ἐπόησε τρίχας ἔχειν.

[11] *CIL* XI 1305 = *ILS* 3135; for discussion of the epigraphic evidence for this sanctuary, see Sauer, 1996.

[12] Luke 22.50–1. See Hamilton, 2012, p. 4, for a selection of other examples.

[13] See, for example, Cilliers and Retief, 2013.

of restored body parts – whether extremity, eye, or hair – by referring to prostheses.[14] Thus, the man supposedly operated on by Cosmas and Damian was in actual fact given an extremity prosthesis, the man who claimed that Asklepios restored his lost eye was in actual fact given a prosthetic one (after all, no mention is made of his vision having been restored, just his eye), and the man who claimed that Asklepios restored his lost hair was in actual fact given a wig or hairpiece. This potential connection between ancient healing miracles and prostheses can be traced through the use of so-called 'anatomical' votives – that is, votive offerings in the form of body parts both external (such as fingers, hands, arms, toes, feet, legs, etc.) and internal (such as viscera, uteri, etc.) made from substances including, but not limited to, precious and semi-precious metal, marble, ivory, terracotta, and wood. The traditional interpretation of these objects is that they served as a representation of the part of the body that was ill, injured, or impaired in some way; they were offered to the god either in the hope that the god would heal the afflicted part, or as thanks for the afflicted part having been healed. See, for example, Figure I.2: this marble votive relief found near the Enneakrounos fountain in Athens, originally from the sanctuary of the hero-physician Amynos and dating from the late fourth century BCE.[15] It was dedicated by Lysimachides, son of Lysimachos, from Acharnai, and depicts him holding what appears to be an anatomical votive leg displaying a prominent varicose vein, with two anatomical votive feet on the left-hand side. Ever after, or at least until the sanctuary was cleared out and the votives ritually disposed of, the votive body part remained with the god, a visual representation both of the dedicant's faith in the god and the god's power.[16] The isolated body part contrasted with the now whole real body of the dedicant.[17] However, it has been suggested that anatomical votives can be viewed as an attempt to signify the metaphorical representation of the body in illness and pain.[18] In this way, they were used to represent the fragmentation or disaggregation of the ailing body of the person who was dedicating them, with the healing process conceived of as the reintegration of the fragmented parts leading to the reconstitution of the body of the person who was dedicating them.[19] One example of this

[14] See, for example, Walter, 2016 for discussion of the 'miracle of the black leg' in relation to medieval theories of prosthesis. However, on occasion, explicit mention is made of an individual using a prosthesis before undergoing miraculous healing which thereby renders the prosthesis obsolete – see Gregory of Tours, *VM* 3.9, 4.41.

[15] National Archaeological Museum of Athens inv. 3562.

[16] For discussion of this practice, see Glinister, 2000. She refers to this material as 'sacred rubbish'.

[17] Pazzini, 1935; Rynearson, 2003, pp. 9–10. [18] Hughes, 2008, p. 226.

[19] Hughes, 2008; this argument is expanded in Hughes, 2017, pp. 25–61.

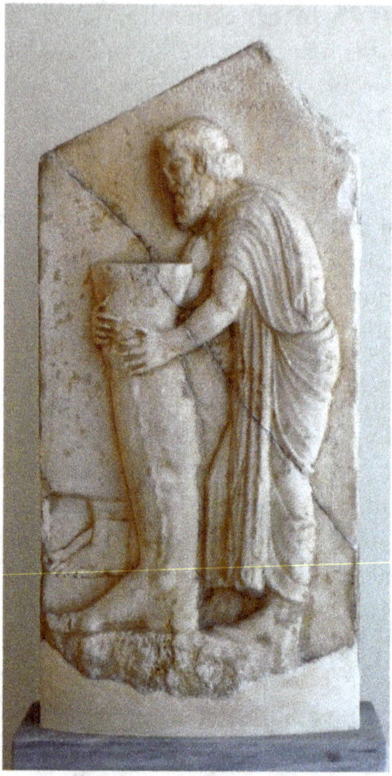

Figure I.2 Greek votive relief. National Archaeological Museum of Athens inv. 3562. Image courtesy of Alamy.

process can be seen on a votive relief found in the Asklepieion at Athens and dating from the fourth century BCE.[20] It depicts what appears to be the offering of anatomical votives to Herakles Menytes by a female dedicant; if all of the disparate parts on display were put together, they would form a complete female body.[21] It has been interpreted as 'a kind of "non-amputation" underscoring the integrity of the absent, cured dedicant'.[22] In some cases, anatomical votives represented an amputated part.[23] They have been considered to serve as 'ritual prostheses, deployed to render the body whole and healthy again'.[24] They have also been described as 'a psychological prosthesis ... an aid to feeling whole ... an aid to the healing

[20] National Archaeological Museum of Athens inv. 7232.
[21] See van Straten, 1981, p. 106, n. 1.1 for this observation.
[22] Rynearson, 2003, p. 10.
[23] van Straten, 1981, p. 76.
[24] Adams, 2017, p. 199.

process'.[25] It has been observed that anatomical votives rarely depict the illness, injury, or impairment; rather, they usually represent the body part in its normal or desired state.[26] Interestingly, a documentary papyrus from Egypt dating to around 118 CE can be seen as making this link explicit through its reference to a maker of artificial limbs manning a healing shrine.[27]

But what of actual prostheses in classical antiquity?[28] While literary, documentary, archaeological, and bioarchaeological evidence for congenital and acquired amputation of various parts of the body in ancient Greece and Rome is plentiful, evidence for prostheses, prosthesis use, and prostheses users is somewhat harder to come by, and the evidence that exists is open to debate. The earliest surviving mention of a prosthesis in Graeco-Roman literature can be found in Pindar's recounting of the myth of Pelops in the first *Olympian Ode* (circa 522–433 BCE), but this is obviously a mythological rather than an historical episode, and so we should proceed with caution when using this as a source for the lived experience of an actual ancient person in possession of a physical impairment.[29] While the finer details of the myth vary from source to source, ancient authors are generally in agreement regarding the main points: Pelops' father Tantalus wished to make a suitable offering to the gods of the Olympian pantheon, so he killed his son, cut him up, and cooked him in a stew, which he then served to them.[30] All of the gods except for Demeter declined the stew, but since she was distracted by the loss of her daughter Persephone following

[25] Adams, 2017, p. 200.

[26] Petsalis-Diomidis, 2006, pp. 210, 220. As a result, attempts have been made to argue that individual healing sanctuaries specialised in healing particular parts of the body, or particular health problems, based on the proportion of particular types of anatomical votives found at them. For example, since 40 per cent of the anatomical votives found at the sanctuary of Asklepios in Athens are eyes, it follows that the sanctuary specialised in healing eye problems; for this, see Oberhelman, 2014.

[27] *P.Giss.* 20. Draycott, 2014; for further discussion of this papyrus and its contents, see Chapter 4.

[28] Parts of this section of the Introduction use material from Draycott, 2019b as a starting point.

[29] Somewhat confusingly, Pindar's account first relates and then refutes that Pelops' ivory shoulder was a prosthesis, and yet still retains this as a key feature of the myth, arguing that he was born with it as a sort of birthmark rather than he somehow acquired it later in life. According to Paley, 1868, p. 3 n. 2, since the name Pelops means 'dark faced', this could be seen to refer to a pale shoulder that is revealed when clothing is removed. According to Gerber, 1982, p. 58, since Pelops' ivory shoulder is one of the most consistent and conspicuous features of the myth, whatever it actually was, it was probably considered to be a mark of beauty. For further discussion of this, see Noel, 2019. This is not, however, the earliest mention of prostheses in world literature: that honour belongs to the iron leg of Vishpala, which is referred to in the *Rig Veda* (*circa* 1200–900 BCE): see 1.118.8; Vishpala is mentioned in several other places in the *Rig Veda*: see 1.112.10, 1.117.11, and 10.39.8. For similarities between the Greek of Pindar and the Sanskrit of the *Rig Veda*, see Watkins, 2002.

[30] Lycoph. *Alex.* 149; Ov. *Met.* 6.405; Sen. *Thyestes* 145; Apollod. *Bibl.* 2.1–3; Hyg. *Fab.* 83; Eugentius, *Mythologies* 2.15.

her abduction by Hades, she ate the portion she was offered, and it so happened that this portion contained Pelops' left shoulder. Upon discovering what Tantalus had done, the gods reassembled and resurrected Pelops, replacing his missing shoulder with an ivory prosthesis. However, the earliest mention of a prosthesis in Graeco-Roman literature that can be classed as historical and attributed to a genuine historical figure can be found slightly later than Pindar's *Olympian Odes* in Herodotus' *Histories* (circa 485–484 BCE).[31] According to Herodotus, Hegesistratus of Elis, the most distinguished soothsayer from among the Telliads, a Greek clan renowned for their knowledge of prophecy, was captured and imprisoned by the Spartans and, in an attempt to avoid the torture and execution which they undoubtedly had in store for him, amputated enough of his foot to enable him to remove his shackles. He then broke through the wall of his cell and escaped to the safety of Tegea. Once his wound healed, he acquired a wooden foot and continued to work against the Spartans, actions which led to his subsequent recapture and execution after the battle of Plataea.[32]

Precisely how useful either of these episodes are as a source of information on any aspect of ancient prostheses, prosthesis use, or prostheses users is debatable.[33] Yet while there are some obvious differences in the fine details of these two accounts, there are also some notable similarities. Both the myth of Pelops and the account of Hegesistratus demonstrate an individual losing a body part and subsequently replacing it with an artificial substitute; ancient authors emphasise the fact that their incomplete bodies are rendered complete through these actions, thus contextualising and rationalising the decision to do it.[34] They demonstrate a particular emphasis being placed upon the material from which the prosthesis is manufactured; Pelops' prosthesis is made from the exotic and luxurious imported substance ivory; ever after, this ivory shoulder serves to distinguish its bearer by its gleaming, shining and glowing, while Hegesistratus' prosthesis is made from ubiquitous, utilitarian, hardy wood, a material that was readily available even in wartime.[35] They demonstrate that subsequently these prostheses are what they are famous for (in the case of Pelops, reference to his prosthesis

[31] Hdt. 9.37; some details of this episode are also included in Plut. *Mor. De frat. amor.* 3.1.

[32] Hdt. 9.38. For discussion of Hegesistratus, see Dillery, 2005.

[33] See Draycott, 2019b for discussion.

[34] Pelops: Ov. *Met.* 6.405; Hyg. *Fab.* 83. Hegesistratus: Hdt. 9.37; Plut. *Mor. De frat. amor.* 3.1.

[35] Pelops: Pind. *Ol.*1.37; Tib. 1.4.63–4; Philostr. *Imag.* 1.30.7–11. According to Lorimer, 1936, pp. 32–3, the gods utilise ivory because, when suddenly called upon to provide a spare part, they can only produce one made from their own substance. According to Kenna, 1961, p. 100 n. 10, this could be an allusion to a seal stone worn either around the neck or on the upper arm that, due to being made from a tusk, resembled a shoulder blade. For discussion of the origin of the elephant or possibly

serves almost as a heroic epithet; in the case of Hegesistratus, his act of self-mutilation is described in the language of heroic accomplishment and his prosthesis is an eternal indicator and reminder of that act).[36]

The English term 'prosthesis', which is used today to refer to an artificial device that replaces or augments a missing or impaired part of the body – whether lost or impaired because of trauma, disease, or a congenital condition – is a compound of the Greek preposition πρός ('on the side of') and noun θέσις ('setting' or 'placing'). It seems to have first entered the English language in 1533, and at that time was used in a grammatical capacity to designate the addition of a syllable to the beginning of a word; it was not until 1704 that it seems to have been first used in a medical capacity, and only in the middle of the nineteenth century that it came to mean this almost exclusively.[37] Despite its Greek origins, it is not a term that was readily utilised by ancient authors, or at least not quite in the way that we use it today.[38] When the word πρόσθεσις ('application') is used in Greek literature, it indicates the application of an object for a specific purpose, as in the application of a medicinal remedy such as a pessary or a piece of medical equipment such as a cupping vessel, both of which would have been temporary.[39] No ancient Greek or Latin medical treatise mentions what we would recognise as prostheses, however; clearly, the application of a prosthesis to the body for the purpose of replacing a missing part, whether temporary in the sense of applying it for a period of time each day, or permanent in the sense of applying it every day for the remainder of one's life, was not considered a medical remedy. The nearest any ancient Greek or Latin medical writer gets to this is recommending that gold wire be utilised to fix loose teeth in place; there is, however, no mention of the possibility of utilising a dental prosthesis to replace these loose teeth if the gold wire is unable to secure them and they are lost.[40] Whereas in the twenty-first century we tend to refer to prostheses using the noun 'prosthesis' or the adjective 'prosthetic', whatever the type of

hippopotamus ivory utilised in Bronze Age Greece, the time that Pindar was writing about, see Hayward, 1990.

36 Pelops: Verg. *G* 3.7; Hegesistratus: Plut. *Mor. De frat. amor.* 3.1.

37 Wills, 1995, p. 218; Davis, 2013, p. 68.

38 One occasion on which it is used that is perhaps relevant to our purposes here is in reference to the wings that Daedalus made for himself and Icarus to facilitate their escape from Crete; see Palaephatus, *On Unbelievable Things*, p. 12. Intriguingly, there seems to have been an ancient proverb in which the term 'the wings of Daedalus' was used to describe those who employ delay as a tactic because they lack a prosthesis; see the *Suda*, delta,109; Diogenianus 4.25.

39 Pessary: Hippoc. *Mul.* 1.11, and Hippoc. *Nat. mul.* 11; cupping vessel: Arist. *Rhet.* 1405b3.

40 See Hippocrates, Hippoc. *Art.* 33.9–10; Celsus, *Med.* 6.12.1; this process is discussed in more detail in Becker and Turfa, 2017 and Turfa and Becker, 2019.

prosthesis under discussion, when prostheses are referred to in ancient literature, they are described in a very different way, which involves using the combination of the substitute body part and the substance from which it is made. So, for example, Pelops has a shoulder of ivory (ὦμος ἐλεφάντου or *umerus eburno*), Pythagoras has a thigh of gold (μηρός χρυσοῦ), Hegesistratus has a foot of wood (πούς ξυλίνου), Marcus Sergius Silus has a hand of iron (*manus ferrea*), and Statyllius has the hair belonging to another (ἀλλότριος πλόκαμος).[41]

Prostheses in the Twenty-First Century

In a monograph dedicated primarily to the subject of prostheses, prosthesis use, and prosthesis users in classical antiquity, it would be helpful at the outset to clarify to what am I referring when I use the term 'prosthesis'. What, exactly, *is* a prosthesis?[42] To the twenty-first-century reader, a prosthesis is a device that replaces a missing body part, usually (but, crucially, as we shall see, not always) designed and assembled according to the individual's appearance and functional needs, and usually (but, again, crucially, not always) as unobtrusive and as useful as possible so as to maximise the chances of their acceptance of it.[43] The missing body part can be missing due to a congenital or an acquired impairment, although in the case of the former scenario it could be argued that the individual is not, in their opinion at least, impaired as they have never known any different.[44] Studies have shown that if an individual both mentally and physically accepts their prosthesis and is satisfied with it, they will be more likely to use it: the prosthesis needs to 'fit', in all senses of the word, its user.[45] A user is more inclined to accept a prosthesis that is aesthetically pleasing to them than not and consequently considerable effort is expended on the part of

[41] Interestingly, the first well-known modern prosthesis user, Gottfried von Berlichinger, a German knight who lost his right hand at the siege of Landshut at the age of twenty-five, was likewise referred to in this way, as '*Götz mit der eisernen Hand*' ('Götz with the iron hand'). During the Second World War, the 17 SS Panzer Grenadier Division, was named after him and used an iron hand as its emblem.

[42] This section of the Introduction uses material from Draycott, 2019b as a starting point.

[43] Murray, 2005.

[44] On the relationship between parts of the body and the whole body, and the extent to which the body can be fragmented or considered fragmented, see Adams, 2017; on the issue of whether individuals born with a condition such as deafness are, in fact, impaired or disabled, see Adams, 2019.

[45] The reasons why individuals abandon their prostheses are complex and are as much to do with the individuals themselves (for example, age, sex, gender, ethnicity, level of education, etc.) as the prostheses, but studies have made the importance of comfort and functionality in successful prosthesis use clear; see, for example, Murray and Fox, 2002; Pezzin et al., 2004; Biddiss and Chau, 2009.

the prosthetist to match skin tone, hair colour, etc., or to design and create something unusual and truly unique if that is what the user desires.[46] A user is also, understandably, more inclined to accept a prosthesis that makes their life easier than one that makes their life harder.[47] Thus, it is necessary to consider each contemporary prosthesis as having a dual role, one aspect of this being its form and another being its function, although these aspects can and do also overlap, as we shall see. The nature of these forms and functions varies from prosthesis to prosthesis. A contemporary extremity prosthesis such as a finger, hand, or arm not only resembles the missing finger, hand, or arm but can also restore some (but not all) of its functionality, whereas in the not too distant past someone who lost a hand or an arm was required to choose between a prosthesis shaped like a hand but impractical, or one shaped like a hook but practical.[48] A facial prosthesis – or cosmesis, as examples of this type are sometimes designated – such as an eye or a nose resembles the missing eye or nose and, while it does not restore the lost sense of sight or smell, it does enable the user to 'pass', if that is what they wish to do.[49] And, indeed, the precise form of a prosthesis can be its primary function, if it is designed first and foremost with its appearance in mind, and its function is to be seen and to make a statement on behalf of its user, whatever its owner wishes that statement to be. In this sense, it may be said that its function is not to be practically useful to its user but to be impractically useful to its user. It depends entirely upon one's perspective.

Yet this was not always the case, and it would be helpful to summarise briefly how we got to this point. How far can utilising contemporary prostheses, prosthesis use, and prosthesis users as points of comparison assist us in our attempt to understand their ancient equivalents? It is important to remember that not only is our contemporary understanding of impairment and disability not necessarily applicable to ancient societies, but also that our contemporary understanding of assistive technology

[46] Sansoni et al., 2014.

[47] Studies have shown that the sooner after the amputation the prosthesis is fitted, the more likely the user is to accept the prosthesis and use it successfully; see Pezzin et al., 2004. Of course, someone is under no obligation to use or even attempt to use a prosthesis (although terminology such as 'accept' and 'reject' may imply otherwise), however surprising this might be to individuals who are themselves without impairments; see Goggins, 2021, p. 124.

[48] Benhamou, 1994, p. 845.

[49] A recent study has shown that facial prosthesis users tend to prefer implanted prostheses over adhesive prostheses, as the users of the latter type feel more self-conscious; see Wondergem et al., 2016. As far as the functionality of facial prostheses is concerned, in recent years, scientists have had some success in developing a prosthetic retina that has partially restored the sight in mice; see Nirenberg and Pandarinath, 2012.

might not necessarily be either. While, as we shall see over the course of this monograph, congenital and acquired amputation has always been present in human history, prosthesis use seems to have been relatively static from our first available archaeological evidence of it from Italy and China in the third century BCE until the sixteenth century, a period of some 1,800 years.[50] The French surgeon Ambroise Paré seems to have been the first maker of prosthetic limbs to explore the possibilities of mechanics.[51] However, the contemporary prosthesis in all its variability is the result of almost three centuries of medical and surgical advances, such as the development of anaesthesia, antiseptic, and amputation techniques, in conjunction with recognition of the necessity of dealing with the after-effects of modern warfare.

We first see prostheses come to prominence, albeit on a small scale, in the wake of the Napoleonic Wars (1803–15). Henry William Paget, the first Marquess of Anglesey, was shot in the right knee at the Battle of Waterloo, and his right leg was amputated.[52] He was subsequently fitted with a prosthetic leg designed and patented by James Potts of London, the world's first articulated prosthetic leg, that comprised a wooden shank and socket, and a foot that could be controlled by catgut tendons running from the knee to the ankle. Flexion of the knee caused dorsiflexion of the foot, and extension of the knee caused plantar flexion of the foot. Even though this type of leg had first been manufactured in 1800, it came to be known as the 'Anglesey Leg' after its most famous user. He ultimately came to possess several different prosthetic legs, examples of which can be seen at Plas Newydd in Anglesey, the Household Cavalry Museum in London, and the Musée de l'Armée in Paris.[53] The amputation did not spell the end of his

[50] For an example of a skeleton of an elderly man dating to the Neolithic period, circa 4900–4700 BCE, at Buthiers-Boulancourt near Paris in France, which appears to have undergone amputation of the lower left arm, see Buquet-Marco et al., 2007. Two other Neolithic and two Palaeolithic skeletons have been suggested as bearing signs of amputation but none of these have been definitively proven.

[51] See Thurston, 2007 for a brief overview of the history of prostheses since the sixteenth century; see Hernigou, 2013 for more detail on Paré's prostheses.

[52] For a recreation of the event, see the painting 'Imaginary Meeting of Arthur Wellesley, Duke of Wellington (1769–1852) and Henry William Paget, 2nd Earl of Uxbridge, later 1st Marquess of Anglesey (1768–1854) after the Amputation of his Leg in 1815', by Constantin-Fidèle Coene, at Plas Newydd, Anglesey, National Trust inv. NT 1175944. The amputated leg was initially buried in the garden of the house at the entrance to the village of Waterloo where the Marquess was operated on. The owner of the house, a Monsieur Hyacinthe Joseph-Marie Paris, asked if he might bury the leg in his garden, and proceeded to inter it in a tiny coffin and set up a monument over it with the following inscription: 'Here lies the Marquess of Anglesey's leg, pray for the rest of his body we beg.' The spot subsequently became something of a tourist attraction.

[53] Science Museum/Wellcome Collection inv. A500465.

military career; he went on to become a Field Marshall, Knight of the Garter, Lord Lieutenant of Ireland, and Master-General of the Ordinance. In fact, the amputation and the adoption of an extremity prosthesis made the Marquess, who came to be known as 'One-leg', something of a celebrity in Victorian society, and both his original leg and his prosthetic leg likewise became celebrities.[54] It is worth noting, though, that he was in a privileged position as a member of the British aristocracy, being wealthy enough to afford to purchase multiple technologically advanced prosthetic legs, and having been operated on by a surgeon competent enough to leave him with a stump that enabled him to wear them. Many contemporaneous amputees had to make do with simple peg-legs, or even just a pair of crutches. In some cases, the 'social condition' of a patient was considered by the surgeon performing the amputation, who was of the view that while a wealthy individual would be in a position to avail themselves of the highest-quality prosthesis, which necessitated providing them with a suitable stump, a poor individual would not, so it did not.[55]

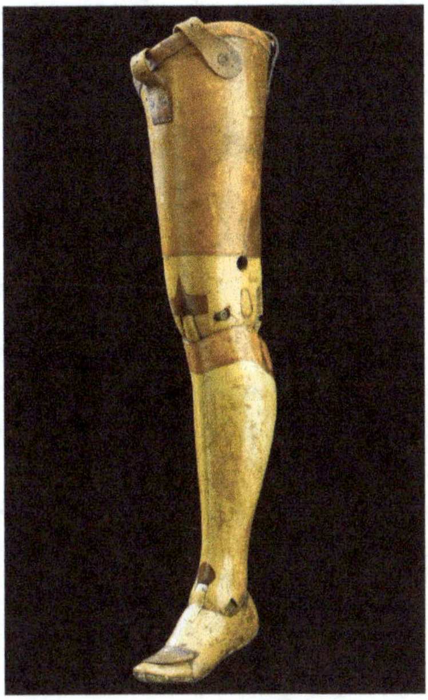

Figure I.3 Anglesey Leg. Science Museum/Wellcome Collection inv. A500465. Image courtesy of the Science Museum, London.

[54] Warne, 2008, p. 29; see also Anglesey, 1961. [55] Warne, 2008, p. 31.

In the wake of the United States of America's Civil War (1861–5), during which an estimated 60,000 limbs were amputated, a concerted effort was made by private companies to develop prosthetic technology to cater to the unprecedented demand for it, and these drew upon the 'Anglesey Leg' for inspiration.[56] This relationship between warfare and prosthesis manufacture continued in the wake of the First World War (1914–18) and other wars fought in the twentieth century, such as the Second War (1939–45), the Vietnam War (1955–75), and the wars in Afghanistan and Iraq (2001–present).[57] It has been suggested that the soldiers who returned from these wars posed a problem: the 'crippled soldier problem'.[58] In order to reintegrate veterans into society, it was considered necessary to restore not only the former soldier's economic productivity and thus prevent him from proving a drain on national resources, but also his masculinity, endangered by his new-found frailty and vulnerability. Anxiety about a former soldier's or sailor's ability to return to their previous occupation or at the very least earn a living was profound.[59] This anxiety was not only felt by the soldier or sailor in question, but also by society at large, which saw the primary problem with the veteran being not the impairment but the possibility that it would result in them becoming a burden on post-war society, crippling (and here I use that pejorative word deliberately) the nation's economic growth and well-being.[60] This was a problem that needed to be solved. Consequently, cooperation between surgeons who performed amputations and prosthetists who designed and manufactured prostheses increased. Alternatively, we could consider these soldiers to be 'broken soldiers' rather than 'crippled', 'wounded', or 'injured', because what is 'broken' can be 'fixed', and it is clear that a concerted effort was made to 'fix' these 'broken soldiers' by crafting them prostheses of varying types.[61] In this period, the preferred prosthesis was one that was facilitated easy and natural motion; appeared realistic; and was durable, lightweight, and affordable.[62] It promised its user the 'fiction of wholeness'.[63] While there was a certain amount of pride felt about a wound received in service to one's country, which could be viewed a sign of martial valour and manly courage, broadly speaking nineteenth and twentieth century society tended to stigmatise impaired bodies and characterise them as economically burdensome, psychologically unstable, and socially objectionable.[64]

[56] Figg and Farrell-Beck, 1993; Hasegawa, 2012, p. xiii.
[57] On American prostheses, see Hermes, 2002 and Hasegawa, 2012; on German prostheses, see Neumann, 2010.
[58] Brown, 2002. See also Kinder, 2015, p. 3, for the 'problem of the disabled veteran'.
[59] Hasegawa, 2012, pp. 3–4. [60] Kinder, 2015, p. 9. [61] Hasegawa, 2012, p. ix.
[62] Hasegawa, 2012, pp. 3–4. [63] Kinder, 2015, p. 35. [64] Kinder, 2015, p. 30.

Concurrent with the development of the prosthesis industry during the nineteenth and early twentieth centuries was the rise of mechanical surgery – that is, treatment with apparatus such as trusses and other types of 'technologies of the body'.[65] This resulted in a complex relationship between bodies, machines, instruments, and mechanics, and an equally complex relationship between their effects upon an individual's appearance, image, and identity.[66] For perhaps the first time, it was thought that errant nature could be corrected.[67] Purveyors approached their target audience as customers rather than patients, and claimed that their approaches would succeed where medicine had failed, deliberately creating a link between medicine and scientific instruments and gadgets.[68]

Just as the Marquess of Anglesey popularised prostheses in Victorian society, the increasingly high profile of prostheses in western Europe during the early twenty-first century is the result of the high profile – one might say celebrity status, even – of veterans of the wars in Afghanistan and Iraq and participants in the Paralympic Games, particularly the London 2012 Olympic Games. Personalised prostheses are becoming more popular, particularly among younger prosthesis users. Thus, we might speak of 'aesthetic prosthetics' or 'proAesthetics'.[69] Notable here is the work of Sophie Oliveira Barata at the Alternative Limb Project, where 'alternative' prostheses are designed and constructed in consultation with the client and their prosthetist according to the client's specific tastes and preferences, with prices for an 'alternative' prosthesis starting at £1,000 (the Alternative Limb Project also offers 'realistic' prostheses; prices for these start at £700 and can go up to £6,000).[70] Other companies, such as Limbitless Solutions, aim to utilise 3D printing to create bionic prostheses for children at affordable cost, and a promotional short film for the company featured the actor Robert Downey Jr, in character as the Marvel superhero Tony Stark/Iron Man, presenting a 3D printed prosthesis to a young boy with a partially developed right arm.[71]

Bespoke prostheses such as those made by Sophie Oliveira Barata are intentionally simultaneously prostheses and works of art, and have been exhibited accordingly, demonstrating recognition of the growing

[65] Hasegawa, 2012, p. 11; see also Withey, 2016. The term 'body-equipment' has also been used; see Vainshtein, 2012, p. 143.

[66] Withey, 2016, p. 5. [67] Withey, 2016, p. 93.

[68] Withey, 2016, pp. 6–7. For discussion of a possible link between prostheses, scientific instruments and gadgets in antiquity, see Chapter 4.

[69] O'Sullivan, cited in Vainshtein, 2012, p. 146.

[70] www.thealternativelimbproject.com/ (accessed January 2021).

[71] https://limbitless-solutions.org/ (accessed January 2021). This stunt was subsequently critiqued by Smith, 2016.

importance of the form of a prosthesis in addition to its function, and the way that this form can be enlisted as a means of self-expression, just like any other accessory.[72] In 2017, the exhibition 'Prosthetic Greaves' ran from 14 to 29 October at the Glasgow School of Art, and exhibited the outcomes of the Glasgow School of Art's 'Prosthetic Greaves' research project.[73] Two researchers, Jeroen Blom and Tara French, developed a method for digitally designing bespoke limb-shaped models that can be customised according to an amputee's body shape and preferences, and these models could then be used to create craft-specific templates that suit the materials and techniques. Using this method as a basis, the creative design process between artisans and amputees could focus on creating a shared background and deep understanding of the needs that can be translated into the designs of the lower limb prosthesis covers. Since research has found that many amputees prefer a different aesthetic than the common prosthetic design choices of either a foam limb-shaped cover or a bare pole, the 'Prosthetic Greaves' research project sought to deliver a beautiful crafted aesthetic for lower limb prothesis covers – 'greaves' – by having artisans work in collaboration with amputees.[74] Three unique prosthesis covers were created and subsequently displayed in conjunction with information about the design and production process. The first, made by Karen Collins from Naturally Useful, a willow weaving company, used different types and colours of willow and wove them into a beautiful, strong, and lightweight shape. The 'greave' sought to embody the connection to nature using naturally grown materials woven by hand, and the prosthesis user took part in practicing the weaving of willow, strengthening the personal connection with the final product. The second, made by Scott Gleed from Gleed3D, a company that specialises in model-making, combined casting techniques of white metal and crystal-clear resin to create a seamless integration of materials. The front of the 'greave' showed a pattern of stockings and the rear combined metal and resin to create the seam of the stocking. The rear also had an angular design, so it has its own unique shape rather than mirroring a human limb. The third, made by Roger Milton from Auldearn Antiques, an antiques company that also restores items and creates its own unique pieces of furniture, used

72 See, for example, the discussion of glasses/spectacles and how they have gone from being assistive technology to 'eyewear', at Pullin, 2009, pp. 16–23.

73 www.gsa.ac.uk/life/gsa-events/events/p/prosthetic-greaves/ (accessed January 2021); www.gsa.ac.uk/life/gsa-events/events/p/prosthetic-greaves/ (accessed August 2022).

74 The extent to which ancient prosthesis users would have collaborated with artisans during the process of designing, commissioning, and manufacturing protheses, or even designed and manufactured their own, will be discussed further in Chapter 4.

carefully selected timber, highlighting the imperfection of the burls on the material to emphasise its unique character. Burls occur due to 'illness' of the tree, and the pattern that it creates is something truly unique to the tree and highly sought after by woodworkers. The resultant beautiful imperfection of the 'greave' signified the beautiful 'imperfection' of the human body through amputation, creating unity between the 'greave', the prosthesis, and the prosthesis user. This approach to the problem of the undesirability of the form of the contemporary basic prosthesis, essentially providing a desirable form for a cover for the prosthesis, is potentially a very flexible – not to mention cost-effective – solution.

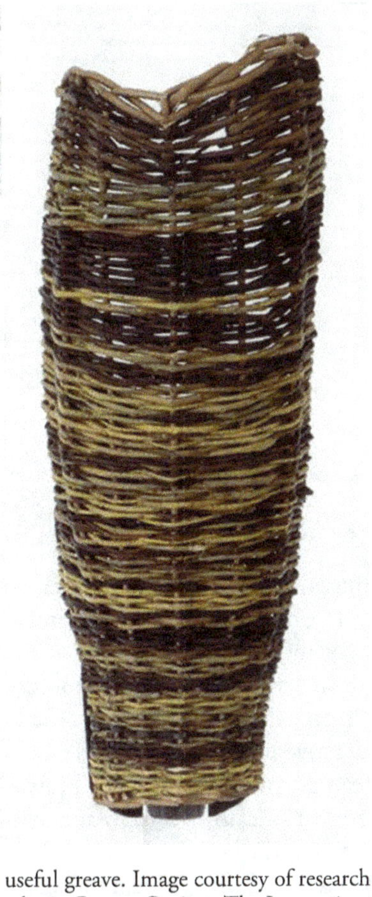

Figure I.4 Naturally useful greave. Image courtesy of research fellows Jeroen Blom and Tara French, Prosthetic Greaves Project, The Innovation School, GSA. http://radar.gsa.ac.uk/6990/3/Aesthetics%20of%20Prosthetic%20Greaves.pdf.

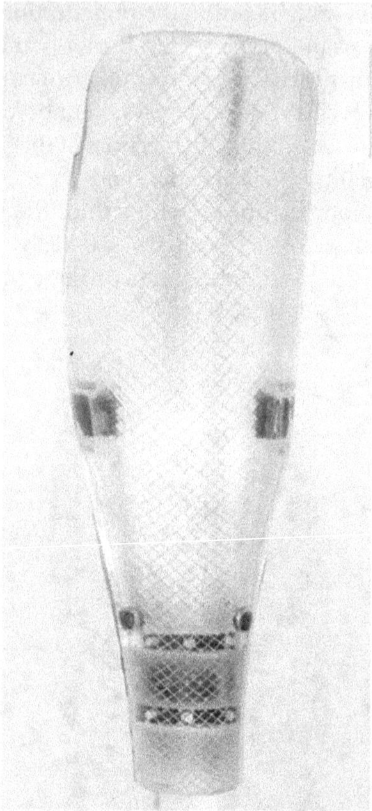

Figure I.5 Gleed 3D greave. Image courtesy of research fellows Jeroen Blom and Tara French, Prosthetic Greaves Project, The Innovation School, GSA. http://radar.gsa.ac.uk/6990/3/Aesthetics%20of%20Prosthetic%20Greaves.pdf.

Two recent major museum exhibitions at the Victoria and Albert Museum in London, the world's leading museum of art and design, have included prostheses, and have raised the profile of prostheses as works of art even further. In fact, both exhibitions' advance publicity and promotional material featured the prostheses heavily. In 2018 the exhibition 'Frida Kahlo: Making Herself Up' ran from 16 June to 4 November and displayed more than 200 of Kahlo's possessions that had been discovered in the Blue House in 2004, having been locked away since the artist's death in 1954. Among these possessions were several of her 'technologies of the body', a number of medical corsets that she wore to support her spine after a traffic accident she was in at the age of eighteen displaced three of her vertebrae, and a prosthetic leg that she wore after she

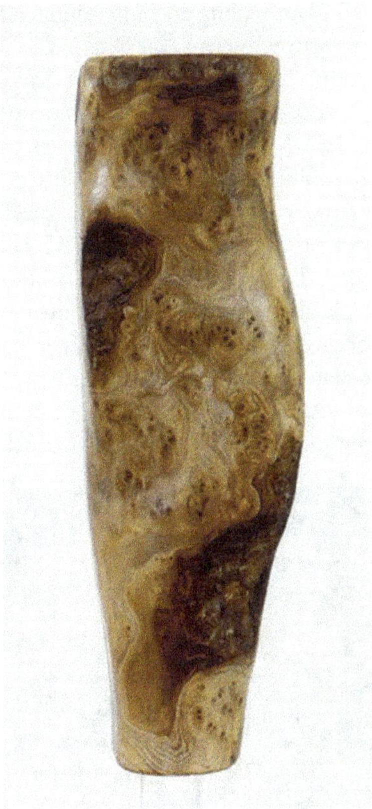

Figure I.6 Auldearn Antiques greave. Image courtesy of research fellows Jeroen Blom and Tara French, Prosthetic Greaves Project, The Innovation School, GSA. http://radar.gsa.ac.uk/6990/3/Aesthetics%20of%20Prosthetic%20Greaves.pdf.

contracted gangrene and her right leg was amputated in 1953.[75] The prosthetic leg is set into a red leather boot embroidered with fantastical creatures and strung with bells that would jingle as she walked. Kahlo designed and decorated these items herself, reclaiming these medical objects as a means of self-expression and using them to communicate her own feelings about her physical condition. Her relationship with these objects has been described as 'one of support and need – her body was dependent on medical attention – but also one of rebellion'.[76] By personalising her 'technologies of the body' through decorating and adorning them, Kahlo was presenting herself as having explicitly chosen to wear them, rather than having to wear them.[77] Moreover, they served

[75] For discussion, see Henestrosa, 2018, pp. 78–80.
[76] Henestrosa, 2018, p. 80.
[77] Henestrosa, 2018. p. 80.

as a means of simultaneously revealing and concealing her disabilities, allowing her to present herself on her own terms.[78]

In 2015, the exhibition 'Alexander McQueen: Savage Beauty' ran from 14 March to 2 August and served as the first retrospective of the fashion designer's life and work.[79] McQueen has been described as 'the designer [who] has most meaningfully worked with disability and disabled bodies'.[80] In his work, 'there is an understanding of and willingness to see disability as an aesthetic possibility, something which can be worked with, rather than disguised'.[81] His thirteenth fashion show, n° 13, for spring/summer 1999, was opened by the Paralympic athlete and double amputee Aimee Mullins, and to do so she wore a pair of prosthetic legs that McQueen had designed especially for her.[82] They had collaborated the previous year for the September 1998 'Fashion-Able' issue of *Dazed & Confused* magazine and its 'Access-Able' editorial, and McQueen subsequently aimed to create three different pairs of

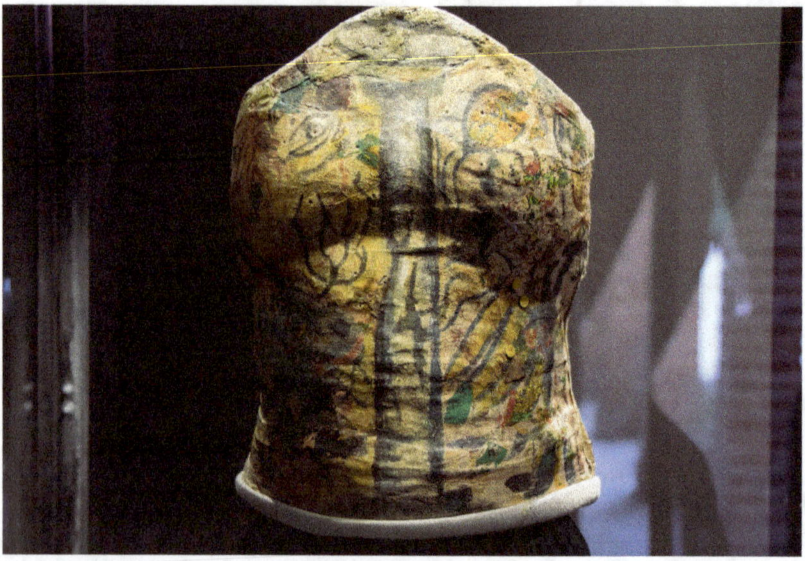

Figure I.7 Medical corset belonging to Frida Kahlo. Image courtesy of Alamy.

[78] It is worth noting, however, that Kahlo did not actually wish to have such private possessions displayed in public, see Adams, 2021b, p. 90. For discussion of how museums struggle with the issue of exhibiting technologies of the body such as prostheses, see Goggins, 2021.

[79] For the V&A's online Museum of Savage Beauty, see www.vam.ac.uk/museumofsavagebeauty/ (accessed January 2021).

[80] Smith, cited in Allwood, 2015.

[81] Smith, cited in Allwood, 2015.

[82] The Museum of Savage Beauty has a specific entry for Aimee Mullins' prosthetic legs: www.vam.ac.uk/museumofsavagebeauty/mcq/prosthetic-legs/ (accessed January 2021).

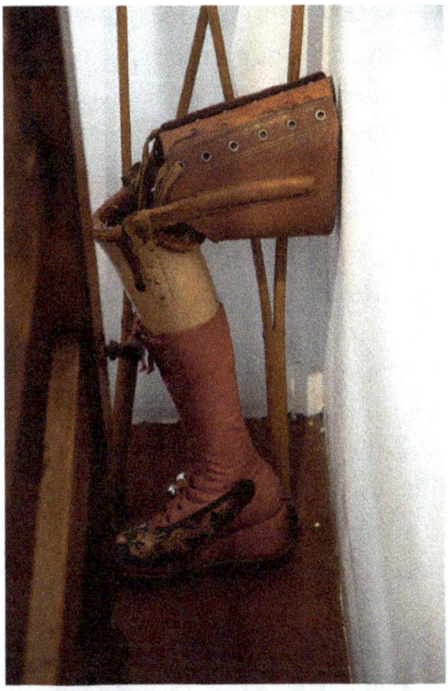

Figure I.8 Prosthetic leg belonging to Frida Kahlo. Image courtesy of Alamy.

legs for her to wear in his show. The first of these was to be glass, the second Swarovski crystal, and the third wood, although ultimately only the wooden pair was produced. The legs were designed to resemble a pair of Victorian knee-length boots with Louis heels, pointed toes, and slim ankles (McQueen was fascinated by Victorian literature, particularly the works of Charles Dickens), and inspired by a Louis XIV style table and contemporary wood carvers such as Grinling Gibbons.[83] They were made from ash wood for two reasons: the first being that the strength of the wood was sufficient to bear Mullins' weight, and the second that it could be elaborately carved.

Most recently, in the autumn of 2018 the National Museum of Scotland acquired the 'Vine Arm', a prosthetic arm made by Sophie Oliveira Barata at the Alternative Limb Project for the model Kelly Knox, to display in its Technology by Design exhibit.[84] Knox was born without her lower left arm and chooses not to use a functional prosthesis; rather, she uses prostheses as

[83] Most of Charles Dickens' works include references to prosthetic legs: for example, *The Pickwick Papers* (1937), *The Old Curiosity Shop* (1840), *Barnaby Rudge* (1841), *Martin Chuzzlewit* (1844), *David Copperfield* (1850), and *Our Mutual Friend* (1865). However, these portrayals are not positive; they 'repeatedly associate prostheses with ignorance, intemperance, and greed'; see Warne, 2008, p. 32; O'Connor, 2000, p. 130; Carey, 1973, p. 91.

[84] National Museum of Scotland inv. T.2018.1. For discussion of the genesis of this exhibition, see Goggins, 2021.

accessories to express her personality and explore aspects of her identity.[85] According to Knox, 'I want to change the way society perceives disability – showing disability can be cool, fashionable, beautiful and powerful . . . it's like my body is a canvas and when wearing an Alternative Limb, I become art.'[86] The 'Vine Arm' comprises a botanical tentacle which contains twenty-six individual vertebrae that allow movement in the arm to be fluid and curve around objects, and this is controlled by round sensors worn in Knox's matching shoes, underneath her big toes, that enable her to move the Vine from side to side and to curve it. By pressing on the sensors with different pressure, she can control the speed and direction of the Vine's movement.[87] In this context, Knox is not simply wearing a prosthesis; rather, she is wearing an entire outfit. The form of the 'Vine Arm' is its entire function.

According to Sophie Oliviera Barata, the Alternative Limb Project's mission statement is to use 'the unique medium of prosthetics to create highly stylised art pieces. As with fashion, where physical appearance

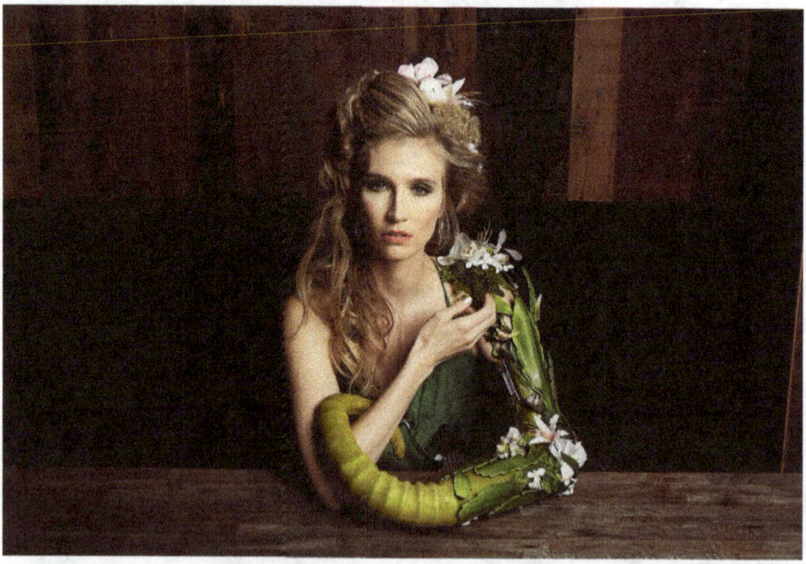

Figure I.9 Vine Arm designed by the Alternative Limb Project for Kelly Knox. National Museum of Scotland inv. T.2018.1. Image courtesy of the Alternative Limb Project, photograph taken by Omkaar Kotedia.

85 Knox was the winner of BBC3's Britain's Missing Top Model competition in 2008.
86 www.nms.ac.uk./explore-our-collections/stories/science-and-technology/vine-arm/ (accessed January 2021).
87 For a demonstration, see https://youtu.be/jBSqG5DTeqU (accessed January 2021).

becomes a form of self-expression, [we see] the potential of prosthetics as an extension of the wearer's personality.'[88] Testimonials from the Alternative Limb Project's clients support this. Jo-Jo Cranfield says the following of her 'alternative' prosthetic arm:

> I've never seen the interest in having a prosthetic arm, they are heavy, uncomfortable and not at all practical. I like to be different and I love the fact that having one arm makes me effortlessly different to the majority of people – however, an alternative limb is something entirely different; I wanted people to have to look at me twice with amazement. My alternative limb is so different to any other prosthetic limb I have ever had. I wear it with pride. I've never seen a two armed person with snakes crawling into their skin, and even if I did I don't think it would be so comfy! My alternative arm makes me feel powerful, different and sexy![89]

Kiera Roche notes the fundamental importance of her prostheses in coming to accept her new life as an amputee, and says the following of her prosthetic leg:

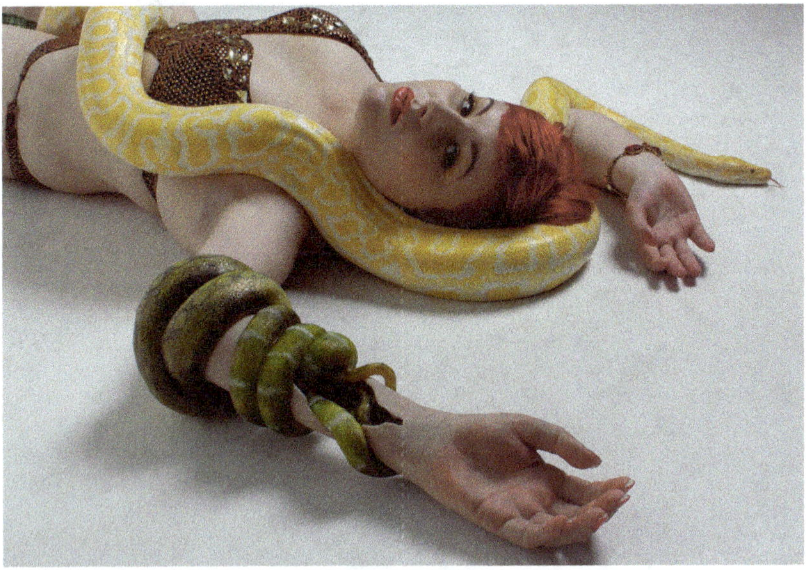

Figure I.10 Snake Arm designed by the Alternative Limb Project for Jo-Jo Cranfield. Image courtesy of the Alternative Limb Project, photograph taken by Rosemary Williams.

88 https://thealternativelimbproject.com/about/ (accessed August 2022).
89 https://thealternativelimbproject.com/limbs/snake-arm/ (accessed August 2022).

> My attitude to being an amputee and wearing an artificial limb has changed with time. To begin with one is very aware of being different, of being disfigured, but as time moves on one adjusts and changes perspective. In the first few years my focus was on trying to be normal, wearing clothes that hid the fact that I was an amputee, but over the years I have become more comfortable with who I am and I now embrace having different legs for different activities and different occasions. I think losing a limb has a massive impact on one's self esteem and body image. Having a beautifully crafted limb designed for you makes you feel special.[90]

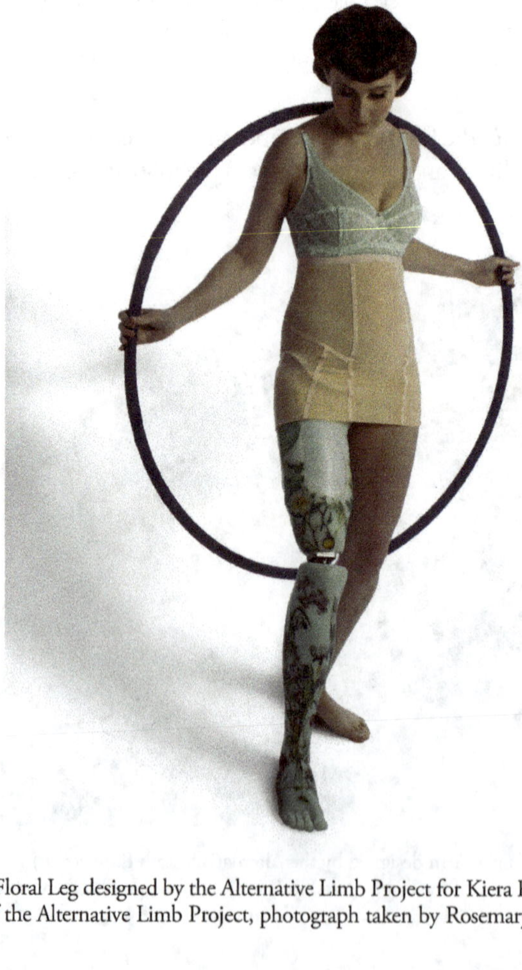

Figure I.11 Floral Leg designed by the Alternative Limb Project for Kiera Roche. Image courtesy of the Alternative Limb Project, photograph taken by Rosemary Williams.

90 https://thealternativelimbproject.com/limbs/floral-leg/ (accessed August 2022).

How applicable are these aspects of the recent history of prostheses, prosthesis use, and prosthesis users to their ancient historical equivalents? They are more applicable than one might first think. Let us bear the statements from users of Alternative Limbs in mind as we consider the Turfan Limb, an extremity prosthesis only very recently recovered from a grave at Turfan in China that has been dated to approximately 300–200 BCE, making it one of the two oldest known functional prostheses in the world.[91] It is roughly the same age as the famous Capua Limb, an extremity prosthesis recovered from a tomb at Capua in Italy that has been dated to approximately 300 BCE, which will be discussed later.[92] The skeleton of the deceased prosthesis user was present in the grave alongside the prosthesis, a relatively unusual occurrence when it comes to ancient assistive technology, and this has enabled bioarchaeologists to undertake a detailed examination not just of the prosthesis but of its user as well.[93] The deceased was a man aged between fifty and sixty-five years old at the time of his death, and he lived with a severe case of tuberculosis that froze his left knee joint in a bent position and consequently rendered walking unaided impossible. Since during this period traditional Chinese law decreed that mutilation punishment (*xing*) was to be meted out for a range of transgressions, impaired individuals experienced a considerable amount of stigmatisation, whether their impairments were the result of mutilation punishment or not.[94] The cultural and social context in which the deceased was living might therefore explain why he chose to supplement his impaired limb with a prosthesis rather than undergo surgical amputation of his left leg above the knee and then replace his lost leg with a prosthesis. It is, of course, equally possible that he simply did not have access to a surgeon who could or would have performed the operation had he requested it. But we should also bear in mind that the unusual nature of his impairment meant that he did not have to submit to what would undoubtedly have been a dangerous and extremely unpleasant procedure; he was able to use a prosthesis to restore his lost functionality regardless.

[91] Li et al., 2013.

[92] See Bourguignon and Henzen, cited in Sudhoff, 1917; von Brun, 1926 for the announcement of the discovery and early discussion and analysis of it.

[93] See Li et al., 2013, pp. 338–9 for discussion of the skeleton and palaeopathology.

[94] See Milburn, 2017 for discussion of impairment and disability in ancient China. Two cases of individuals with mobility impairments using prostheses without first undergoing amputations to remove their impaired leg or foot are also known from Late Antique Gaul (see Gregory of Tours, *VM* 3.9 and 4.41), but it should be born in mind that these are accounts of miraculous healing, with the impaired limbs being restored to full functionality after sufficient prayer, something that would obviously not have been possible had either individual undergone an amputation.

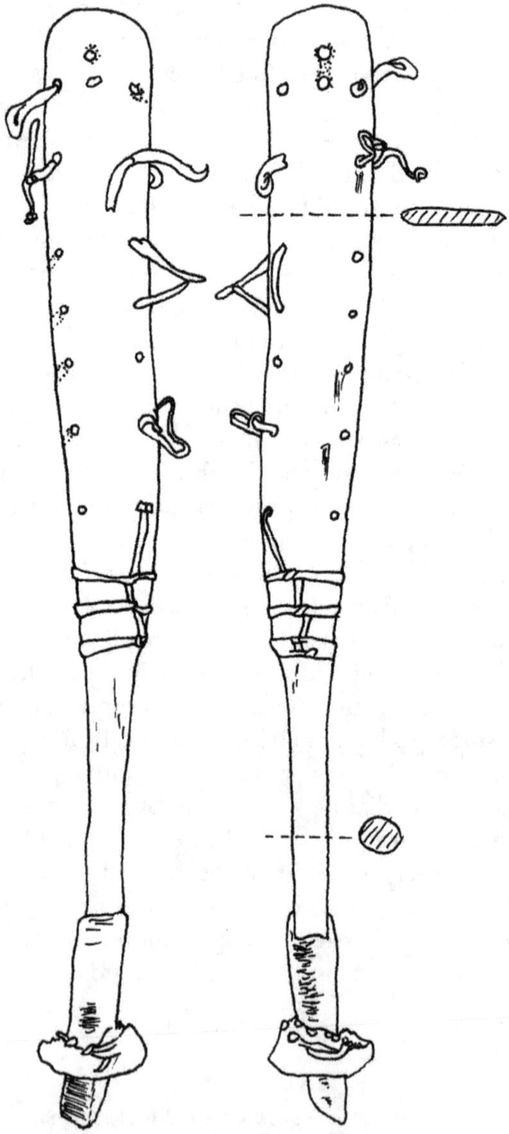

Figure I.12 Turfan Limb. Image courtesy of the German Archaeological Institute.

The Turfan Limb was made from leather, sheep or goat horn, and the hoof of a horse or an Asiatic ass.[95] It comprised a plate that was fastened to

[95] See Li et al., 2013, p. 339, for discussion of the technical aspects of the prosthesis.

the left thigh by leather straps and which tapered into a peg-leg. No attempt was made to carve the peg-leg to resemble the human limb that it was supplementing; on the contrary, the peg-leg terminated in a hoof which may, in fact, have rendered the prosthesis easier to use. There is no indication that the deceased used crutches in conjunction with his prosthesis in the manner of several other ancient prosthesis users that we shall meet later. Since the deceased was not buried in isolation but was only one burial in a cemetery, it is possible to gain a degree of understanding of this community and its circumstances. The population were relatively poor, and the goods recovered from the deceased's grave do not indicate that he was in any way unusual as far as wealth or social status were concerned.[96]

The owner of the Turfan Limb was seemingly determined not to allow his impairment to become a disability in a culture and society where impairments were viewed as highly undesirable at best, punishment for a major transgression at worst, but either way were responsible for ensuring that those experiencing them were stigmatised and treated as pariahs. As a member of a relatively poor community with no access to prestige materials such as gold, silver, bronze, iron, etc., he elected to use materials that were in plentiful supply in his agrarian and pastoral society to create his prosthesis. These materials were the animal products of leather, horn, and even a hoof, and while the materials that his prosthesis comprised and the form that his prosthesis took can be seen as entirely practical, even utilitarian, a means of stabilising him as he moved around, it is also possible that his choice of an animalistic rather than humanoid limb was influenced by his Subeixi culture's interaction with the Pazyryk culture of the Scythian communities in the nearby Altai mountains.[97]

This leads us to an aspect of ancient prostheses, prosthesis use, and prosthesis users that it is necessary to take into account that dovetails nicely with the aims of the Alternative Limb Project: since each ancient prosthesis was entirely unique and designed and manufactured in isolation by the user, one artisan (for example, a carpenter), or a team of artisans (for example, a carpenter, a metal-worker, and a leather-worker), ancient prostheses can, perhaps, give us an insight into ancient cultures and societies and their users' places within those, in addition to telling us something about the individuals themselves. Regarding the finished product, how influential was the consumer? How influential were the artisans? Whether the prosthesis is cosmetic, functional, or a combination of both, how far are the substance or substances from which it is made and the way

[96] See Li et al., 2013, p. 336 for discussion of the archaeological context.

[97] Li et al., 2013, p. 341.

in which it is made (for example design, craftsmanship, etc.) intended to serve an additional purpose related to conspicuous consumption to either demonstrate or enhance the status and prestige of its wearer?[98] Should we view ancient prostheses as having been akin to clothing and jewellery, and approach them as a type of 'bodywear' by which the ancient prosthesis user could show off his or her personal style or fashion sense?[99] Or should we view them as having been akin to a scientific gadget, such as the Antikythera Mechanism or the portable sundial, and approach them as a means by which the ancient prosthesis user could show off his or her intellectual and technical sophistication?[100]

Literature Review

To date, relatively little scholarship has focused specifically on prostheses, prosthesis use, and prosthesis users, or any type of assistive technology at all, in classical antiquity.[101] Until 2018, the only reasonably comprehensive work on the subject was Lawrence Bliquez's contribution to one of the volumes dedicated to medicine in the *Aufstieg und Niedergang der römischen Welt* series, entitled 'Prosthetics in Classical Antiquity: Greek, Etruscan, and Roman Prosthetics' (1996).[102] This piece selectively curated a certain amount of literary and archaeological examples, not all secure, of ancient prostheses, but the analysis and discussion of the subject was relatively limited. Then, in 2019, the edited volume *Prostheses in Antiquity*, the proceedings of a workshop held in 2015 and funded by the Wellcome Trust, was published. It comprised eight papers, each one dealing with a different type of prosthesis (e.g. facial, extremity) or an issue relevant to the subject (e.g. care).[103]

As far as discussions of impairment and disability in classical antiquity are concerned, discussions of prostheses, prosthesis use, and prosthesis users play a relatively minor role. The first monograph devoted to the subject, Robert Garland's *The Eye of the Beholder: Deformity and Disability*

[98] For the role that certain types of prosthesis played in demonstrating social status through their material, see Turfa and Becker, 2019; Draycott, 2019c; Lehmhaus, 2019. For conspicuous consumption in relation to prostheses in later historical periods, see Kwass, 2006; Warne, 2009.

[99] Pullin, 2009, pp. 16–23, discusses spectacles as 'eyewear'; should we perhaps consider prostheses as 'bodywear'?

[100] On gadgets in antiquity, see Wikander, 2008. On the Antikythera Mechanism, see most recently Jones, 2017. On portable sundials, see Talbert, 2017.

[101] For a cursory overview of the staff in antiquity, see Loebl and Nunn, 1997; for a more detailed study, see Draycott, in press b. There has been some discussion of the staff in its capacity as a symbolic object: see De Waele, 1927. For studies of the iconography, see Couvret, 1994; Brule, 2006.

[102] This was inspired by an earlier piece on the subject written for a general audience: Bliquez, 1983.

[103] Wellcome Trust Small Grant 108557/Z/15/Z.

in the Graeco-Roman World (first edition 1995, second edition 2010), included a brief reference to the famous story of the Persian diviner Hegesistratus of Elis in a chapter focusing on medical diagnosis and treatment, noting simply that it was possible for an ancient amputee to utilise a prosthesis.[104] The second, Martha L. Rose's *The Staff of Oedipus: Transforming Disability in Ancient Greece* (first edition 2003, second edition 2013), and the first attempt to integrate the relatively new discipline of Disability Studies into Classics, devoted slightly more space to the subject in the opening chapter of the work, an effort to set the scene in advance of a series of studies focused on particular aspects of impairment and disability in the ancient Greek world.[105] Like Bliquez, Rose curated some literary and archaeological examples, concluding that 'it is difficult to believe that any prosthetic device would have been practical as well as cosmetic'.[106] The third, Christian Laes' *Beperkt? Gehandicapten in het Romeinse Rijk* (*Restricted? The Handicapped in the Roman Empire*) (2014), contains an entire chapter on mobility impairments but prostheses are mentioned only in passing.[107] The English translation, a slightly updated version of the original Dutch text, *Disabilities and the Disabled in the Roman World: A Social and Cultural History* (2018), follows suit. Discussions of impairment and disability in the classical world are more frequently found in the form of edited volumes, and accordingly one might expect to find rather more discussion of prostheses here. Unfortunately, these likewise do not devote more than a sentence or two to the subject.[108] Prostheses, prosthesis use, and prosthesis users in other historical periods and contexts are equally understudied, although this is beginning to change.[109] There is, however, a considerable amount of scholarship on these subjects in the contemporary world and utilising this material as a source of comparative evidence is a distinct possibility.[110]

[104] Garland, 1995 reissued 2010, p. 126; the story of Hegesistratus appears in Hdt. 9.36–7; it is also referred to in Plut. *Mor. De frat. amor.* 3.1.

[105] Rose, 2003, pp. 26–7. [106] Rose, 2003, p. 26. [107] Laes, 2014.

[108] See, for example, Collard and Samama, 2010; Breitwieser, 2012; Laes, Goodey, and Rose, 2013; Krötzl, Mustakallio, and Kuuliala, 2015; Laes, 2017. A recent exception is Adams, 2021a, in which two chapters on prostheses can be found: Draycott, 2021 and Goggins, 2021.

[109] See, for example, Porter et al., 2017, although this work focuses on notions of prosthesis in medieval and early modern theological debate rather than prostheses as assistive technology. Forthcoming work by Richard Godden will focus on assistive technology, including prostheses, in the medieval period (personal communication).

[110] See, for example, Ott et al., 2002; Smith and Morra, 2006.

Methodology

As mentioned, no surviving ancient medical treatise mentions prostheses. No surviving ancient scientific or technical treatise mentions them either. Nor do we have any examples of ekphrasis the way that we do for other lost medical, scientific, or technical objects of antiquity.[111] Yet, due to the scattered and fragmentary nature of the surviving literary, documentary, archaeological, and bioarchaeological evidence that attests that a variety of different types of prostheses were used by Greeks and Romans (broadly defined) to replace various missing body parts, the subject of prostheses, prosthesis use, and prosthesis users in classical antiquity lends itself to a 'mosaicist' approach. If we trust that the literary and documentary evidence provides a true representation of the way that the Greeks and Romans referred to prostheses in their daily lives, it becomes apparent that no uniform umbrella term, such as the adjectives 'prosthetic', 'artificial', or 'false', for example, was used. Perhaps the closest ancient authors come is referring to prosthetic hair and teeth using variations on the verb 'to purchase' (Greek πρίαμαι, Latin *emo*). As stated earlier, ancient authors more commonly refer to prostheses using a combination of the substitute body part and the substance from which that substitute has been made. Consequently, searching for ancient literary and documentary references to prostheses necessitates the extremely time-consuming process of entering numerous combinations of adjectives and nouns into bibliographic search engines such as the *Thesaurus Linguae Graecae* and the *Thesaurus Linguae Latinae*, and, when that fails, simply reading ancient literary and documentary texts from all historical periods and all historical genres. In Bliquez's initial study, he admittedly focused his attention rather selectively:

> The scope of this investigation was confined to those devices attached to the human body which had some practical as well as cosmetic purpose; that is to say, I was interested in dental appliances and false limbs, as opposed to wigs and bodily padding of the sort detailed by comic poets and satirists.[112]

I have discussed what I consider to be the issues with Bliquez's differentiation between what he perceived to be practical and impractical prostheses elsewhere.[113] As discussed, it is extremely difficult to separate a prosthesis' form from its function. The binary opposition between practical and

[111] That such a thing might have occurred is not entirely implausible; for ekphrasis applied to medical machines and automata, see Roby, 2016.

[112] Bliquez, 1996, p. 2641. See Draycott, 2019c on why wigs and hair pieces should be classed as functional rather than cosmetic prostheses.

[113] Draycott, 2019c, pp. 71–2.

cosmetic assumes that there is nothing practical about a cosmetic prosthesis; but what may seem impractical to one person is highly practical to someone else. In any case, using this rationale, he collated sixteen ancient literary references to prostheses, comprising eleven dental prostheses and five extremity prostheses (three feet, one leg, one hand). To date, I have found 107 ancient literary references to prostheses, and these include references to prosthetic hands, shoulders, feet, legs, thighs, eyes, noses, teeth, and hair (see Table I.1); due to the nature of the search, even this is not necessarily exhaustive.[114] It is possible to differentiate between factual and fictitious references in the sense that prostheses appear in both ancient works of non-fiction such as Pliny the Elder's encyclopaedia *Natural History* and fiction such as Petronius' novel *Satyricon*, and between real and mythological references in the sense that prostheses are used by real individuals such as Hegesistratus of Elis and by mythological figures such as Pelops (see Table I.2). And yet, while at first glance we might be tempted to dismiss some, perhaps many, of these references on the grounds that they are not sufficiently 'historical', whether factual or fictitious, whether real or mythological, to a degree, archaeological and bioarchaeological evidence supports their veracity. Examples of prosthetic toes, feet, legs, teeth, hair, and a hand that seem to correspond rather closely with those referred to by ancient authors have been recovered from tombs and graves around the ancient and late antique Mediterranean (see Table I.3). Consequently, this data set can be used to elucidate a substantial amount of information about prostheses in classical antiquity, and the ways in which they were viewed in ancient Mediterranean cultures and societies.

It is crucial, however, that the ancient literary and documentary references to prostheses be treated critically.[115] Regarding ancient literature, references to prostheses can be found in a variety of different genres, but it is notable that the information provided about prostheses, and the ways in which they are presented, varies considerably depending upon the genre in which the reference is found.[116] For example, both men and women are presented as using prostheses (see Table I.4).[117] However, there are

[114] See, for example, Draycott, 2021 – at the time of writing that piece of work, I had found 102.

[115] For a good example of how ancient literature can be mined for information regarding the living conditions of the impaired and disabled in antiquity, see Laes, 2011.

[116] For discussion of how 'the medium' affects 'the message' regarding the transmission of scientific and technical information, see Taub, 2017, p. x.

[117] To date, I have found no references to children using prostheses, although that is not to say that they did not, simply that no one thought to record it; see Laes, 2008 and 2013 on evidence for impaired and disabled children in antiquity. There are, however, depictions in art of children using wheeled walking frames to assist with their physical mobility.

Table I.1 *All ancient literary references to prostheses found to date*

Body Part	References	Total
Finger		
Hand	Stat. *Theb.* 94–97 (1); Dio Chrys. *Or.* 8.28 (2); Plin. *HN* 7.29 (1)	4
Arm	Diod. Sic. 3.52 (1?)	1(?)
Shoulder	Pind. *Ol.* 1.37 (1); Hyg. *Fab.* 83 (1); Ov. *Met.* 6.405 (1); Mart. 12.84 (1); Verg. *G* 3.7 (1); Philostr. *Imag.* 1.30 (2); Luc. *De Salt.* 54 (1); Tib. 63–64 (1); Plin. *HN* 28.6.24 (1); Nonnus, *Dion.* 15.24–30 (1); Sext. Emp. *Math.* 255–256 (1); Paus. 5.13.4–6 (1); Dio Chrys. *Or.* 8.28 (1)	14
Toe		
Foot	Hdt. 9.36–37 (1); Plut. *Mor. De frat. amor.* 3.1 (1); Luc. *Ind.* 6 (2); Babylonian Talmud Yebamot 102b–103a (1)	5
Thigh	Arist. On the Pythagoreans Fr. 191 (1); Porph. *Pyth.* 28 (1); Diog. Laert. Pythagoras 11 (1); Plut. *Vit. Num.* 65 (1); Luc. *Alex.* 40 (1); Ael. *VH* 4.17 (1); Ael. *VH* 2.26 (1); Luc. *Dial. mort.* 416 (1); Amm. Marc. 22.21 (1)	10
Leg	Erycius, *Greek Anthology* 9.233 (1); Mart. 10.100 (1); Babylonian Talmud Chagiga 3a (1); Mishnah Shabbat 6.8 (1); Tosefta Shabbat 5:1–2 (1); Talmud Yerushalmi Shabbat 8:8, 8c (1); Babylonian Talmud Yoma 78b (1); Gregory of Tours, *VM* 3.9 (1); Gregory of Tours, *VM* 4.41 (1)	9
Eye	Dio Chrys. *Or.* 8.28 (2); Palestinian Talmud/Yerushalmi Nedarim 9.8 (1); Luc. *Ver. hist.* 1.25 (1)	4
Nose	Theophanes, Chronographia (1)	1
Teeth	*Laws of the Twelve Tables* 10.8–9 (1); Hippoc. *Art.* 33.9–10 (1); Celsus, *Med.* 6.12 (1); Hor. *Sat.* 1.8.47–50 (1); Mart. 14.46 (1); Mart. 12.23 (1); Mart. 1.72 (1); Mart. 9.38 (1); Mart. 5.43 (1); Luc. *Rhet.* 24 (1); Macedonius the Concul, *Greek Anthology* 11.374 (1); Lucilius, *Greek Anthology* 11.310 (1); Mishnah, Shabbat 6.5 (2); Palestinian Talmud, Shabbat 6.5 (2); Palestinian Talmud/Yerushalmi Nedarim 9.8 (1); Babylonian Talmud Nedarim 66a–b	21
Hair	Hor. *Sat.* 1.8.47–50 (1); Mart. 12.23 (1); Mart. 9.38 (1); Mart. 12.45 (1); Mart. 6.12 (1); Lucilius, *Greek Anthology* 11.310 (1); Lucilius, *Greek Anthology* 11.68 (1); Luc. *Dial. meret.* 11 (4); Avienus, *Fables* 11.7–12 (1); Luc. *Alex.* (1); Arist. *Thesm.* 258 (1); Suet. *Calig.* 11 (1); Suet. *Ner.* 26 (1); Suet. *Oth.* 12 (1); Joseph. *Vit.* 47 (1); Juv. 6.120–122 (1); Herodian, *History of the Empire* 4.7.3 (1); Ael. *VH* 1.26 (1); Ath. 10.415a–b (1); Apul. *Met.* 11.8 (1); Xen. *Cyr.* 1.3.2 (1); Ov. *Met.* 14.654–660 (1); Cass. Dio 80.2 (1); Polyb. 3.78 (1); Philostr. *Ep.* 22 (1); Myrinus, *Greek Anthology* 6.254 (1); Petron. *Sat.* 110 (2); Mishnah, Shabbat 6.5 (2)	33
Eyebrows	Petron. *Sat.* 110 (2); Mart. 3.38 (1)	3
Phallus	Luc. *Ver. hist.* 1.22 (2)	2
Total		107

Table I.2 *Types of prostheses mentioned in ancient literature, and natures of prosthesis users*

Body Part	Fact	Fiction	Hypothetical	Total	Historical Figure	Mythological Figure
Finger						
Hand	1	1	2	4	1	1
Arm	1(?)			1(?)	1(?)	
Shoulder		14		14		14
Toe						
Foot	2	2	1	5	2	
Thigh	9	1		10	8	
Leg	3		6	9	3	
Eye		1	3	4		
Nose	1			1	1	
Teeth	6	2	13	21		
Hair	18	10	2	33	12	1
Eyebrow	1	2		3		
Phallus		2				
Total	41	35	24	107	28	16

Table I.3 *Types of prostheses mentioned in ancient literature, and genders of prosthesis users*

Body Part	Male User	Female User	Unspecified	Total
Finger				
Hand	4			4
Arm	1(?)			1(?)
Shoulder	14			14
Toe				
Foot	5			5
Thigh	10			10
Leg	6		3	9
Eye	2	1	1	4
Nose	1			1
Teeth		18	3	21
Hair	16	17		33
Eyebrow	2	1		3
Phallus	2			2
Total	63	37	7	107

Table I.4 *Materials the prostheses mentioned in ancient literature are made from*

Body Part	Gold	Silver	Bronze	Iron	Wood	Ivory	Bone	Horn	Diamond	Malachite	Leather	Hair	Textile	Unspecified	Total
Finger															
Hand	1			1		2									4
Arm											1(?)				1(?)
Shoulder						14									14
Toe															
Foot					4									1	5
Thigh	9										1				10
Leg					6									3	9
Eye	1								1	1				1	4
Nose	1														1
Teeth	8	1					1	1						10	21
Hair											1	4		28	33
Eyebrow														2	3
Phallus					1	1									2
Total	20	1		1	11	17	1	1	1	1	3	4		45	107

significant differences not only in the types of prosthesis that they are presented as using, but also in the ways in which these stories are told, and whether their prosthesis usage is a positive or a negative thing. There are also significantly more examples of men using prostheses than women. Why is this? Is it simply a result of the generally gendered nature of ancient literary sources? Very possibly, for while it is notable that the references are found in both prose and poetry across a range of genres, certain types of references are found in specific genres. The references to men using prostheses are found in all literary genres, but the references to women using prostheses are concentrated in satirical poetry and prose.[118] Men are presented as utilising extremity prostheses (i.e. feet, legs, hands), while women are presented as utilising facial prostheses (i.e. teeth, hair). Why is this? Were men more likely to lose limbs while women were more likely to lose facial features? Although realistically it is likely that both genders could lose any number of body parts in any number of ways – accidents do happen, after all – in literature men lose their body parts through military or agricultural activity, while women lose their body parts through mutilation or the natural ageing process. For men undertaking military activity, the loss of the right hand (the sword hand) and one or both eyes (due to lack of appropriate protective gear) seem to have been particularly common, while for men undertaking agricultural activity, the feet or legs were at risk from accidents with agricultural tools or bites from venomous creatures.[119] Women seem to have been particularly at risk of facial mutilation that occurred as the result of interpersonal violence, carried out purposefully to spoil their beauty and, in doing, so make them less attractive to men and therefore less valuable, and the female natural ageing process that resulted in the loss of teeth and hair receives much more commentary from ancient writers than the male one, again because of the effect that this had on a woman's beauty, her attractiveness to men, and her intrinsic value.[120] Interestingly, in ancient Jewish literature, facial prostheses are recommended specifically to

[118] See for example Hor. *Sat.* 1.8.47–50; Juv. 6.120–2; Mart. 1.72, 5.43, 9.38, 12.23, 12.45, 14.56, Lucillius, *Greek Anthology* 11.68, 11.310; Macedonius, *Greek Anthology* 11.374; Luc. *Rhet.* 24.

[119] Loss of the right hand during military activity: Plin. *HN* 7.29; Plut. *Vit. Cam.* 142; Luc. *Tox.* 10, 62; Amm. Marc. 17.10; Nonnus, *Dion.* 2.427–35, 22.196–202. Loss of one or both eyes during military activity: Dion. Hal. *Ant. Rom.* 5.23.2–25; Plut. *Vit. Sert.* 4.2; Caes. *BCiv.* 3.53.4; Suet. *Iul.* 68.4; Lucan, *Pharsalia* 6.213–16. Loss of the foot or the leg during agricultural activity: Erycius, *Greek Anthology* 9.233.

[120] Loss of facial features through mutilation: Plaut. *Aul.* 188–9; Diod. Sic. 1.78.4–5; Hermesianax, *Fragments* (*Leontion*) 2.4. Loss of teeth and hair through the natural ageing process: Cokayne, 2003; Parkin, 2003.

restore a woman's physical attractiveness and make her a more desirable potential bride.[121] But perhaps there was some sort of visible imbalance in prosthesis use in ancient societies and this fed into existing stereotypes and bolstered them. It could be simply that male bodies were more visible in ancient Greek and Roman society than female ones, so male extremity prosthesis use was apparent to the casual observer in a way that female extremity prosthesis use was not.[122] And, yet again, archaeological and bioarchaeological evidence supports these demarcations (see Table I.5).

Table I.5 *Archaeological and bioarchaeological evidence for ancient prostheses*

Body Part	Archaeological Evidence	Total
Finger		
Hand	Povegliano Hand (Italy)	1
Arm		
Shoulder		
Toe	Greville Chester Toe (Egypt); Cairo Toe (Egypt)	2
Foot	Bonaduz Foot (Switzerland)	1
Thigh		
Leg	Capua Leg (Italy); Hemmaberg Leg (Austria); Griesheim Leg (Germany)	3
Eye		
Nose	Unknown (Egypt) (1)	1
Teeth	Etruria (Italy) (1); Bisenzio (Italy) (1); Lake Bolsena (Italy) (1); Orvieto (Italy) (2); Chiusi (Italy) (1); Populonia (Italy) (1); Tarquinia (Italy) (5); Vulci (Italy) (2); Valsiarosa (Italy) (1); Teano (Italy) (1); Praeneste (Italy) (1); Satricum (Italy) (1); Bracciano (Italy) (1); Tanagra (Greece); Sardis (Turkey); Sidon (Lebanon) (2); Alexandria (Egypt) (1); El-Qatta (Egypt) (1); Tura El-Asmant (Egypt) (1); Eretria (Greece) (1); Rome (Italy) (1); Jersualem (Israel) (4)	32
Hair	Les-Martres-de-Veyre (France) (3); Rainham Creek (England) (1); York (England) (1); Vindolanda (England) (1); Newstead (Scotland) (1); Dush (Egypt) (2); Gurob (Egypt) (1); Harit (Egypt) (1); Unknown (Egypt) (2); Rome (Italy) (2)	15
Eyebrow		
Phallus		
Total		55

[121] Palestinian Talmud, tractate Nedarim 9.41c; Babylonian Talmud, Nedarim 66b. For discussion, see Lehmhaus, 2019, pp. 112–13. Interestingly, it was also considered acceptable in ancient Jewish society for women to wear cosmetics as a means of enhancing their natural beauty; see Orizaga, 2013.

[122] On the clothing of Greek and Roman women, see Lee, 2015; Olson, 2012.

Of the extremity prostheses that have survived from classical antiquity (broadly defined), all but one of those found in situ were found in the tombs and graves of men.[123] These include the third century BCE Capua Limb and the sixth century CE 'Hemmaberg Limb'. Of the facial prostheses that have survived from classical antiquity, all of those found in situ were found in the tombs and graves of women, and the size of those that are unprovenanced indicates that they belonged to women too.[124]

It is likewise crucial that archaeological and bioarchaeological evidence for prostheses be treated critically.[125] While some of the surviving ancient prostheses, such as the 'Hemmaberg Limb' and the 'Povegliano Veronese Hand', have been discovered only very recently, and as a result have been excavated carefully and scientifically analysed as rigorously and comprehensively as possible, most surviving ancient prostheses were discovered a century or more ago, and little, if anything, is known about their provenances.[126] In the case of the Capua Limb, while the prosthesis was excavated, recorded, photographed, and sketched carefully, it was subsequently destroyed in an air raid during the Blitz and only a partial replica survives today. Where possible, I have visited museums and examined both original and replica prostheses, and, where it exists, their accompanying documentation, to get a sense of the objects themselves. This has provided me with insights regarding their design, creation, and usage that I would not otherwise have had, and I have applied these insights to what follows.

Outline

This monograph will examine the prostheses, prosthesis use, and prosthesis users of classical antiquity from several different angles. My aim is to answer the following questions: How common – or uncommon – were prostheses in classical antiquity? Who made

[123] The exception is the Cairo Toe, a prosthetic right toe that belonged to Tabaketenmut, the daughter of the priest Bakamon. For discussion, see Finch, 2019.

[124] Becker and Turfa, 2017, pp. 113–14.

[125] For what archaeology can contribute to the study of disability, see Southwell-Wright, 2013.

[126] The 'Hemmaberg Limb' was discovered in 2013; see Binder et al., 2016. The 'Povegliano Veronese Hand' was discovered in 1985 but only made public recently; see Micarelli et al., 2018. It is entirely possible that more prostheses will be discovered in the future, as exploratory and rescue archaeological excavations are undertaken in, for example, the United Kingdom and Italy in response to large-scale infrastructure building projects.

them? How did they make them? Why did they make them? Who used them? How did they use them? Why did they use them? How were they – and their prostheses – viewed by other members of ancient society as a result? I shall do this by focusing on each type of prosthesis that we have ancient evidence – literary, documentary, archaeological, bioarchaeological – for in turn. Where relevant, I shall also consider evidence for other types of assistive technology, such as walking sticks, canes, crutches, and walking frames that were used in conjunction with prostheses.

The first chapter, Extremity Prostheses and Assistive Technology, will explore the numerous ways in which extremities ranging from fingers, hands, and arms to toes, feet, and legs could be lost, and how prostheses were utilised as a means of substitution. It will survey the ancient literary evidence for extremity amputation and prosthesis use, and study in detail the archaeological remains of extremity prostheses and the bioarchaeological remains of individuals who utilised them. The second chapter, Facial Prostheses, will explore the numerous ways in which parts of the face – eyes, nose, teeth – could be lost, and how or even if prostheses were utilised as a means of substitution. Unlike with extremity prostheses, the evidence for facial prostheses, particularly prosthetic eyes and noses, is limited and enigmatic. The third chapter, Hair Prostheses, will explore the type of ancient prosthesis for which the evidence is most plentiful: the wig or hairpiece. Yet, although wigs and hair pieces are so well attested in the classical world, that is not to say that their interpretation is straightforward. It will survey the ancient literary evidence for wig and hairpiece use, and study in detail the archaeological remains of wigs and hair pieces and the bioarchaeological remains of individuals who utilised them. The fourth chapter, Design, Commission, and Manufacture of Prostheses, will survey the evidence for the process of commissioning, designing, and manufacturing a prosthesis, and consider the materiality of ancient prostheses and other types of assistive technology. The fifth chapter, Living Prostheses, will consider the extent to which other people, primarily the enslaved, and animals, such as dogs or apes, served as 'living prostheses', and either supplemented prosthesis use or rendered it unnecessary.[127] It will explore how this process of requisitioning the body of another entity was rationalised.

[127] For the phrase 'living prostheses' used in reference to human caregivers, see van Schaik, 2019.

Ultimately, the aim of this monograph is to fill the current gap in scholarship and offer a new insight into the lived experience of the impaired and disabled in classical antiquity, thereby contributing to the study of impairment and disability in classical antiquity, the history and archaeology of medicine in antiquity, and social and cultural history.

CHAPTER 1

Extremity Prostheses and Assistive Technology

Introduction

A small terracotta figurine, thought to originate from Corinth, that is currently housed in the collection of the Musée d'art et d'histoire in Geneva offers us what is perhaps one of our first views of an ordinary as opposed to a mythological impaired individual in classical antiquity.[1] I say 'perhaps' because the figurine is enigmatic. Does it depict someone with congenital limb amputations, specifically a condition called ectromelia, as suggested by Mirko Grmek and Danielle Gourevitch?[2] Or is the way that the man is portrayed simply a stylistic quirk? This figurine is emblematic of the difficulty in attempting to retrospectively diagnose medical conditions suffered by individuals in classical antiquity, let alone attempting to access the lived experiences of the impaired and disabled.[3]

Potentially somewhat more straightforward, for our purposes, is a passage from Cassius Dio's *Roman History*. In his account of the events of the year 20 BCE, Dio records that an embassy from India came to Samos to visit the emperor Augustus:

> The people of India, who had already made overtures, now made a treaty of friendship, sending among other gifts tigers, which were then for the first time seen by the Romans, as also, I think by the Greeks. They also gave him a boy who had no shoulders or arms, like our statues of Hermes. And yet, defective as he was, he could use his feet for everything, as if they were hands: with them he would stretch a bow, shoot missiles, and put a trumpet to his lips. How he did this I do not know; I merely state what is recorded.[4]

[1] Musée d'art et d'histoire inv. HM 79. [2] Grmek and Gourevitch, 1998, p. 278.

[3] For medical conditions in classical works of art, see Grmek and Gourevitch, 1998; Mitchell, 2013; Mitchell, 2017; Trentin, 2017.

[4] Cass. Dio. 54.9.8–9 (trans. E. Cary): οἱ Ἰνδοὶ προκηρυκευσάμενοι πρότερον φιλίαν τότε ἐσπείσαντο, δῶρα πέμψαντες ἄλλα τε καὶ τίγρεις, πρῶτον τότε τοῖς Ῥωμαίοις, νομίζω δ' ὅτι καὶ τοῖς Ἕλλησιν, ὀφθείσας. καί τι καὶ μειράκιόν οἱ ἄνευ ὤμων, οἵους τοὺς Ἑρμᾶς ὁρῶμεν, ἔδωκαν. καὶ μέντοι τοιοῦτον ὂν ἐκεῖνο ἐς πάντα τοῖς ποσὶν ἅτε καὶ χερσὶν ἐχρῆτο, τόξον τε αὐτοῖς ἐπέτεινε καὶ βέλη ἠφίει καὶ ἐσάλπιζεν, οὐκ οἶδ' ὅπως· γράφω γὰρ τὰ λεγόμενα. This embassy is also referred to in Aug. *RG* 31.1.

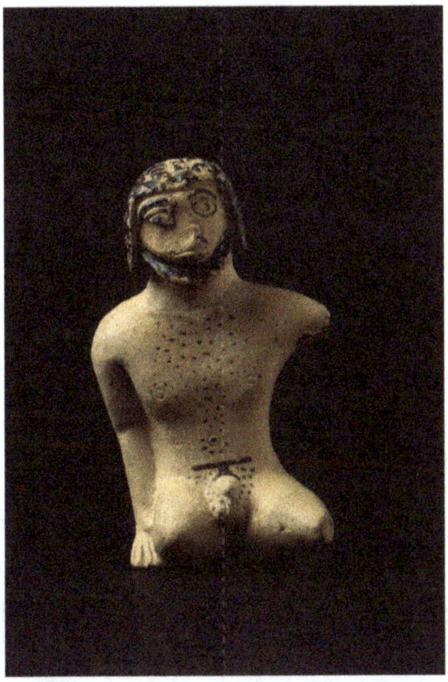

Figure 1.1 Terracotta figurine. Musée d'Art et d'Histoire inv. HM 79. Image courtesy of © Museum of Art and History, City of Geneva, Prêt de l'Association Hellas et Roma, photograph taken by Flora Bevilacqua.

The way that Dio describes the boy suggests that he was someone with congenital limb amputations rather than someone who had undergone surgical limb amputations. For the boy to be considered a suitable gift for such an eminent figure, first by the Indians and subsequently by the Romans and Greeks on Samos, he had to be something out of the ordinary. Someone who had undergone a surgical procedure that was, after all, rather familiar to both the Romans and the Greeks would hardly have been impressive, although the young age of the patient might have been considered noteworthy.[5] Yet Dio considers him worth mentioning in conjunction with the first sighting of tigers in the ancient Mediterranean! But then, it is clear that the boy's condition was only the introduction to the spectacle. The main event was the way in which he had adapted and compensated for his lack of arms and hands by using his legs and feet instead. No mention is made of mundanities, but if the boy were capable of shooting an arrow and playing a trumpet, it is probable that he could also

[5] On paediatric medicine in antiquity, see Dean-Jones, 2013 and Bradley, 2005. On impaired and disabled children in antiquity, see Laes, 2008 and 2013.

do things such as feed and groom himself. Additionally, no mention is made of the use of prostheses, again something that was familiar to the Romans and Greeks and consequently less impressive. Considering Augustus' reported distaste for 'freaks of nature' (*ludibria naturae*) and his belief that they were bad omens, it is worth considering what his response to such a gift was, not to mention what ultimately became of the boy.[6] Perhaps he was passed on to the emperor's stepson Tiberius, who does not seem to have shared Augustus' feelings and apparently had a number of people with dwarfism present at his court.[7]

The story of the Indian boy begs the question: would an individual born with a congenital limb amputation or deficiency seek to use a prosthesis, or would they, like him, adapt?[8] In the contemporary world, individuals born with apodia (absence of hand or foot), hemimelia (absence of the distal part of the hand or foot), amelia (absence of the arm or leg), or phocomelia (foreshortening of arms or legs) are strongly encouraged to utilise prostheses and aids, in part due to the perceived desirability of 'passing' for 'normal'.[9] It is unlikely that this would have been possible in classical antiquity, where such an individual would have been set apart from birth due to their condition and viewed as something akin to a prodigy.[10] Further to that, would an individual who lost a limb later in life seek to replace the lost limb with a prosthesis, or would they too seek to adapt in some way? In this chapter, I examine the literary, archaeological, and bioarchaeological evidence for limb loss in classical antiquity before assessing the role that extremity prostheses played in impairment and disability in this period. I also consider how other types of assistive technology, such as walking sticks, canes, crutches, and walking frames, were used in conjunction with prostheses.

Limb Loss in Classical Antiquity

The loss of a body part and any associated functionality was recognised as being permanent in classical antiquity. According to Aristotle, 'from possession you may pass to privation but not from the latter to the former.

[6] Suet. *Aug.* 83. See Trentin, 2011 on deformity in the Roman imperial court.

[7] Suet. *Tib.* 61.6. For bioarchaeological evidence of dwarves in Ancient Rome, see Minozzi et al., 2013.

[8] To my knowledge, there is no bioarchaeological evidence for congenital limb amputation or deficiency in classical antiquity; see Mann et al., 1998 for discussion of this condition in the archaeological record.

[9] Yet, as we saw in the Introduction with the case of Kelly Knox, this is not necessarily something that they choose to do.

[10] On teratology in classical antiquity, see Gevaert and Laes, 2013.

A man who has once become blind never finds that his sight is restored, as a man who has once become bald never after recovers his hair and a man who has once lost his teeth never after can grow a new set.'[11] An individual who lost a body part was considered mutilated (*kolobos* in Greek, *colobos* in Latin) and thus curtailed and incomplete. According to Aristotle, 'a man is not mutilated if he loses flesh or his spleen, but if he loses some extremity; and not every extremity, but only such as cannot grow again when completely removed'.[12] Under normal circumstances, a finger or toe, hand or foot, arm or leg would certainly not grow back again, nor could it be reattached if severed completely. The fact that several tall tales recording the opposite survive perhaps reflects the anxiety people felt about the finality of losing a body part that could not be replaced or have its function replicated. Diodorus Siculus records the voyage of Iambulus to an island where the inhabitants used the blood of a creature similar to a tortoise as glue with which to reattach severed limbs. Directly contradicting Aristotle, he says that 'even if a hand or the like should happen to have been cut off, by the use of this blood it is glued on again, provided that the cut is fresh, and the same thing is true of such other parts of the body as are not connected with the regions which are vital and sustain the person's life'.[13] This is an interesting detail for Diodorus to include in his presentation of this island utopia that offers an insight into the ancient mind when presented with the ability to rewrite the natural order of things: in a perfect world, lost body parts could and would be reattached with relative ease.[14] Ancient accounts of miraculous healing events at sanctuaries indicate that it was believed that only through divine intervention could such an affliction be cured, and it is notable that in even in these cases some sort of substance (*pharmakon*) was applied to the body.[15]

As far as the 'type' of amputation is concerned, contemporary surgeons distinguish between disarticulation or 'amputation in contiguity', which is removal of the extremity through an articulation or joint without dividing the bone; 'guillotine amputation', which is complete transection of the

[11] Arist. *Cat.* 10.13a (trans. H. P. Cook): ἀπὸ μὲν γὰρ τῆς ἕξεως ἐπὶ τὴν στέρησιν γίνεται μεταβολή, ἀπὸ δὲ τῆς στερήσεως ἐπὶ τὴν ἕξιν ἀδύνατον. οὔτε γὰρ τυφλὸς γενόμενός τις πάλιν ἀνέβλεψεν, οὔτε φαλακρὸς ὢν πάλιν κομήτης ἐγένετο, οὔτε νωδὸς ὢν ὀδόντας ἔφυσεν.

[12] Arist. *Metaph.* 5.27.4 (trans. H. Treddenick): ὁ ἄνθρωπος οὐκ ἐὰν σάρκα ἢ τὸν σπλῆνα, ἀλλ᾽ ἐὰν ἀκρωτήριον, καὶ τοῦτο οὐ πᾶν ἀλλ᾽ ὃ μὴ ἔχει γένεσιν ἀφαιρεθὲν ὅλον.

[13] Diod. Sic. 2.58.4 (trans. C. H. Oldfather): ἂν ἀποκοπεῖσα χεὶρ ἢ ὅμοιον εἰπεῖν τύχῃ, δι᾽ αὐτοῦ κολλᾶσθαι προσφάτου τῆς τομῆς οὔσης, καὶ τἄλλα δὲ μέρη τοῦ σώματος, ὅσα μὴ κυρίοις τόποις καὶ συνέχουσι τὸ ζῆν κατέχεται.

[14] Pinheiro, 2006.

[15] See also the miraculous healing accounts from Epidauros: Epidaurian iamata A9 (eyeball) and Epidaurian iamata A 19 (hair).

extremity, cutting both skin and bone at the same level; 'instinctive amputation', which is the cutting off of extremities *in extremis*, particularly associated with entrapment and often done by the individual themselves; and 'traumatic amputation or avulsion', which is the complete or near complete removal of the extremity with great force.[16] However, identifying the type of amputation that occurred does not necessarily provide an explanation as to why that amputation occurred. Examination of bioarchaeological evidence comprising human skeletal remains showing evidence of limb amputation, whether healed or unhealed, can be informative regarding the ways in which limbs were lost. Simon Mays has suggested that this evidence can be interpreted as showing that limbs could be lost in one of three ways: through amputation as surgical intervention following disease or trauma to the extremity; through amputation as judicial punishment; and through amputation by means of injury with a sharp blade.[17] Survival for less than a week following the amputation ensures that no discernible healing takes place.[18] However, the more time that passes between the initial amputation and the death of the individual, the harder it is to assess the type of instrument used to perform the amputation due to the formation of osteophytes at the amputation site.[19] This means that contextual information such as sex, gender, and age have to be utilised as a means of making an estimation.

However, using literary evidence in conjunction with bioarchaeological evidence facilitates a more nuanced view of the phenomenon of acquired limb loss in classical antiquity. Once literary evidence is taken into account, it is possible to differentiate five different ways in which limbs could be lost. Lennard Davis has argued that, prior to the middle of the nineteenth century, people in western society lacked a concept of 'normalcy' and so did not fetishise the 'normal' body but rather the 'ideal' body, which meant that since the majority of human beings fell below that standard, they existed in various states of imperfection.[20] Drawing on bioarchaeological evidence from a number of Roman cemeteries, Emma-Jayne Graham has argued that 'the "normal" body of the Roman world was one that was far from completely able, far from modern concepts of "normal" . . . disparity was actually the norm'.[21] On the contrary, she has suggested that there was 'a sliding scale of impairment', and that impairment was ordinary rather than extraordinary.[22] Certainly, the sheer frequency with which acquired limb loss is mentioned in ancient literature,

[16] Kirkup, 2007, pp. 2–4. [17] Mays, 1996, p. 107.
[18] Aufderheide and Rodriguez-Martin, 1998, p. 30. [19] Mays, 1996, p. 107.
[20] Davis, 2002, pp. 100–1. [21] Graham, 2013, p. 258. [22] Graham, 2013, p. 268.

particularly within certain contexts and happening under particular circumstances, suggests that it was fairly common. It is possible that the manner in which a limb was lost influenced the amputee's choice of whether to attempt to use a prosthesis or not; the quality of the amputation would certainly have influenced whether the amputee was physically able to use a prosthesis or had to resort to another type of assistive technology, such as a walking stick, a cane, or either one or two crutches.

Amputation Through Surgical Intervention

An indication of what it would have been like to suffer from a debilitating wound and gangrenous infection can be found in Sophocles' tragedy *Philoctetes*. The eponymous hero is bitten on the foot by a snake as a punishment for trespassing in a sacred grove, and the wound becomes infected and refuses to heal. His crew mates, unable to bear his cries of pain or the stench of the wound, abandon him on an island for ten years. At one point in the play, he begs Neoptolemus to amputate his leg with his sword.[23] Pliny the Elder describes a statue crafted by Pythagoras of Rhegium that, judging by the description, may have been of Philoctetes: 'At Syracuse there is his Lame Man, which actually makes people looking at it feel a pain from his ulcer in their own leg.'[24] It has been suggested that Sophocles' portrayal of Philoctetes and his wound was inspired by the veterans of the Peloponnesian War.[25] Thus, it is not surprising to find surgical amputation being attested from the Classical period onwards, although it seems to have been utilised as a measure of last resort. The equipment required was relatively simple: a small plain-toothed saw (*priwn* in Greek, *serrula* in Latin) for sawing through bone and a block (*epikopon* in Greek, *epikopon* in Latin) to provide a firm surface upon which to cut, saw, and chop.[26] Examples of these instruments have been found in a variety of locations around the ancient Mediterranean, including temples, forts, houses, surgeries, tombs, and graves.[27]

The Hippocratic treatise *On Joints*, dating to the second half of the fifth century BCE, tells us that in cases of accident, frostbite, or gangrene, extremities such as fingers or toes, or even hands or feet, should be

[23] Soph. *Phil.* 743–50.
[24] Plin. *HN* 34.59 (trans. H. Rackham): *Syracusis autem claudicantem, cuius ulceris dolorem sentire etiam spectantes videntur*. For artistic representations of Philoctetes, see *LIMC* s.v. Philoctetes.
[25] Rose, 2003, p. 19. See also Edwards, 2012.
[26] Bliquez, 2014, p. 38, pp. 183–4. Science Museum inv. A9219.
[27] On bone surgery and surgical instruments, see Jackson, 2005.

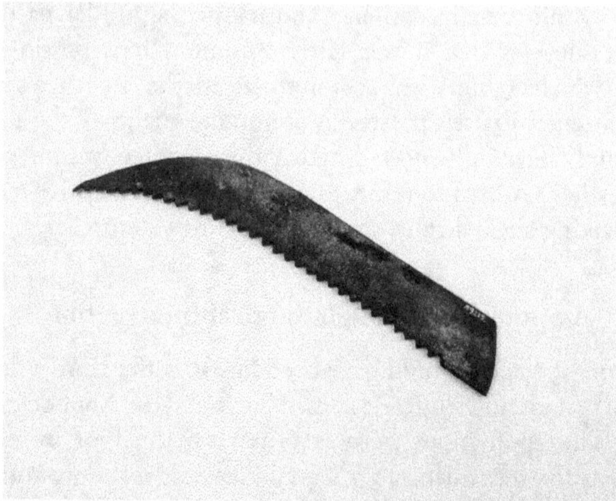

Figure 1.2 Roman bone saw. Science Museum/Wellcome Collection inv. A9219. Image courtesy of the Science Museum, London.

amputated at the joint.[28] The treatise differentiates between amputation of the fingers and toes at the joint, which the writer considers not usually dangerous, and more extensive amputation which might be accompanied by loss of consciousness and fever.[29] It instructs that in cases of gangrene the amputation should occur above the point at which the gangrene begins, and warns that cutting into sound flesh causes the patient considerable pain, which is itself dangerous and can result in death.[30] However, the surgeon's role here seems to be simply facilitating the removal of necrotic tissue and tending to the stump rather than surgically removing the extremity. It has been proposed that it was only in the Hellenistic period that surgical practitioners based in Alexandria discovered how to ligate blood vessels, and this discovery resulted in the development of more extensive surgical procedures, which accounts for the more sophisticated techniques detailed by the medical writers of the Roman period.[31] This potentially also accounts for the increasing frequency with which amputation is mentioned in ancient literature outside of medical literature from the Roman Republic onwards.[32]

Aulus Cornelius Celsus, writing in the early first century CE, goes much further than the Hippocratic writer and provides a detailed description of

[28] Hippoc. *Art.* 68–9. [29] Hippoc. *Art.* 68. [30] Hippoc. *Art.* 69. [31] Majno, 1975, p. 328.

[32] Discussion of amputation appears frequently in the political sphere, where it is used as a simile or a metaphor; see, for example, Cic. *Off.* 1.38; Cic. *Phil.* 8.15; Quint. *Inst.* 8.3.75.

the process by which a surgeon should amputate a limb. He acknowledges that the procedure is dangerous and can itself lead to death, but states that 'it does not matter, however, whether the remedy is safe enough, since it is the only one'.[33] He instructs that the amputation should not occur at the actual joint, as additional bone and skin is needed to create the stump, and the most important thing is that the amputation should occur in sound flesh, as all traces of the disease should be removed.[34] While Celsus does not mention ligating blood vessels here, he does refer to it elsewhere in the treatise in a section dealing with wounds and haemorrhage, stating that they should be tied in the first instance but cauterised as a last resort, so it is clear that he was familiar with the technique.[35]

Heliodorus, writing later in the first century CE, warns that the higher up the extremity amputation is attempted, the more dangerous the procedure due to the risk of haemorrhage from large blood vessels.[36] He states that some of his peers prefer to amputate the limb in its entirety and then deal with the blood vessels rather than proceeding methodically and dealing with them vessel by vessel. He recommends using a ligature above the amputation site to slow the blood flow, then using a scalpel to cut through the skin and blood vessels before sawing through the bone. He advises leaving sufficient skin so as to create skin flaps to cover the remaining bone, and suggests using bandages with sponges attached.

Archigenes, writing in the late first and early second centuries CE and practising in Rome during the reign of the emperor Trajan, advises the surgeon to consider whether or not the patient is strong enough for the procedure.[37] He likewise disagrees with the Hippocratic writer that amputation should take place at or near the joint. He instructs his reader to either tie or sew the blood vessels and apply cold water to the area to slow the blood flow, and to apply a circular band to the extremity to protect the skin and provide a template for the incision. Perhaps he was referring to an object akin to one currently held in the Wellcome Collection that is described as a 'thigh tourniquet'.[38] There are references in other works of medical literature to the use of a tourniquet (*telamon*) for procedures such as venesection, phlebotomy, and snakebite, but these appear to have been cloth.[39] Once the surgeon

[33] Celsus, *Med.* 7.33.1 (trans. W. G. Spencer): *Verum hic quoque nihil interest, an satis tutum praesidium sit, quod unicum est.*

[34] Celsus, *Med.* 7.33.1. [35] Celsus, *Med.* 5.26.1.

[36] Adams, 1846, p. 411 cited in Kirkup, 2007, p. 111.

[37] Adams, 1846, p. 411 cited in Kirkup, 2007, p. 57.

[38] Science Museum/Wellcome Collection inv. A63014.

[39] Venesection: Oribasius, *Medical Collection* 7.9.1; phlebotomy: Paul of Aegina, *Medical Compendium* 6.40.3; Aetius in Cornarius 13.25. For discussion, see Bliquez, 2014, pp. 271–2.

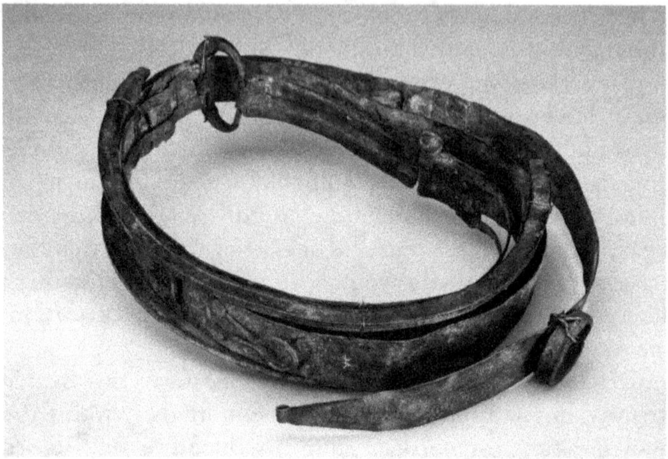

Figure 1.3 Roman tourniquet. Science Museum/Wellcome Collection inv. A63014. Image courtesy of the Science Museum, London.

reaches the bone, the bone is to be scraped and sawn through and the blood vessel cauterised. Upon completing the surgical part of the procedure, the surgeon is to apply a medicament containing leeks, bread, and salt to the stump.

While Galen, writing in the late second and early third centuries CE, does not specifically discuss surgical amputation, in his commentary on the Hippocratic treatise *On Joints* he agrees with the writer that they should be undertaken at the joint rather than elsewhere.[40] He also cautions that sometimes amputees can experience an evacuation of blood through the intestines, indicating that he undertook a certain amount of aftercare, or at the very least patient observation, following the procedure.[41]

Paul of Aegina, writing in the seventh century CE and compiling information found in earlier medical treatises that are now lost, offers several detailed descriptions of amputations. He states that Leonidas, writing in the late second and early third centuries CE, instructs his readers to amputate methodically, starting at an easy place before working down through the skin to the bone, stopping to cauterise and medicate blood vessels.[42]

Outside of medical literature, ancient authors refer to surgical amputation both literally and figuratively, emphasising the necessity of removing what is useless or diseased, whether from the human body, the family, or

[40] Gal. *Hipp. Art.* 18A.667–83K. [41] Gal. *Nat. Fac.* 3.13.192.
[42] Paul of Aegina, *Medical Compendium* 84.

even from the body politic, and the importance of taking considerable care while doing so. Xenophon states that not only do men have surgeons amputate and cauterise their 'useless and unprofitable' limbs, but that they thank them and pay them for the service.[43] Quintilian states that just as surgeons amputate diseased limbs, so must a family cut off a member who is wicked and dangerous.[44] Cicero states the necessity of removing what is diseased through cutting or cauterisation in order to save the rest, equating the human body with the body politic, while acknowledging that it is a harsh remedy.[45] Strabo, when discussing the preparation of his treatise *Geography*, critiques the work of his predecessor Eratosthenes by equating the necessity of undertaking a methodical geographical survey with the necessity of undertaking a methodical surgical amputation.[46] These types of references emphasise the seriousness with which amputation was taken in classical antiquity.

Unequivocal bioarchaeological evidence for surgical amputation is found on the skeleton of an adult male aged 20–30 years old recovered from a cemetery in Ephesus, the stump of whose amputated right leg displays marks from the blade of a saw, although since there is no evidence of healing, it is thought that he died soon after the operation was performed.[47] There are other examples of amputation in the bioarchaeological record of Italy and Britain that have been attributed to surgical intervention, although these attributions have been made due to the site and quality of the amputations rather than the presence of surgical saw marks on the bones. A young adult male recovered from the Arlington Avenue cemetery in Dorchester was found to have had his right arm amputated at the middle of the humerus, and as in the case of the man from Ephesus, no evidence of healing suggests that he died soon after the operation was performed.[48] An adult male aged at least 35–40 years old recovered from the Lankhills cemetery, dating to circa 390–410 CE, was found to have had parts of both feet amputated, possibly the left foot having been treated prior to the right, and it has been suggested that this was surgical intervention to treat some sort of underlying disease or injury such as trench foot.[49] Unlike the other two examples, this man survived his operations for some time. Finally, an adult left femur recovered from a collective burial at the cemetery of Isola Sacra in Italy, dating from

[43] Xen. *Mem.* 1.54 (trans. E. C. Marchant and O. J. Todd): τι ἂν ἀχρεῖον ᾖ καὶ ἀνωφελές.

[44] Quint. *Inst.* 8.3.75. [45] Cic. *Phil.* 8.16. [46] Strabo, *Geog.* 2.30.

[47] Kanz and Grossschmidt, 2009, p. 216. [48] Redfern, 2010, p. 464.

[49] Stuckert and Kricun, 2011, pp. 114–15. Similar surgical intervention has been found on two mummies from Egypt: see Dupras et al., 2010.

the second–third centuries CE, shows signs of surgical intervention, but the individual survived for months, perhaps even years, after the procedure was performed.[50]

Amputation Through Participation in Military Activity

Works of both poetry and prose attest frequent instances of limbs lost as a result of participation in military activity. Most often, the limb lost is the right hand – the sword hand – and it is lost either in single combat or in the course of pitched battle.[51] In works of poetry, the right hand frequently continues to move after it is severed, a rather gruesome detail that serves to underline its dexterity and its significance.[52] The severing of the right hand was often a precursor to death in descriptions of battle, the act leaving the individual incapacitated and unable to defend themselves and thus driving them to even greater heroics in their final moments. Lucan tells the story of a soldier who sacrificed himself to save his twin brother and their comrades:

> Twin brothers fought there, the pride of a fertile mother; but the same womb gave them birth for different deaths. The cruel hand of death made distinction between them; and the wretched parents, no longer puzzled by the likeness, recognised the one survivor but found in him a source of unending sorrow; for he keeps their grief ever present and recalls his lost brother to their mourning hearts. One of these twins dared to catch hold of a Roman ship from his own deck, when the oars were entangled and overlapped each other. The hand was lopped off by a heavy downward blow; but still it clung with the effort of its first grip and, holding on with strained muscles, stiffened there in death. His valour rose with disaster; mutilated, he displays yet more heroic ardour. Fiercely he renews the fight with his left hand and leans forward over the water to rescue his right hand; the left hand also and the whole arm were cut off. Then bereft both of shield and sword, not hiding away in the bottom of the ship but full in view, he protects his brother's shield with his own bare breast, standing firm, though pierced with many a point, and, although he had amply earned his death already, stopping missiles that would in their fall have made an end of many. Then the life that was departing through many wounds he gathered together into his spent frame, and bracing his limbs with all his remaining strength, he sprang on board the Roman ship; his sinews had lost their power, and his only weapon was his weight.[53]

[50] Weaver et al., 2000, p. 686.

[51] On right- and left-handedness in ancient Greece and Rome, see Wirth, 2010.

[52] See, for example, Nonnus, *Dion.* 2.427–35, 22.196–202.

[53] Lucan, *Pharsalia* 3.603–26 (trans. J. D. Duff): *Stant gemini fratres, fecundae gloria matris, quos eadem variis genuerunt viscera fatis. Discrevit mors saeva viros, unumque relictum agnorunt miseri sublato*

The loss of a hand, whether the right or the left, was potentially survivable; one of the most famous examples of extremity prosthesis use in classical antiquity comes from a man who suffered just such a wound in the Second Punic War:

> Nobody, in my judgement at all events, can rightly rank any human being above Marcus Sergius, albeit his great-grandson Catiline diminishes the credit of his name. Sergius in his second campaign lost his right hand; in two campaigns he was wounded twenty-three times, with the result that he was crippled in both hands and both feet, only his spirit being intact; yet although disabled, he served in numerous subsequent campaigns. He was twice taken prisoner by Hannibal (for it was with no ordinary foe that he was engaged), and twice escaped from Hannibal's fetters, although he was kept in chains or shackles on every single day for twenty months. He fought four times with only his left hand, having two horses he was riding stabbed under him. He had a right hand of iron made for him and going into action with it tied to his arm, raised the siege of Cremona, saved Piacenza, captured twelve enemy camps in Gaul.[54]

Although Marcus Sergius Silus' prosthetic hand does not survive, a depiction of him using it can be found on a series of silver denarii issued by his descendent, also named Marcus Sergius Silus, who used his authority as quaestor to do so in the year 116–115 BCE.[55] The obverse face of the coin depicts the goddess Roma; the reverse face of the coin depicts the earlier Marcus Sergius Silus on horseback, and what is interesting about this depiction is that where a Roman soldier would ordinarily be depicted holding his sword in his right hand and his shield strapped to his left arm,

errore parentes, aeternis causam lacrimis; tenet ille dolorem semper et amissum fratrem lugentibus offert. Quorum alter mixtis obliquo pectine remis ausus Romanae Graia de puppe carinae iniectare manum; sed eam gravis insuper ictus amputat; illa tamen nisu, quo prenderat, haesit deriguitque tenens strictis inmortua nervis. Crevit in adversis virtus: plus nobilis irae truncus habet fortique instaurat proelia laeva rapturusque suam procumbit in aequora dextram: haec quoque cum toto manus est abscisa lacerto. Iam clipeo telisque carens, non conditus ima puppe sed expositus fraternaque pectore nudo arma tegens, crebra confixus cuspide perstat telaque multorum leto casura suorum. Emerita iam morte tenet. Tum volnere multo effugientem animam lassos collegit in artus membraque contendit toto, quicumque manebat, sanguine et hostilem defectis robore nervis insiluit solo nociturus pondere puppem.

54 Plin. *HN* 7.29 (trans. H. Rackham): *M. Sergio, ut equidem arbitror, nemo quemquam hominum iure praetulerit, licet pronepos Catilina gratiam nomini deroget. secundo stipendio dextram manum perdidit, stipendiis duobus ter et vicies vulneratus est, ob id neutra manu, neutro pede satis utilis, animo tantum salvo, plurimis postea stipendiis debilis miles. bis ab Hannibale captus – neque enim cum quolibet hoste res fuit, bis vinculorum eius profugus, in viginti mensibus nullo non die in catenis aut compedibus custoditus. sinistra manu sola quater pugnavit, duobus equis insidente eo suffossis. dextram sibi ferream fecit, eaque religata proeliatus Cremonam obsidione exemit, Placentiam tutatus est, duodena castra hostium in Gallia cepit.* On Marcus Sergius Silus, see Beagon, 2002; Beagon, 2005, pp. 293–7; Laes, 2011, pp. 921–5.

55 *RCV* I 163; *RSC* 1; Crawford 286/1.

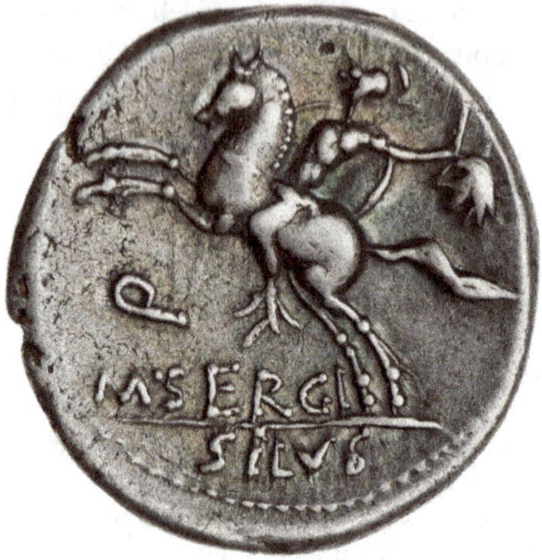

Figure 1.4 Silver denarius, Rome, 116–115 BCE. American Numismatic Society inv. 1941.131.92. Image courtesy of the American Numismatic Society.

Marcus Sergius Silus is holding his sword and a severed head in his left hand and has his shield strapped to his right arm instead.[56] This depiction accords with the scenario described by Pliny the Elder and indicates the high regard in which Marcus Sergius Silus was held by his family almost a century later.

However, the scenes of wounding in battle that proliferate in non-medical literature are problematic when it comes to attempting to utilise them for information regarding loss of limbs because ancient writers included such scenes with a specific purpose in mind – the construction of a heroic image – with the scenes of wounding or the treatment of the wound used as a device to emphasise the hero's excellence.[57] What is clear is that wounds received in battle were frequently used as physical proof of bravery and valour, sometimes years after they were originally received.[58]

It is difficult to differentiate between surgical amputation and martial amputation of extremities when examining human skeletal remains, since both are done with a sharp blade and, in point of fact, a limb could be lost through military activity and then subjected to surgical intervention, such as in the case of the gladiator from Ephesus discussed earlier. Potentially,

56 According to Wirthe, 2010, p. 223, being rendered left-handed because of an injury to one's right hand was considered preferable to being naturally left-handed.

57 Salazar, 2000, p. xxiv.

58 Leigh, 1995; Evans, 1999.

the location of the amputation site can be informative since, as we have seen, medical treatises instructed surgeons to amputate at the joint whereas war wounds could occur at any point on the limb. There is some disagreement as to whether ancient blades were sharp enough to affect a complete transection of the skin and bone as opposed to simply causing severe injury.[59] It is thought that it would have been more likely for a soldier to have been severely injured by a spear or a missile than a blade.[60]

Amputation as Judicial Punishment

Numerous ancient civilisations utilised amputation as judicial punishment for a range of infractions through the principle of *ius talionis*; the Babylonian Code of Hammurabi from Mesopotamia (circa 1754 BCE), the Hindu Laws of Manu from India (circa 200 BCE–200 CE) and the Zoroastrian Zend-Avesta from Persia (224–651 CE) all attest to the practice. There is a considerable variety in the ways in which amputation of an extremity was utilised as a punishment in classical antiquity and, depending upon the context, the practice could be viewed as either entirely appropriate – a case of the punishment fitting the crime, so to speak – or as completely excessive and indicative of tyranny on the part of the individual responsible for decreeing it. There seems to have been a preference for amputating the body part that was considered to bear responsibility for the initial transgression, and presumably this not only served as an example and a deterrent to anyone else considering committing a similar crime, but also a means of preventing reoffending in the future. This is articulated by Diodorus Siculus, and seems to have occurred fairly consistently:

> In the case of those who had disclosed military secrets to the enemy the law prescribed that their tongues should be cut out, while in the case of counterfeiters or falsifiers of measures and weights or imitators of seals, and of official scribes who made false entries or erased items, and of any who adduced false documents, it ordered that both their hands should be cut off, to the end that the offender, being punished in respect of those members of his body that were the instruments of his wrongdoing, should himself keep until death his irreparable misfortune, and at the same time, by serving as a warning example to others, should turn them from the commission of similar offences.[61]

[59] Salazar, 2000, p. 13; James, 2010. [60] Salazar, 2000, p. 13.

[61] Diod. Sic. 1.11.3 (trans. C. H. Oldfather): καὶ τῶν μὲν τὰ ἀπόρρητα τοῖς πολεμίοις ἀπαγγειλάντων ἐπέταττεν ὁ νόμος ἐκτέμνεσθαι τὴν γλῶτταν, τῶν δὲ τὸ νόμισμα παρακοπτόντων ἢ μέτρα καὶ σταθμὰ παραποιούντων ἢ παραγλυφόντων τὰς σφραγῖδας, ἔτι δὲ τῶν γραμματέων τῶν ψευδεῖς χρηματισμοὺς γραφόντων ἢ ἀφαιρούντων τι τῶν ἐγγεγραμμένων, καὶ τῶν τὰς ψευδεῖς συγγραφὰς ἐπιφερόντων, ἀμφοτέρας ἐκέλευσεν ἀποκόπτεσθαι τὰς χεῖρας, ὅπως οἷς ἕκαστος μέρεσι τοῦ

As with martial amputation, the body part that is lost most frequently is the hand.[62] So those responsible for forgery, whether it is done in writing, such as Josephus' friend Justus' brother, who forged letters at the outbreak of hostilities, or by other means, have their hands cut off.[63] Thieves, no matter what they steal or how they steal it, have their hand(s) cut off. Thus, a dishonest moneylender is punished in the same way as a soldier discovered stealing rations.[64] In extreme cases, the hands, once severed, are displayed publicly.[65]

It was recommended that if a man beats his father, a crime which was viewed in the same light as parricide by the Romans, both hands should be cut off, and this should be done whether the man was the biological or adoptive father.[66] Even in a hypothetical situation where one man comes to an arrangement with another that they should beat each other's fathers, they should still both lose both hands.[67] However, it would appear that a father seeking to have the penalty applied to his son was subject to a certain amount of criticism, as Quintilian describes how such an individual might seek to justify himself:

> The young man, gentlemen, the worst of criminals, ungrateful because thanks to me he received the daylight and a father both, is a parricide twice over, once in my house, again in the Forum. If anyone is still going to doubt how richly he deserved to lose his bloody hands, let him behold: he beats me again in your sight and, mutilated now and crippled, whole only in his rage, he rushes at a poor old man. What if he had hands? In case anybody should think him subdued by the penalty, he has become even more audacious: he sets his heart on crippling me and directs his anger especially at that part of my body through which he is alive. I confess, gentlemen, yes I confess that these hands should have been cut off – but when they took him up! I am not ashamed, gentlemen, to be reviled (the least to be expected from him) and even accused of cruelty. Let him call me cruel by all means, so long as he shows himself: I am not afraid that this charge against me may be found credible when my adversary is himself a living memorial of my compassion.[68]

σώματος παρενόμησεν, εἰς ταῦτα κολαζόμενος αὐτὸς μὲν μέχρι τελευτῆς ἀνίατον ἔχῃ τὴν συμφοράν, τοὺς δ' ἄλλους διὰ τῆς ἰδίας τιμωρίας νουθετῶν ἀποτρέπῃ τῶν ὁμοίων τι πράττειν.

62 Wirthe, 2010, p. 148. 63 Joseph. *Vit.* 177; Suet. *Claud.* 5.

64 Suet. *Galb.* 9; Frontin. *Str.* 4.17.

65 See for example Suet. *Galb.* 9. This recalls the display of Cicero's hands on the rostra.

66 Quint. 358. 67 Quint. 362.

68 Quint. 372 (trans. D. R. Shackleton Bailey): *Sceleratissimus omnium, iudices, iuvenis, ingratus vel quia lucem beneficio meo accepit vel quia [in] patrem, bis parricida est, semel domi, iterum in foro. Quam merito cruentas perdiderit manus si quis adhuc dubitabit, aspiciat: iterum me in conspectu vestro pulsat, et iam truncus ac debilis, sola rabie integer, in miserum senem incurrit. Quid si haberet manus? Ac ne quis illum coercitum poena putet, etiam audacior factus est: debilitatem meam concupiscit, et ei praecipue corporis parti irascitur per quam vivit. Fateor, iudices, fateor praecidendas fuisse has manus,*

This type of punishment is carried out publicly and used to send a message, whether the individual being punished is a civilian or a soldier. This seems to have been considered particularly important when transgressions occurred in military contexts. In cases of punishments for desertion or cowardice, the guilty man has his right hand cut off, rendering him no longer able to participate in military activities, or at the very least making it significantly more difficult for him to do so. This begs the question of whether, or how, it was possible to differentiate a hero who had lost his right hand in battle and a coward who had lost his as a punishment.[69]

It would appear that this method of punishment was not always considered an acceptable one. According to Xenophon, during the Peloponnesian War the Athenians voted to cut off the right hands of any prisoners of war.[70] Plutarch's later account blames the general Philocles specifically.[71] When recounting the Athenian legislation regarding cutting off the thumbs of prisoners of war from Aegina so that they could no longer hold oars and possess a navy powerful enough to challenge the Athenian one, both Cicero and Valerius Maximus are critical of it. Cicero calls the legislation a 'cruel wrong', while Valerius Maximus states that it was a 'decree unworthy of [Athens'] glory', before going on to say 'I do not recognize an Athens that would borrow a remedy for fear from cruelty.'[72]

Amputation as Extra-Judicial Punishment

As with judicial amputation, there is a considerable variety in the ways that amputation was utilised as an extra-judicial punishment and, in extreme cases, as a means of torture at the apparent whim of a powerful individual in classical antiquity, whether that individual was Greek, Roman, Carthaginian, or Persian. Thus, there are many accounts of tyrants ordering the mutilation of their subjects.[73] This could be utilised as a means of humiliating a specific individual and undermining their credibility, such as in the case of Valentinian's mutilation of his rival John.[74]

sed cum istum tollerent. Nec erubesco, quod ab isto minimum est, male audire et crudelitatis quoque reus fieri. Sane crudelem me vocet, dum se ostendat: non timeo ne istud in me crimen credibile sit cum misericordiae meae adversarius ipse monumentum sit.

69 For discussion of the ambiguous attitudes displayed towards Roman soldiers with physical impairments resulting from their military service, see Van Lommel, 2015.

70 Xen. *Hell.* 2.1.31. 71 Plut. *Vit. Lys.* 9.

72 Cic. *Off.* 3.11 (trans. W. Miller): *durius*; Val. Max. 9 External 8 (trans. D. R. Shackleton Bailey): *non agnosco Athenas timori remedium a crudelitate mutuantes.*

73 Diod. Sic. 33.14.3. 74 Procop. 3.3.9.

As we have seen, in some cases the mutilation of prisoners of war can be classed as judicial punishment. However, there are many examples of prisoners of war having their hands cut off with no reference to formal legislation.[75] Frequently prisoners would have their hands cut off just prior to their release, and would be sent back to their camp or city with a message, of which their mutilation was one part.[76] In some cases, prisoners were mutilated in full view of their comrades, such as in the case of Hasdrubal, angry at the sacking of Megara, leading his Roman prisoners out onto the city wall and mutilating them in full view of their comrades in an attempt to make reconciliation between Carthage and Rome impossible.[77] This tactic seems to have relied on the fact that mutilation was considered abhorrent. Even individuals who were not technically prisoners of war might be treated in this way. Julius Caesar recounts that some couriers on their way from Corduba to Pompey's camp wandered into his by mistake, and he had their hands cut off before allowing them to continue on their way.[78] It would appear that certain prominent historical generals set a precedent for this. Thus, Gaius Scribonius Curio Burbuleius' example when campaigning in Dardania in 73 BCE was later followed by Theodosius when suppressing the revolt of the Moorish chieftain Firmus in the fourth century CE.[79]

Depending upon the context and the identity and status of the amputee, this was seen either as appropriate or as inappropriate, excessive, and potentially tyrannical. For example, on one occasion Alexander the Great ordered the mutilation of Bessus as a punishment for treachery, leading Arrian to insert his opinion regarding this into the narrative: 'For my part, I do not approve of this excessive punishment of Bessus; I regard the mutilation of the extremities as barbaric, and I agree that Alexander was carried away into imitation of Median and Persian opulence and of the custom of barbarian kings not to countenance equality with subjects in their daily lives.'[80] Polybius considered this sort of behaviour to be damaging to the soul.[81] While extra-judicial amputation might be utilised, like judicial amputation, as a means of preventing future transgressions, there

[75] Joseph. *BJ* 5.455; Frontin. *Str.* 3.15.4; Amm. Marc. 29.31.

[76] Caes. *BHisp.* 12; Joseph. *BJ* 5.455; Quintus Curtius, *History of Alexander* 3.16.

[77] App. *Hann.* 8.118. [78] Caes. *BHisp.* 12.

[79] Curio: Livy, *Epit.* 95; Theodosius: Amm. Marc. 29.5.22.

[80] Arr. *Anab.* 4.7.3–4 (trans. P. A. Brunt): καὶ ἐγὼ οὔτε τὴν ἄγαν ταύτην τιμωρίαν Βήσσου ἐπαινῶ, ἀλλὰ βαρβαρικὴν εἶναι τίθεμαι τῶν ἀκρωτηρίων τὴν λώβην καὶ ὑπαχθῆναι Ἀλέξανδρον ξύμφημι ἐς ζῆλον τοῦ Μηδικοῦ τε καὶ Περσικοῦ πλούτου καὶ τῆς κατὰ τοὺς βαρβάρους βασιλέας οὐκ ἴσης ἐς τοὺς ὑπηκόους ξυνδιαιτήσεως.

[81] Polyb. 1.81.

seems to have been an aspect of it that was entirely vindictive: that leaving an individual alive but mutilated was more satisfying than killing them.

Amputation as Self-Mutilation or Deliberate Mutilation

The mutilation of oneself or of another for a specific purpose or to make a point is attested quite rarely and was clearly done as an extreme measure. One might amputate a limb or part of a limb as a means of removing restraints and escaping captivity, as in the case of Hegesistratus of Elis, the Persian diviner who was imprisoned by the Spartans during the Persian War, which necessitated him amputating part of his own foot at the instep in order to remove his leg-irons.[82] Attested more often is the removal of a digit in order to avoid military service; Ammianus Marcellinus states that this practice was popular in Italy and that those who did it were called *murci*, 'cowards'.[83] It is true that the examples that survive are all from Roman Italy. Gaius Vettianus amputated two fingers from his left hand in an attempt to avoid participating in the Italian War, but when found out the Senate ordered that his property was confiscated and he was sentenced to life in chains.[84] The possibility of severe punishment for such an act did not necessarily serve as a deterrent; a subsequent case that occurred under the reign of the emperor Augustus saw a father amputate the thumbs of his two sons in order to render them unfit for military service; upon being found out, he was sold into slavery before being freed and banished from Rome.[85] More admirable, perhaps, was a woman who amputated her brother's thumb while he was asleep in order to prevent him from fighting as a gladiator.[86]

Rather than self-mutilate in a clandestine way, one might do so publicly in order to make some sort of statement, as in the case of Theron of Thessaly, who drew his sword and cut off his left thumb in order to prove his love to the object of his affection, before challenging his rival to do the same thing.[87] So too one might mutilate oneself as part of a religious ritual or as a sign of religious devotion, and offer the severed digit as tribute. However, this type of self-mutilation had serious consequences for the mutilator and their position in ancient Roman society. For the Romans, the thumb was viewed independently of the fingers and a particular

[82] Hdt. 9.37–8. [83] Amm. Marc. 15.3. For discussion of this practice, see Wierschowski, 1995.
[84] Val. Max. 6.3. [85] Suet. *Aug.* 24.1. [86] Quint. *Inst.* 8.5.2.
[87] Plut. *Mor. De frat. amor.* 761C.

significance was attached to it; there was an etymological connection between the thumb and political power.[88]

The Practicalities of Limb Amputation

As has been demonstrated, ancient literary evidence attests to a wide variety of ways in which fingers and toes, hands and feet, arms and legs could be lost, but this begs the question of how, exactly, they were lost. Who was responsible for removing them? In the case of surgical intervention in order to treat disease, trauma, or frostbite, it would have been a physician (*iatros* in Greek, *medicus* in Latin). Greek and Roman medical treatises attest to the fact that surgery was recognised as one part of general medicine rather than a specialty in its own right. While some physicians might have been called upon to amputate limbs more often than others – military physicians, for example – it is clear that there was a certain amount of expectation that they would know how to do it.[89]

In the case of martial amputation, it would have been a soldier wielding a bladed weapon of some kind. In the case of judicial and extra-judicial amputation, the situation is less clear. Was a physician enlisted to undertake as competent an amputation as possible? In the case of judicial and extra-judicial amputation undertaken in military contexts, perhaps the military physician was utilised. However, that suggests a degree of concern on the part of those handing down the punishment regarding the current and future welfare of those they were punishing. In some cases, the texts give details regarding the process, which involved amputation followed by cauterisation or searing. According to Suetonius, the emperor Claudius 'insisted that an executioner be summoned at once with knife and block' in order to amputate the hands of a man convicted of forgery.[90] Yet today it is recognised that the skill of the surgeon and the care with which the amputation is undertaken affects the nature of the stump and the possibility of using a prosthesis. Perhaps this is why there are relatively few references to extremity prostheses in classical antiquity, despite the fact that there are numerous references to limb loss, and rather more to cosmeses such as wigs and dental appliances. Potentially incompetent

88 Corbeill, 2004, p. 42, pp. 6–7.

89 See, for example, Eutyches, the occupant of the House of the Surgeon at Rimini, an individual who, due to his vast collection of orthopaedic surgical instruments, is thought to have been a retired military surgeon.

90 Suet. *Claud.* 5 (trans. J. C. Rolfe): *Proclamante quodam praecidendas falsario manus, carnificem statim acciri cum machaera mensaque lanionia flagitavit.*

amputations rendered stumps unsuitable for prosthesis use, leaving people to utilise alternatives such as walking sticks, canes, or crutches for locomotive purposes, for which there is ample literary, archaeological, and bioarchaeological evidence.[91]

Extremity Prostheses

In cases where the use of an extremity prosthesis is recorded in ancient literary evidence, what was the nature of the prosthesis? There is no ancient evidence for the use of prosthetic fingers; perhaps the loss of a finger or two was not considered to be sufficiently debilitating or disfiguring to require a prosthesis. There is one detailed historical account of a prosthetic hand, the iron hand of Marcus Sergius Silus, described by Pliny the Elder in his *Natural History*, and discussed earlier.[92] However, Statius refers to the hero Pelops as having an ivory hand in his epic poem *Thebaid*, a departure from the traditional version of the myth in which Pelops is equipped with an ivory shoulder blade, and, when discussing Pelops' ivory shoulder blade, Dio Chrysostom refers to gold and ivory hands, so it is possible that individuals other than Marcus Sergius Silus were equipped with prosthetic hands and references to them have not survived, if they were ever made in works of literature in the first place.[93] Unfortunately, no prosthetic hand has survived in the archaeological record from classical antiquity and we can only speculate as to how they were crafted and the extent to which they could be utilised. Marcus Sergius Silus is described as fighting on with his left hand, presumably bearing his shield on his right arm, so his prosthetic right hand must have included some way of fixing the shield in place. If we consider the specific function of this particular prosthetic hand, it seems to have been intended as a way of holding or at least supporting a shield rather than anything else, so we might imagine a simple cap placed over the stump to hold the shield in place once the arm had been placed through the straps. There is some archaeological evidence for extremity prostheses being designed with combat in mind: the recent archaeological discovery of a skeleton of a male aged between forty and fifty years old from a Longobard necropolis at Povegliano Veronese in the Veneto in Northern Italy, dating from the sixth to eighth centuries CE, who had undergone the amputation of his right forearm and seems to have utilised an iron knife as a prosthesis demonstrates how an individual could weaponise their extremity prosthesis if necessary.[94] The knife was attached to his right forearm with

[91] For bioarchaeological evidence for crutch use, see Belcastro and Mariotti, 2000.
[92] Plin. *HN* 7.29. [93] Stat. *Theb.* 94–7; Dio Chrys. *Or.* 8.28. [94] Micarelli et al., 2018.

a leather strap and buckle, and the considerable wear on his right upper second incisor shows that he used his teeth in conjunction with his left hand to attach and adjust it.[95] It is also possible that a prosthetic hand might be made entirely from leather; the Hellenistic historian Dionysius bore the nickname Schytobrachion – 'leather-arm' – and this may have been a reference to a prosthetic arm.

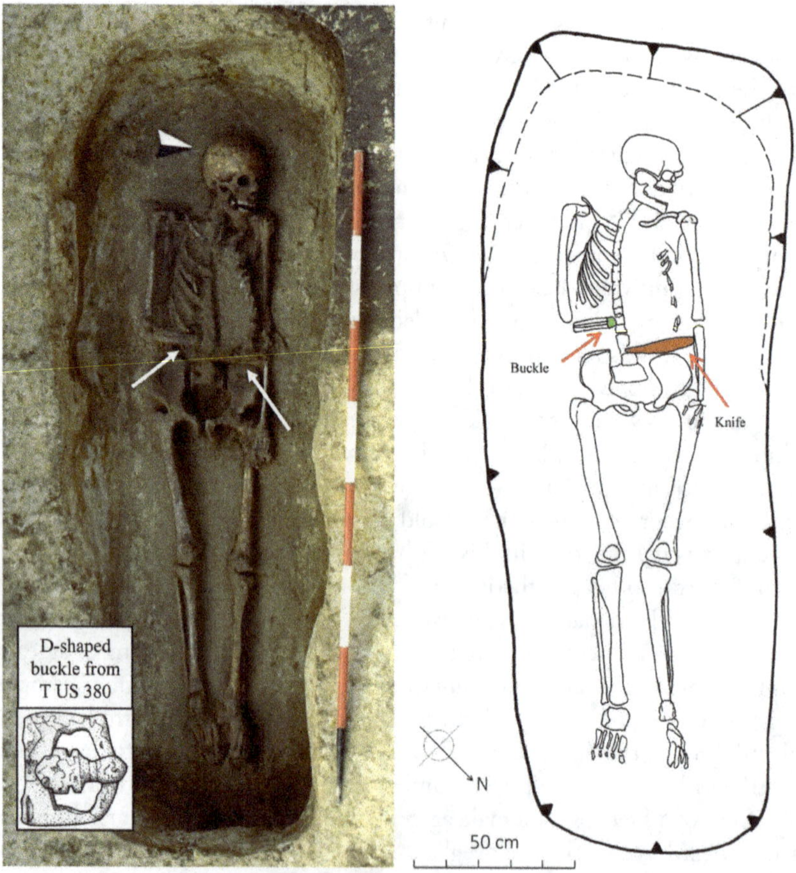

Figure 1.5 Longobard knife prosthesis, sixth–eighth century CE. Image courtesy of Micarelli, I., Paine, R., Giostra, C., Tafuri M. A., Profico, A., Boggioni, M., Di Vincenzo, F., Massani, D., Papini, A., Manzi, G. 2018. 'Survival to Amputation in Pre-Antibiotic Era: A Case Study From a Longobard Necropolis (6th–8th centuries AD)', *JASs Journal of Anthropological Sciences*, 96, pp. 185–200.

[95] Micarelli et al., 2018, p. 6, p. 8, p. 12.

There are rather more literary references to prosthetic legs and feet, and a variety of these have survived in the archaeological record.[96] The most detailed literary reference is found in an epigram attributed to Erycius that is included in the *Greek Anthology*.[97] It details how a man called Mindon was cutting down a tree and was bitten on the left foot by a spider. The bite became infected and turned gangrenous, necessitating the amputation of Mindon's leg. However, he replaced it with a prosthetic leg made from olive wood. Olive wood was frequently utilised for the making of tools, partly because of its ready accessibility around the Mediterranean but also partly because of its properties (such as malleability), so it is not surprising that it should be utilised to make a prosthetic leg.[98] Martial also mentions a wooden leg, although he does not specify the type of wood, using it as a metaphor in a piece of literary criticism delivered to someone plagiarising his verses.[99] He equates his verses to the leg of a man called Laedas, presumably a man renowned for his speed, and the verses of his imitator to a wooden leg, which allows us to speculate on the speed with which someone could move when utilising such a thing – presumably not very quickly, hence Martial's metaphor. It is also worth considering the role that an individual's gait played in their self-image.[100] For members of the social and political elite, moving in a way considered correct was extremely important, and the extent to which a prosthetic leg or foot either facilitated or obstructed this could have had a significant impact upon an individual's public persona.[101]

As we have seen, Hegesistratus of Elis amputated part of his own foot and replaced it with a wooden prosthesis of his own creation.[102] Lucian describes a man who lost both of his feet to frostbite after walking through snowdrifts and replaced them with wooden prostheses, continuing to get about with the assistance of the enslaved.[103] Lucian is critical of the man's preference for wearing expensive golden shoes on his wooden feet in much the same way that Dio Chrysostom is critical of using substances such as gold and ivory to make a prosthetic hand, or diamond or malachite to make a prosthetic eye. Several examples of prosthetic toes survive from Egypt, with wear on their bases indicating that they were worn during the

96 Whether the daimonic creature Empusa's leg, which is described variously as bronze, brass and copper, can be considered a prosthesis is debatable; see Arist. *Ran.* 294 and *Eccl.* 1094.

97 Erycius, *Greek Anthology* 9.233.

98 There is a potential reference to lime wood being used as a splint for an impaired leg in Arist. *Aves.* 1378–9; on this, see also Cinesias, *Testimonia* 10.

99 Mart. 10.100.

100 O'Sullivan, 2011; Corbeill, 2004, pp. 107–39.

101 For discussion of the ways in which an individual's physical appearance could be incorporated into invective, see Corbeill, 1997, particularly pp. 14–56.

102 Hdt. 9.36–7.

103 Luc. *Ind.* 6.

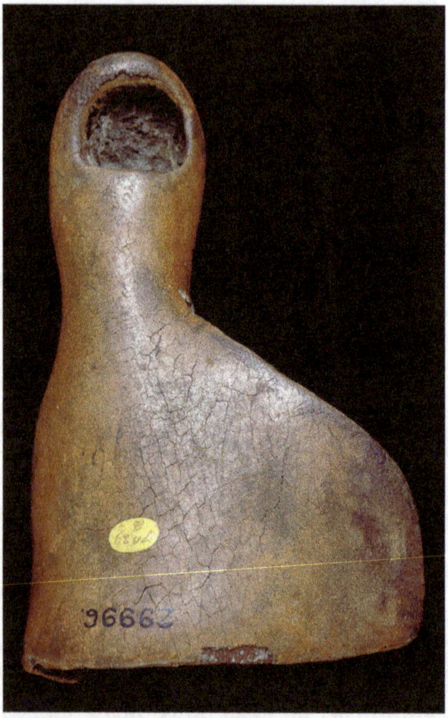

Figure 1.6 Greville Chester Toe, prior to 600 BCE. British Museum inv. EA 29996. Image courtesy of the British Museum.

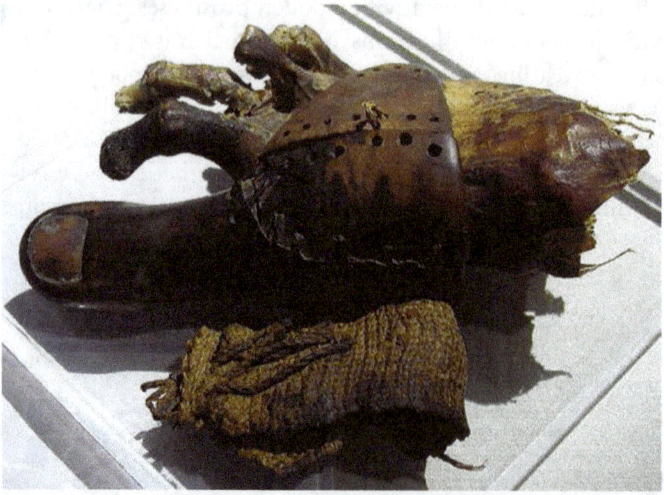

Figure 1.7 Cairo Toe, Cairo Museum inv. 453. Image courtesy of the University of Basel, Project *Life Histories of Theban Tombs*, photograph taken by Matjaž Kačičnik.

lives of the individuals who owned them rather than just incorporated into their mummies after death.[104] Experimental archaeological research has demonstrated that these objects were not only extremely functional, but also comfortable when worn with a sandal.[105] The Greville Chester Toe is made from cartonnage composed of linen and animal glue, the top covered in a layer of light brown gesso (a mix of plaster, glue, and red ochre), the bottom covered in a red resin, and modelled after the lost toe so faithfully that it originally included an inset toe nail, although this is now lost.[106] Eight small circular holes indicate that it would have been laced and tied onto the foot of its wearer.[107] The Cairo Toe is made from wood and leather, and was found fitted to the foot of a woman aged 50–60 years old in a tomb complex in the necropolis of Thebes-West (Sheik Abdel-Gurna).[108] The section of the tomb complex where the remains were found has been dated to the 21st–22nd Dynasty (1065–740 BCE).[109] The prosthesis consists of three sections attached to each other by leather strings and fastened with marline hitches.[110] These prostheses show the variety possible even in the smallest prosthetic device.

To date, the only extremity prosthesis known to have survived from classical antiquity is the famous Capua Limb, a Roman prosthetic right leg recovered from a tomb in Capua dating to approximately 300 BCE that was, prior to the recent discovery of the Turfan Limb in China, the oldest known functional prosthetic limb in the world.[111] The Capua Limb was made from wood and bronze, and it is probable that leather featured too in the form of some sort of padded cup at the point where the stump would come into contact with the prosthesis, and at the point where the prosthesis would have come into contact with the ground. The main part of the prosthesis consisted of a wooden core that was covered in bronze sheeting, and it seems to have been worn in conjunction with a leather and bronze belt to hold it in place. If the prosthesis could be securely fastened at the thigh and the waist, it would have enabled its user to achieve a limited amount of movement, although this likely required the additional assistance of a staff, a walking stick or a crutch or perhaps even two crutches.[112] Unfortunately, the original Capua Limb was destroyed in an air raid during the Blitz so for information regarding it we are reliant on the

[104] Finch, 2019. [105] Finch, 2019, pp. 42–3.
[106] British Museum inv. EA 29996; Finch, 2019, p. 33. [107] Finch, 2019, p. 33.
[108] Cairo Museum inv. 453. [109] Finch, 2019, p. 33. [110] Finch, 2019, p. 34.
[111] See Bourguignon and Henzen in Sudhoff, 1917; von Brun, 1926 for the announcement of the discovery and the early discussion and analysis of it. For the Turfan Limb, see Li et al., 2013.
[112] See Bliquez, 1996, pp. 2669–71 for discussion of the prosthesis' functionality.

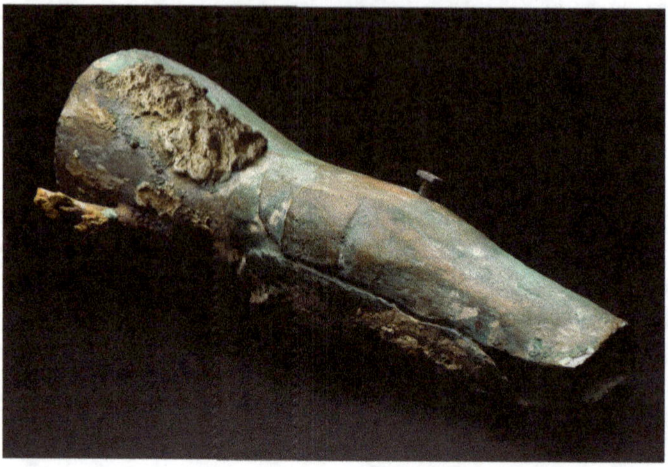

Figure 1.8 Replica of the Capua Limb, Science Museum/Wellcome Collection inv. A646752. Image courtesy of the Science Museum, London.

original excavation reports and a replica that was made of the bronze sheeting and is currently housed in the Science Museum in London.[113] Judging by the materials used in the limb's construction, and by other finds recovered from the tomb, which included a bronze urn and some locally produced red-figure pottery, it was likely owned and worn by an individual of high status or, at the very least, considerable wealth.[114] Even though the sex of the skeleton is not explicitly stated in any of the reports of the find, it has consistently been assumed to be a male skeleton.[115] Its owner was perhaps a veteran of the Second Samnite War (327–304 BCE) or even a retired gladiator, but whoever they were, they did not necessarily have to worry about stigmatisation due to their impairment, since, whether a veteran, a gladiator, or neither, they were an impaired individual in a society with a long history of warfare and were likely surrounded by others who had received equally debilitating injuries.[116] It is also clear from

[113] 'Roman artificial leg of bronze'.

[114] The perceived cost of a prosthesis plays a role in contemporary prosthesis adoption and successful use; users are more likely to adopt and use a prosthesis they perceive to be expensive. See Roeschlein and Domholdt, 1989.

[115] See Bliquez, 1996, p. 2667 n. 47, for assumptions regarding the sex and gender of the deceased. Interestingly, all twenty-one of the ancient literary references to prostheses that survive that specifically mention the gender of the prosthesis user describe them being worn by men (see Table I.3).

[116] See Van Lommel, 2015 for discussion of the variability of attitudes towards wounded veterans in the Roman Republic and Empire.

the materials utilised in the creation of their prosthesis that they were an individual of means, and consequently certainly outsourced the creation of the prosthesis to one or more artisans. Since the bronze sheeting has the appearance of a military greave, this is potentially an indicator of the (former) occupation of the user or perhaps the specialisation of the artisan responsible for the metal components.[117] Since Capua is noted in ancient literature as a city of considerable wealth and luxury and particularly feted for its bronze, it is not surprising that such an object should have been designed, commissioned, and used there.[118]

However, several extremity prostheses dating from Late Antiquity and the early Middle Ages have been found at sites in northern Europe.[119] A skeleton of a man missing a foot and bearing a prosthesis comprising a leather pouch with a wooden sole attached to it by iron nails was excavated at Bonaduz in Switzerland and dated to between the fifth and seventh centuries CE.[120] The pouch was filled with hay and moss, presumably intended to cushion the stump but possibly also to soak up pus from the wound since there is bioarchaeological evidence of minimal healing having taken place and, in any case, the individual lived for a maximum of two years after the amputation. It is debatable whether this prosthesis was functional in the sense of allowing the wearer to walk around since there seems to have been no means of attaching it to the ankle. A skeleton of a man aged 35–50 years old missing his lower left leg and bearing a wood and metal prosthesis in its place has recently been excavated from a Frankish settlement at Hemmaberg in southern Austria and dated to the sixth century CE.[121] Bioarchaeological evidence of osteoarthritis in the knees and shoulders indicates that he used the prosthesis in conjunction with a crutch. A skeleton of a man aged 57–63 missing his lower left leg below the knee and bearing the remains of a wood and bronze prosthesis, probably a wooden peg-leg tipped with bronze, in its place has been excavated from a Frankish cemetery at Griesheim near Darmstadt in Germany from a site dating to the seventh or eighth century CE.[122] In this case, the limb had been ex-articulated – severed at the ankle joint – rather than amputated, and the skeleton's left femur was atrophied,

[117] Bliquez, 1996, p. 2672.

[118] Cato, *Agr.* 135 recommends buying copper vessels from Capua; Plin. *HN* 34.95 highlights the bronze utensils produced in Capua.

[119] For discussion of mobility impairments in the Merovingian period, see Hähn, 2018; and for mobility impairments in Merovingian Gaul, see Laes, 2020.

[120] Baumgartner, 1982. [121] Binder et al., 2016; Eitler and Binder, 2019.

[122] Czarnetzki et al., 1983, pp. 91–4.

indicating that the man had survived for a considerable time after the amputation but had only restricted movement.

The possibility that an individual did not have to have experienced the loss of an extremity to use a prosthetic limb should also be considered. As we saw earlier, during either the third or second century BCE, an adult male aged between fifty and sixty-five years old from Turfan in western China lived with a disease – perhaps a strain of pulmonary tuberculosis – that froze his knee joint, leading to his use of a prosthetic leg which allowed him to remain physically active.[123] It is possible that individuals in the classical world did likewise, and there is some Late Antique literary evidence that suggests as much at that point in time. Gregory of Tours, writing in the late sixth century CE, records two instances of miraculous healing in which men with mobility impairments used wooden and leather peg-legs without first having undergone the amputation of the impaired extremity.[124] The first man, a cleric from Poitiers who remains unnamed, claimed that his mobility impairment had arisen when his foot had been on the receiving end of an attack from a demon which rendered it unusable for nine years, and during that time he had to resort to using an extremity prosthesis attached to his knee.[125] Finally, after three days of prayer, on 4 July 582 CE, he announced that he had been healed and no longer needed his prosthesis. The second man, an enslaved member of the Duke Aginus' household named Maurellus, seems to have been in a similar situation to the man from Turfan, as he had lost the ability to flex one of his knees after some sort of assault and had to resort to using some form of extremity prosthesis to facilitate mobility.[126] Like the cleric, Maurellus prayed for three days in advance of St Martin's Day, 11 November 592 CE (interestingly, Martin had died on 8 November 397 CE and had only been buried three days later), and then on the fourth day his leg was unfrozen and he was able to walk without assistance once more. Despite their inclusion of very specific biographical and temporal details that may have enabled Gregory's contemporary readership to identify the individuals under discussion, both stories are somewhat suspect due to the emphasis placed on the miraculous nature of the healing (the requirement of three days of prayer in advance of both miracles is particularly noteworthy in this respect, considering the significance of this period of time to Christians). This healing was only possible because neither individual had undergone an amputation of their impaired limb, despite that impairment rendering

[123] Li et al., 2013. [124] Gregory of Tours, *VM* 3.9, 4.41. [125] Gregory of Tours, *VM* 3.9.
[126] Gregory of Tours, *VM* 4.41.

them unable to walk without assistance for, in one case, almost a decade (and, realistically, both men would have required extensive rehabilitation for them to build up their withered musculature and learn how to walk again). Yet, literary and religious conventions aside, assuming we take these accounts at face value in their depiction of individuals adapting in the face of potentially debilitating mobility impairments, like the man from Turfan both men may have had their own reasons for choosing not to undergo what was, after all, a potentially hazardous surgical procedure, and this may have been a common scenario: Maurellus' use of a peg-leg is described as having been customary for those with this type of physical impairment.[127] There was not the same stigma attached to limb loss in ancient Greece or Rome as there was in ancient China, so individuals with frozen joints might have been more inclined to undergo surgery if it was presented as an option to them (it is, after all, a repeated refrain in classical literature that the purpose of amputation is to remove something useless), but then again, they might not have. Unfortunately, no archaeological or bioarchaeological evidence to support these accounts has yet been uncovered.

Other Types of Assistive Technology

As stated, there is a vast amount of literary, documentary, archaeological, and even bioarchaeological evidence for the use of walking sticks, canes, and crutches by the physically impaired to provide support and assistance with locomotion. Such objects could be used in conjunction with prostheses, particularly ones like the Capua Limb that extended above the knee, or they could be used instead of prostheses if prosthesis use was not possible. Additionally, it is likely that even individuals who made use of extremity prostheses did not use them all the time, and so potentially alternated between their prosthesis and their walking stick, cane, crutch, or crutches depending upon the circumstances that they were in and the requirements that they had.

The staff seems to have been ubiquitous in ancient Greece, the indicator of a citizen male, but persistent staff use over a prolonged period has been found to cause stress fractures in scapula and the ulna, which then results in a degree of physical impairment.[128] So, somewhat ironically, by utilising staffs their entire adult lives, ancient Greek citizens were causing themselves a higher level of physical impairment in their old age and

[127] Gregory of Tours, *VM* 4.41. [128] Fink-Bennett and Benson, 1984.

inadvertently increasing the extent of their reliance upon the staff or one of its equivalents as a piece of assistive technology in later life. For the physically impaired, the staff was considered to be a 'third foot' or a substitute set of eyes, simultaneously supporting and guiding its user.[129] The elderly, both men and women, are especially associated with physical weakness and with staffs, and so it is appropriate that Geras, the Greek personification of old age, and Senectus, the Roman personification of old age, were depicted as emaciated elderly men, doubled over and leaning on their staffs.[130] Theophrastus recommends that bay be used to make staffs for the elderly because it is lightweight, and presumably the same logic was applied to making staffs or their equivalents for individuals with other types of physical impairment.[131] It is clear that walking sticks, canes, and crutches could vary considerably: the Hippocratic orthopaedic surgery treatises *On Joints*, *On Fractures* and *Instruments of Reduction* recommend a variety of different types depending upon the nature of the individual's physical impairment.[132] Like prostheses, they were personalised and made to measure.

While there is a considerable amount of archaeological evidence for walking sticks, canes, and crutches in ancient visual and material culture, there is unfortunately little archaeological evidence in the form of the objects themselves, probably because most would have been carved from wood and so, like the organic components of prostheses, have not survived. There is, however, some bioarchaeological evidence for their use, and this evidence makes it clear that they were being used specifically for assistance with support and mobility by the physically impaired. A skeleton from the Roman necropolis of Casalecchio di Reno in Bologna, which has been dated to the second or third century CE, attests pathological changes in the upper body, the right-hand side in particular, and these pathological changes are considered to be consistent with crutch use.[133] The deceased, an elderly male, suffered from considerable degeneration of the right hip, and it is likely that his right foot would have been unable to touch the ground, which would have necessitated he

[129] See, for example, Luc. *Pod.* 54–7 (trans. M. D. Macleod): τρίτου ποδὸς. This is a proverb dating back to Hes. *Op.* 51.

[130] On old age in classical antiquity, see Cokayne, 2003; Parkin, 2003. See also Oedipus' answer to the Sphinx's riddle, Diod. Sic. 4.64.3–4; my thanks go to Debby Sneed for the observation that, since Oedipus was himself physically impaired, he would have been more aware than the Sphinx's other victims of different types of physical mobility, leaving him particularly suited to solving this riddle. *LIMC s.v.* Geras, Senectus.

[131] Theophr. *Hist. pl.* 5.7.7. [132] Hippoc. *Art.* 53, 58; Hippoc. *Mochl.* 20, 21, 23, 24.

[133] Belcastro and Mariotti, 2000, p. 532.

use at least one and probably two crutches to enable locomotion.[134] It is even possible that he utilised two different types of assistive technology simultaneously, such as a crutch on the right hand side and a walking stick on the left hand side.[135] A skeleton from the Le Colombier cemetery in Vaison-la-Romaine, which has been dated to the fifth or sixth century CE, attests pathological changes on the right scapula that are considered to be consistent with crutch use.[136] The deceased, a male aged around 50–60 years old who has been tentatively identified as an enslaved individual based on the location of his burial in the cemetery, exhibited a stress fracture on his right scapula, and this indicated that he used a crutch on the right-hand side of his body, perhaps due to osteoarthritis in his right hip. A skeleton from the Shurafa cemetery near Helouan, which has been dated to the Roman period, of a man aged at least thirty years old who suffered from hydrocephalus which resulted in hemiplegia (partial paralysis) of the left-hand side of his body which necessitated the use of some sort of mobility aid. It has been suggested that he used a long staff, held in both hands across the body, as a means of supporting his weaker left-hand side.[137]

The extent to which physically impaired individuals might have utilised assistive technology akin to a wheelchair is unknown; in fact, the existence of wheelchairs in classical antiquity has been categorically denied.[138] There are, however, a few depictions in ancient literature and art of young children using wheeled walking aids similar to modern Zimmer frames (ὁ δίφρος ὑπότροχος in Greek, *sustentaculum* in Latin), although there are none of adults doing something equivalent.[139] Perhaps such aids were considered solely the province of young children learning to walk and not appropriate for impaired adults, and anyone who attempted to do so met with sufficient scorn that they abandoned it.[140] Alternatively, perhaps, like the wheelbarrow, they were simply not necessary in societies that had alternative means of transporting the physically impaired.[141]

134 Belcastro and Mariotti, 2000, pp. 530–1.
135 Belcastro and Mariotti, 2000, p. 538; another individual from the same cemetery shows evidence for crutch use, but this is less clear.
136 Darton 2010. 137 Derry 1913, pp. 455–6.
138 Rose, 2003 reissued 2013, p. 24, goes so far as to say that there is 'absolutely no evidence' for them.
139 Sor. *Gyn.* 1.114. Armstrong, 2014; see also Giuliano, 1981, pp. 73–4, 1985, pp. 472–6; discussed in Langmuir, 2006, pp. 76, 113.
140 British Museum inv. 1910,0615.4; Museo Nazionale Romano inv. 65190. See also British Museum inv. 1996,0712.2 for a terracotta figurine from Egypt dating to the first–second century CE.
141 For discussion of the role that humans and animals played in supporting those with impairments and disabilities, see Chapter 5.

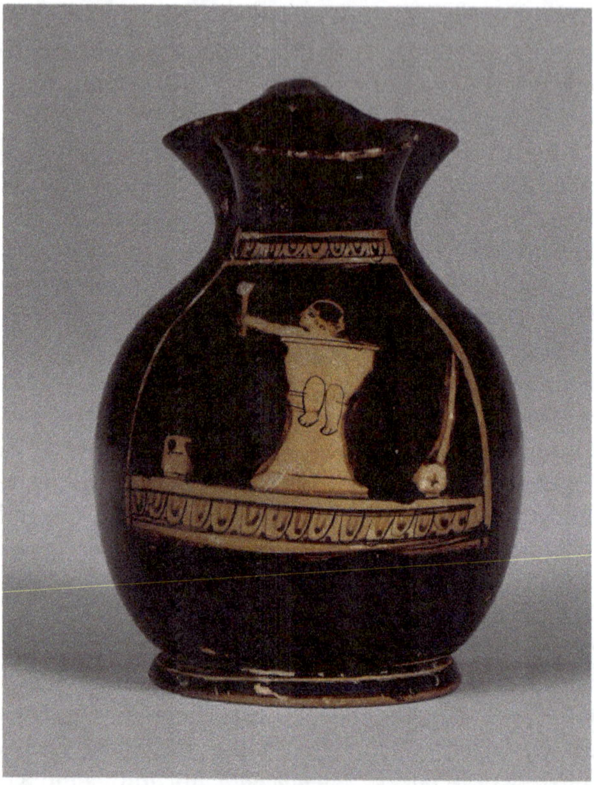

Figure 1.9 Red-figure chous, Attica, circa 440–430 BCE. British Museum inv. 1910,0615.4. Image courtesy of the British Museum.

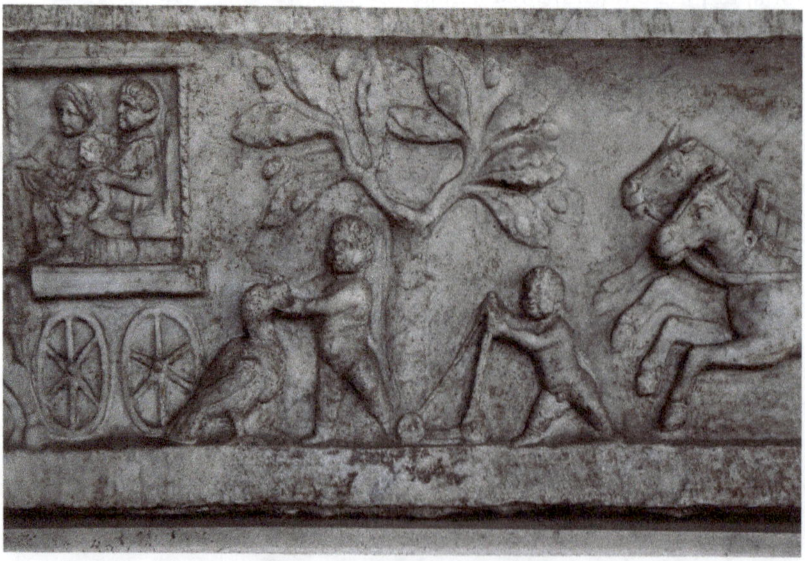

Figure 1.10 Detail from a Roman marble sarcophagus, Museo Nazionale Romano inv. 65190. Image courtesy of Alamy.

Conclusion

While the loss of extremities was relatively common in classical antiquity, extremity prosthesis use was not. There are several possible explanations for this. First, if the loss of a limb or part of a limb was common, coping strategies were clear and the pressure to 'pass' was less. Additionally, in small communities, a member of that community's personal history would be well known by everyone else, rendering attempts to 'pass' ultimately pointless. Second, medical practitioners did not make a habit of treating incurable conditions – in point of fact, they were actively discouraged through peer pressure from doing so; they only treated conditions that they knew they could cure, and even rehabilitation did not seem to have been something that they were generally interested in.[142] So a surgeon might have amputated a limb and monitored the stump until the danger of infection had passed, but that would normally have been the extent of his or her involvement. Additionally, depending upon the quality of the stump, prosthesis use may or may not have been possible or even desirable. Third, the extremity prostheses that survive from classical antiquity are all extremely different, something that makes sense if individuals were responsible for designing, commissioning, and manufacturing their prostheses to suit their own particular needs, and the differences between the surviving prostheses have the potential to be extremely informative regarding individual priorities. Fourth, prosthesis use is not viewed consistently in ancient literature; rather, it has both positive and negative connotations. An extremity prosthesis might be viewed favourably, as in the case of Hegesistratus or Silus, if it enables its user to carry on fighting the Spartans or the Carthaginians, less so if it simply offers its user an excuse to display his or her wealth, as in the case of the man described by Lucian. Fifth, there were a number of alternative and potentially more accessible options for individuals experiencing mobility impairments, such as staffs, sticks, canes, and crutches. Since an individual who used a prosthesis might find themselves also needing to use one or two additional mobility aids in any case, why bother?

One additional point worth considering is that the extremity prostheses that have survived from classical antiquity have done so because they were included in the burials of their users. In all cases, they seem to have been attached to their users' bodies in death as they would have been during life,

[142] See, for example, Hippoc. *Art.* 58, where the author goes to some lengths to justify their focus on the rehabilitation of those who experience injuries or impairments that affect their mobility.

rather than simply included alongside the individual as a grave good. This can perhaps give us an insight into the way that prostheses were viewed by their users, and in turn the way that prostheses and prosthesis users were viewed by their peers, since it would have been their peers that were responsible for undertaking the funerary rites. Since an ancient extremity prosthesis was designed, commissioned, and manufactured specifically for an individual in order to meet their own unique set of needs, it is highly unlikely that one could simply have been reused, such as, for example, an artisan's tools would have been, although one could potentially have been repurposed, particularly the more valuable materials such as metal. So, the fact that this does not seem to have occurred, at least in the cases for which we have evidence, is certainly significant. It would appear that extremity prostheses were viewed, both by their users and by others, as a true substitute or replacement for the individual's missing body part.

CHAPTER 2

Facial Prostheses

Introduction

In Apuleius' novel *Metamorphosis*, the hero Lucius attends a banquet where he encounters a man named Thelyphron who had fallen prey to a coven of witches while travelling through Thessaly.[1] Thelyphron was employed to stand guard over a corpse for the night:

> 'You see, while this very keen-witted watchman was maintaining his intensive vigil over my body, some old witches tried to get at my remains. They had transmuted themselves for the purpose, but to no avail, since in several attempts they were unable to elude his unremitting attentiveness. Finally they threw a cloud of sleep over him and buried him in deep slumber. Then they began calling my name, and kept it up until my sluggish joints and chilly limbs were struggling with slow effort to obey the commands of their magic art. Since, however, the watchman was alive in fact, but only dead asleep, because he had the same name as mine, he unwittingly arose at the sound of his name and walked mechanically like a lifeless ghost. Although the doors to the chamber had been carefully bolted, there was a hole through which he had first his nose and then his ears sliced off; he brought on himself the butchery intended for me. Then, to put the proper finishing touch on their trick, they shaped some wax into ears like the amputated ones and fastened them on him in a perfect fit, and made him a wax nose like his own. And now the poor wretch is standing here, having earned the reward, not of hard work, but of mutilation'. I was terrified at his words and started to test Fortune. I put my hand up and grasped my nose: it came away; I rubbed my ears: they fell off. The crowd were pointing their fingers at me and twisting their heads round to nod at me, and laughter broke out. Dripping with cold sweat, I escaped through the legs of the surrounding mob. I could never afterwards return to my ancestral home so maimed and so ludicrous, but I have let my hair grow long on both sides to hide the scars of

[1] On Thessaly's reputation for witches and witchcraft, see Phillips, 2002.

> my ears, and I have tightly attached this linen bandage for decency's sake to conceal the shame of my nose.[2]

Ancient witches were notorious for wanting to harvest body parts from both the living and the dead, particularly young men, for their spells.[3] While the portrayal of witches in Latin literature is surely exaggerated for horrific or sometimes comedic effect, it is certainly true that many of the curse tablets and voodoo dolls (in Greek: κολοσσοί) that have survived from antiquity include human hair, such as the example in Figure 2.1, originally from Egypt and dating from the period of the first century CE to the third century CE.[4] In this particular passage, it would appear that the witches were after the nose and ears of the deceased, perhaps to use them as ingredients in a potion, but were forced to make do with the nose and ears of the man that stood guard over him, and, having harvested them, they replaced them with prostheses made of wax, the same material that was commonly used to make voodoo dolls. Presumably Apuleius intended their incompetence and its ramifications to be simultaneously amusing and horrifying to the reader. Within the context of the novel, it does not appear that this substitution of wax for flesh was intended to be permanent, and, indeed, it is unlikely that facial prostheses made of wax would have been either convincing or long-lasting. What is useful for our purposes is the way that Thelyphron reacts to his disfigurement, and the potential that this reaction is representative of the ways in which an average individual who experienced some sort of facial disfigurement would react to theirs in antiquity. He refers to it as 'mutilation', and the word used, *debilitatio*, can also be translated as 'weakness'. He perceives himself to be maimed (*debilis*) and ridiculous (*ridiculus*) as a result, although whether this is entirely down

[2] Apul. *Met.* 2.30 (trans. J. A. Hanson): '"*Nam cum corporis mei custos hic sagacissimus exsertam mihi teneret vigiliam, cantatrices anus exuviis meis imminentes atque ob id reformatae frustra saepius cum industriam sedulam eius fallere nequivissent, postremum iniecta somni nebula eoque in profundam quietem sepulto, me nomine ciere non prius desierunt quam dum hebetes artus et membra frigida pigris conatibus ad artis magicae nituntur obsequia. Hic utpote vivus quidem, sed tantum sopore mortuus, quod eodem mecum vocabulo nuncupatur, ad suum nomen ignarus exsurgit, et, in exanimis umbrae modum ultroneus gradiens, quamquam foribus cubiculi diligenter occlusis, per quoddam foramen prosectis naso prius ac mox auribus vicariam pro me lanienam suscitavit. Utque fallaciae reliqua convenirent, ceram in modum prosectarum formatam aurium ei applicant examussim nasoque ipsius similem comparant. Et nunc assistit miser hic, praemium non industriae sed debilitationis consecutus". His dictis perterritus temptare Fortunam aggredior. Iniecta manu nasum prehendo: sequitur; aures pertracto: deruunt. Ac dum directis digitis et detortis nutibus praesentium denotor, dum risus ebullit, inter pedes circumstantium frigido sudore defluens evado. Nec postea debilis ac sic ridiculus Lari me patrio reddere potui, sed capillis hinc inde laterum deiectis aurium vulnera celavi, nasi vero dedecus linteolo isto pressim agglutinato decenter obtexi*'.

[3] See, for example, Hor. *Sat.* 1.8; Hor. *Epod.* 5; Ov. *Her.* 6.83–94; Lucan, *Pharsalia* 6.413–587.

[4] British Museum inv. EA37918.

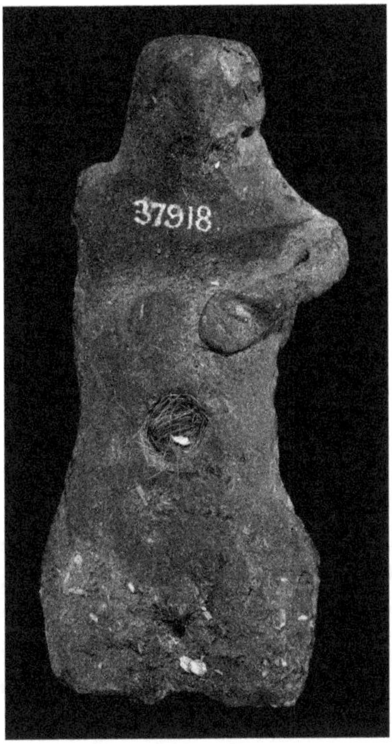

Figure 2.1 Graeco-Roman-Egyptian voodoo doll, Egypt, first –third century CE. British Museum inv. EA37918. Image courtesy of the British Museum.

to his physical appearance or also due to the circumstances under which it happened is not entirely clear. He feels like he cannot go home and so presumably no longer has contact with family or friends. The measures that he has taken to attempt to disguise his disfigurements – growing his hair to cover his missing ears and tying a bandage around his face to cover his missing nose – seem sensible and would have been more accessible to others in a similar position than a set of prosthetic ears or a nose would have been. However, it is worth noting that, particularly in the case of his missing nose, his attempt to disguise it would not have been successful but rather would likely have done the reverse; the bandage covering the obviously missing nose would have drawn the eye and caused anyone encountering him to wonder what had happened and would likely have led them to ask about it. This would, however, have been preferable to someone in Thelyphron's position going about their business with no bandage at all and having to deal with the consequences of that.

People with facial disfigurements have long claimed that people actively avoid them, and studies have been undertaken in response to these reports to attempt to establish whether this is the case and, if so, why this is.[5] Ideally, a facial prosthesis such as an eye or a nose resembles the missing eye or nose to such a degree that it enables the user to 'pass' and allows them to go about their business in relative anonymity.[6] Consequently, such an item is sometimes referred to as a cosmesis. In this chapter, I will examine the literary, archaeological, and bioarchaeological evidence for the use of facial prostheses – eyes, nose, and teeth – in classical antiquity.

Facial Mutilation in Classical Antiquity

Just as there were a variety of means by which limbs could be lost in classical antiquity, there were also a variety of means by which parts of the face could be lost.[7] While the loss of one or both ears could be disguised with relative ease through the use of hair or headgear such as a headwrap or a veil, and the loss of teeth could be disguised simply by closing one's mouth, the loss of an eye or nose was much more difficult to hide. In fact, the loss of an eye or nose was considerably more difficult to hide than the loss of a finger or toe, or even a hand or a foot. Given the face to face nature of ancient society, a facial disfigurement would have been one of the first things – if not the very first thing – that someone noticed about another person upon meeting them.[8] The degree to which someone's face had been mutilated, and the cause of that mutilation, if it were apparent, would have had a significant effect upon their life and most, if not all, of their social interactions.

Loss of a Facial Feature through Surgical Intervention

Someone could experience a variety of different types of trauma (both accidentally and deliberately inflicted) that could result in the need for surgical intervention. As we have seen, several different methods of surgical amputation are attested as having been used from the Classical period onwards, but these methods involve the extremities. Did ancient surgeons

[5] Ryan et al., 2012; Shanmugarajah et al., 2012.

[6] A recent study has shown that facial prosthesis users tend to prefer implanted prostheses over adhesive prostheses; the users of the latter type feel more self-conscious see Wondergem et al., 2016. As far as the functionality of facial prostheses is concerned, in recent years, scientists have had some success in developing a prosthetic retina that has partially restored the sight in mice; see Nirenberg and Pandarinath, 2012.

[7] For discussion of limb loss in classical antiquity, see Chapter 1.

[8] For the practice of physiognomy in antiquity, see Barton, 2002; Swain, 2007.

undertake the amputation of facial features such as eyes, noses, lips, and ears? Did they undertake the extraction of teeth? Facial surgery was practiced by ancient surgeons, but on a relatively limited and superficial basis, and the stated aim of these procedures was to preserve an individual's natural looks and repair damage caused by disease or trauma, as far as such a thing was possible, rather than cause it. Medical writers warn against attempting too ambitious a procedure, as attempting to repair a large defect can potentially do more harm than good, and may even affect the face's function.[9]

Literary evidence in the form of detailed descriptions of various different types of procedures survives in a number of ancient medical treatises, and archaeological evidence, mainly in the form of surgical instruments but also, occasionally, other sorts of material evidence, can provide additional information. Thus, we have accounts of eye operations such as the removal of cataracts, and surgical tools such as cataract needles that indicate that ancient physicians were intimately familiar with the architecture of the eye and were practising a degree of invasive ocular surgery.[10] Courtesy of the Roman medical writer Celsus, we also have an account of a surgical procedure that has been termed a blepharoplasty.[11] This was used to treat the persistent symptoms of an eye disease known as *trachoma*, a result of the sexually transmitted infection *Chlamydia trachomatis*. *Trachoma* is caused by direct contact with infected bodily fluids or an object contaminated with them, leading to the tissue lining the eyelids becoming inflamed between five and twelve days after exposure. If left untreated, the infection can result in the eyelashes turning inwards and rubbing against the cornea, which can cause eye ulcers, scarring and deformity of the eyelids, and even blindness. In classical antiquity, this chronic infection of the eyelid and eye was treated by removing the line of eyelashes and cauterising the places where they had been to prevent them from growing back. It has been suggested that a mummy portrait dating to around 190–210 CE depicts an individual that had undergone this procedure.[12] The portrait is of a relatively young man and it includes a feature which has been identified as a healed surgical scar upon the skin around the subject's right

[9] See, for example, Celsus, *Med.* 9.1; Oribasius, *Medical Collection* 42.25–6.

[10] See, for example, Celsus, *Med.* 6.14. For a set of ancient ophthalmological instruments, see the collection of the oculist Gaius Firmius Severus from Rheims which date to the second century CE, currently held by the Wellcome Collection, inv. 202–308 1936.

[11] Celsus, *Med.* 7.7.8 B.

[12] Metropolitan Museum of Art inv. 09.181.4; the portrait is now displayed with the title 'Portrait of a Youth with a Surgical Cut in the Right Eye'.

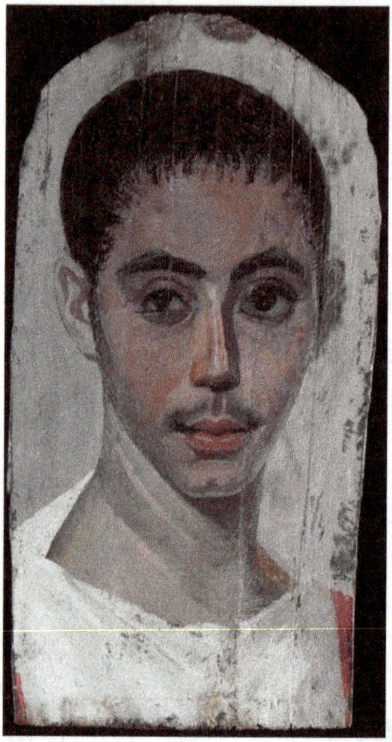

Figure 2.2 Graeco-Roman-Egyptian Mummy portrait. Metropolitan Museum of Art inv. 09.181.4. Image courtesy of the Metropolitan Museum of Art.

eye, the nature of which has resulted in the tentative identification of the blepharoplasty.[13] It has been observed that the way in which the pupil of the right eye has been depicted in comparison to the left eye could be seen to indicate that, unfortunately for the young man, the blepharoplasty failed to save the sight in that eye.[14] However, the operation would certainly have alleviated the pain caused by the chronic infection of his eye and eyelid. The fact that the surgical scar was included in his portrait (if it is in fact a surgical scar) could indicate that he was not ashamed of his condition; perhaps its inclusion could be viewed as an indication that he was proud of the fact that he had been able to afford surgical treatment, or perhaps his ability to withstand the pain of an operation probably undertaken without any kind of anaesthetic. If cataracts were as

[13] Johnson, 2005. [14] Johnson, 2005, p. 31.

common in Roman Egypt as the documentary literature seems to suggest, it is likely that others around him were suffering from similar conditions; perhaps they were unable to afford or even bear the treatment that he could? If this was the case, his scar could have set him apart from them, perhaps even distinguishing him in their opinion. Removal of an entire eye was quite another matter, however. Judging by the numerous literary and documentary accounts of people living with the loss of sight as opposed to the loss of eyes, this was something that would be done only in the direst emergencies, such as when the eyeball was so badly damaged that it was simply unrecoverable. One example of this occurring was after King Philip II of Macedon was shot in the right eye with an arrow during the siege of Methône in 354 BCE. According to Pliny the Elder, the physician Critobulus was worth including in a list of scientific practitioners of renown because he had managed to extract the arrow and remove the damaged eyeball without causing any further disfigurement to Philip's face.[15]

Regarding the definitive removal of parts of the face, the procedure undertaken most frequently would in all likelihood have been the extraction of teeth. Medical authors include information about how to prevent loose teeth from being lost, but presumably these attempts were not always successful.[16] If a tooth needed to be removed, it was grasped with the fingers and wiggled until it was loose, and then pliers or forceps were used for the final stage of the extraction.[17] An electrum vase from Kul'-Oba Kurgan in the Crimea, dating to the fourth century BCE, depicts a procedure of this type.[18] It has been suggested that this vase depicts a figure from Scythian mythology, Agathyrsos, who attempted to draw the bow of Herakles but was unsuccessful; a common result of this sort of failure would be the recoil hitting the would-be archer in the face and breaking a tooth or teeth.[19] Archaeological evidence of professional tooth extraction has been recovered from a taberna set within the podium of the temple of Castor and Pollux in the Forum Romanum.[20] More than eighty teeth, all extensively decayed, and a variety of medical equipment support the identification of the taberna as a dental surgery.

[15] Plin. *HN* 7.37.124. For discussion of the wounding of Philip, see Rigonos, 1994. For discussion of Critobulus' surgery, see Prag, 1990.

[16] Hippoc. *Art.* 33.9–10; Celsus, *Med.* 6.12.

[17] See for example Celsus, *Med.* 12.1 for instructions.

[18] State Hermitage Museum inv. #KO 11–2.

[19] For this interpretation of the scene, see Raevskij, 1982–3. For the mythological episode, see Hdt. 4.8–10.

[20] Becker, 2014.

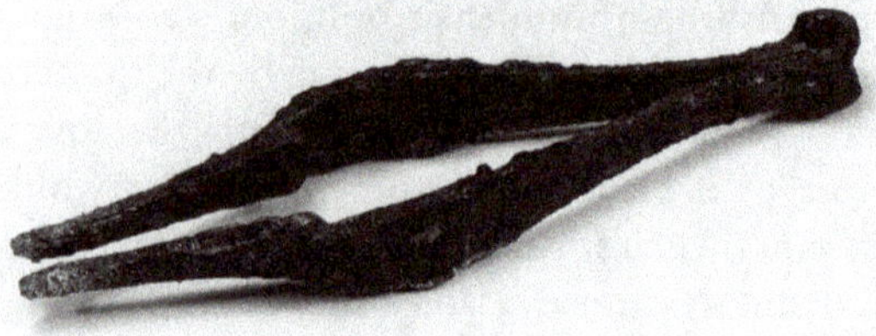

Figure 2.3 Graeco-Roman dental forceps. Image courtesy of the Wellcome Library.

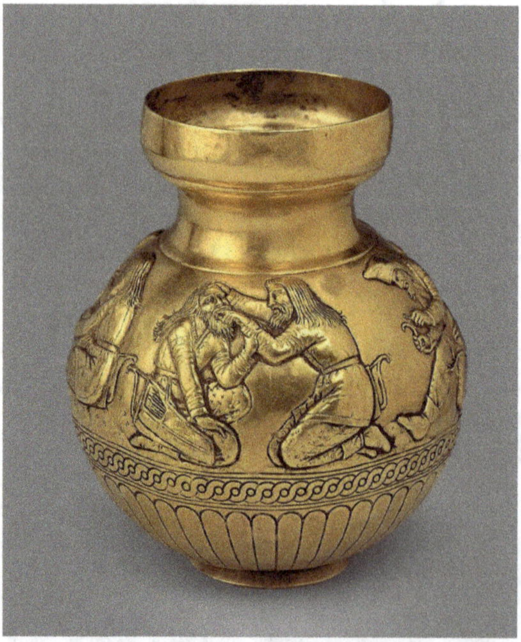

Figure 2.4 Scythian vase, Kul'-Oba Kurgan in the Crimea, second half of the fourth century BCE. State Hermitage Museum inv. #KO 11–2. Image from www.hermitagemuseum.org, courtesy of The State Hermitage Museum, St. Petersburg, Russia.

Loss of a Facial Feature through Participation in Military Activity

Although helmet styles changed over the course of time, they provided minimal protection to a soldier's face, leaving the eyes, nose, and mouth all vulnerable to injury.[21] Soldiers might receive wounds to the face from projectiles such as slingshots, arrows, or spears, or from swords or shields. During the civil war, Julius Caesar reportedly encouraged his soldiers to aim for the faces of his opponent Pompey's forces, as he thought that facial injuries would be more demoralising to the young aristocratic men that comprised his army.[22]

There are numerous examples of prominent historical figures from classical antiquity who lost eyes during the course of their military careers. The Republican heroes Horatius Cocles, who lost his eye either during or prior to the battle against the Etruscans at the Pons Sublicius, and Sertorius, who lost his eye during the Marsic War, indicate that even generals were not safe from severe injuries to their faces.[23] There are also examples of less prominent individuals, such as four centurions from one cohort who lost their eyes during the civil wars that we only happen to know about because Julius Caesar considered it interesting enough to mention in passing, or Cassius Scaeva, who lost an eye to a spear at the battle of Dyrrachium, mentioned by both Suetonius and Lucan.[24] While some soldiers, such as Sertorius, for example, were clearly proud of their wounds, others may have felt considerable embarrassment and shame and subsequently sought to disguise or at least minimise them.[25]

Loss of a Facial Feature through Judicial Punishment

According to Diodorus Siculus, the laws of Egypt declared that anyone who revealed military secrets should have their tongue cut out.[26] He also states that they declared that a married woman who voluntarily committed adultery with a man should have her nose cut off, 'on the ground that a woman who tricks herself out with an eye to forbidden licence should be deprived of that which contributes most to a woman's

[21] See Trentin, 2013, p. 99, for a discussion of Roman helmets and their lack of eye protection.

[22] Plut. *Vit. Caes.* 45.1; Plut. *Vit. Pomp.* 71.4; App. *B Civ.* 2.76.318; Flor. 2.13.50; Frontin. *Str.* 4.7.32; for discussion, see Leigh, 1995, p. 207.

[23] Horatius Cocles: Dion. Hal. *Ant. Rom.* 5.23.2–25; but see also Plut. Vit. *Popl.* 16.4–7. Sertorius: Plut. *Vit. Sert.* 4.2. See also Africa, 1970.

[24] Caes. *BCiv.* 3.53.4; Suet. *Iul.* 68.4; Lucan, *Pharsalia* 6.213–16.

[25] For Sertorius, see Sall. *Hist.* 1.88.

[26] Diod. Sic. 1.78.3.

comeliness'.[27] Thus this would serve not only as a punishment for the original infraction, but a means of preventing it from happening again. Julius Caesar utilised amputation of an eye or both ears as a lesser punishment and deterrent while on campaign in Gaul.[28] Augustine indicates that those who inflicted facial mutilation upon another would themselves be punished with similar treatment.[29]

Loss of a Facial Feature through Extra-Judicial Punishment

The removal of facial features such as the eyes, nose, mouth, tongue, or ears as a means of torture at the apparent whim of a powerful individual in classical antiquity, whether that individual was Greek, Roman, Carthaginian, or Persian, seems to have been rather common in classical antiquity, or at least is presented as being so. Thus, there are many accounts of tyrants ordering the mutilation of their subjects or of individuals that they have in their power.[30] Seneca the Younger discusses the rage of barbarian kings, 'men who had no contact with learning or the culture of letters', before moving on to an example of how even 'civilised' men educated by Aristotle can stoop to those depths.[31] He provides a detailed description of the indignities inflicted upon Telesphorus by King Lysimachus:

> Though Lysimachus escaped by some good luck from the lion's teeth, was he therefore, in view of this experience, a whit more kind when he himself became king? Not so, for Telesphorus the Rhodian, his own friend, he completely mutilated, and when he had cut off his ears and nose, he shut him up in a cage as if he were some strange and unknown animal and for a long time lived in terror of him, since the hideousness of his hacked and mutilated face had destroyed every appearance of a human being; to this were added starvation and squalor and the filth of a body left to wallow in its own dung; furthermore, his hands and knees becoming all calloused – for by the narrowness of his quarters he was forced to use these instead of feet – his sides, too, a mass of sores from rubbing, to those who beheld him his appearance was no less disgusting than terrible, and having been turned by his punishment into a monster he had forfeited even pity. Yet, while he

[27] Diod. Sic. 1.78.4–5 (trans. C. H. Oldfather): τῆς δὲ γυναικὸς τὴν ῥῖνα κολοβοῦσθαι, ὑπολαμβάνοντες δεῖν τῆς πρὸς ἀσυγχώρητον ἀκρασίαν καλλωπιζομένης ἀφαιρεθῆναι τὰ μάλιστα κοσμοῦντα τὴν εὐπρέπειαν. On the frequency with which this particular type of mutilation is weaponised against women, and the rationale behind it, see Skinner, 2014.

[28] Caes. *BGall.* 7.4. [29] August. *Ep.* 34 (*Epistle* 133).

[30] See for example Sen. *Ira* 5.18.1–2 on Sulla; Sen. *Ira* 5.20.1–2 on the king of the Persians; Diod. Sic. 33.14.3 on Diegylis.

[31] Sen. *Ira* 5.17.1 (trans. J. W. Basore): *quos nulla eruditio, nullus litterarum cultus imbuerat.*

> who suffered these things was utterly unlike a human being, he who inflicted them was still less like one.[32]

Often the individual's response in the face of this threat is an opportunity to present their bravery and fortitude. Thus Theodorus, when threatened with torture by King Lysimachus, responds with equanimity:

> And when the king showed him Telesphorus in a cage, his eyes gouged out, his nose and ears lopped off, his tongue cut out, and said: 'To this plight I bring those who injure me', Theodorus replied: 'What cares Theodorus whether he rots above the ground or under it?'[33]

If the powerful individual is a Greek or a Roman, they might come in for criticism for acting like a barbarian tyrant. Thus, Arrian criticises Alexander the Great for ordering that Bessus have his nose and ear lobes cut off prior to being sent to Ecbatana and put to death there in front of an audience composed of Medes and Persians, and goes so far as to accuse him of forgetting himself and getting carried away in his imitation of Median and Persian opulence and excess.[34] Arrian inserts his own personal opinion: 'I regard the mutilation of the extremities as barbaric.'[35]

Procopius details the Byzantine emperor Honoric's cruelty to the Christian community in Libya: he ordered them to convert to Arianism, and when they protested he had their tongues cut out at the throat. However, Procopius adds that, miraculously, this had no effect upon their dissent except in the case of two who also visited prostitutes.[36]

Martial recounts that an acquaintance cut off the nose of a man he found to be having an affair with his wife, asking 'who persuaded you to cut off

[32] Sen. *Ira* 7.3–4 (trans. J. W. Basore): *Numquid ergo hic Lysimachus felicitate quadam dentibus leonis elapsus ob hoc, cum ipse regnaret, mitior fuit? Nam Telesphorum Rhodium amicum suum undique decurtatum, cum aures illi nasumque abscidisset, in cavea velut novum aliquod animal et invisitatum diu pavit, cum oris detruncati mutilatique deformitas humanam faciem perdidisset; accedebat fames et squalor et inluvies corporis in stercore suo destituti; callosis super haec genibus manibusque, quas in usum pedum angustiae loci cogebant, lateribus vero adtritu exulceratis non minus foeda quam terribilis erat forma eius visentibus, factusque poena sua monstrum misericordiam quoque amiserat. Tamen, cum dissimillimus esset homini qui illa patiebatur, dissimilior erat qui faciebat.* See also the experience of Marcus Attilius Regulus when captured by the Sicels: Diod. Sic. 23.16; Cic. *Pis.* 19; Val. Max. 9 External 1; Cass. Dio. 11 Zonaras 8.15. For the process of 'becoming a monster', see Gevaert and Laes, 2013.

[33] Plut. *Mor. On Exile* 606B (trans. P. H. De Lacey and B. Einarson): ἐπιδείξαντος δὲ αὐτῷ Τελεσφόρον ἐν γαλεάγρᾳ, τοὺς ὀφθαλμοὺς ἐξορωρυγμένον καὶ περικεκομμένον τὴν ῥῖνα καὶ τὰ ὦτα καὶ τὴν γλῶτταν ἐκτετμημένον, καὶ εἰπόντος, 'οὕτως ἐγὼ διατίθημι τοὺς κακῶς με ποιοῦντας'· 'τί δὲ Θεοδώρῳ μέλει', ἔφη, 'πότερον ὑπὲρ γῆς ἢ ὑπὸ γῆς σήπεται.

[34] Arr. *Anab.* 4.7.3–4.

[35] Arr. *Anab.* 4.7.3–4 (trans. P. A. Brunt): ἀλλὰ βαρβαρικὴν εἶναι τίθεμαι τῶν ἀκρωτηρίων τὴν λώβην.

[36] Procop. 3.8.4–5.

the adulterer's nose? No offence against you has been committed by this part, my good husband. Idiot, what have you done? Your wife has lost nothing here, since your Deiphobus' cock is safe and sound.'[37] It is possible that this type of punishment was habitually inflicted upon the enslaved, or at least threatened as a possibility; Hermesianax presents a nurse as having the tip of her tongue, her nose, and her fingers cut off by her master and mistress after attempting to facilitate their daughter's (her charge's) love affair.[38]

Alternatively, such a punishment could be inflicted in response to a great outrage: Ovid presents Procne and Philomela as prepared to cut out Tereus' tongue and eyes, or to castrate him, as punishment for his rape and mutilation of Philomela.[39]

Individuals at the mercy of others, such as apprentices or the enslaved, were particularly vulnerable to corporal punishment, the consequences of which could be severe. The *Digest* records a case in which a cobbler struck his young apprentice with a last and put out his eye.[40] The emperor Hadrian once put out the eye of one of his enslaved attendants with a stylus while in a fit of temper.[41]

Loss of a Facial Feature through Self-Mutilation or Mutilation

There are numerous accounts of individuals mutilating themselves as acts of defiance, such as Anaxarchus who, when the tyrant of Cyprus Nicocreon ordered that his tongue be cut out, actually bit it off himself and spat it at him.[42] Valerius Maximus provides a detailed account of this episode:

> Tortured by the tyrant of Cyprus, Nicocreon, no violence could stop him from torturing the tyrant in his turn with lashings of the most wounding insults. At last Nicocreon threatened to cut off his tongue, to which Anaxarchus replied: 'Womanish young man, this part of my body at least will not be in your power', and straight away he cut off his tongue with his teeth, chewed it up, and spat it into the other's mouth, which was open in fury. That tongue had held the ears of many lost in admiration, above all king Alexander's, as it wisely and eloquently expounded the state of the earth, the condition of the sea, the movements of the stars, in fine the nature of the entire universe. But it perished almost more gloriously than it

[37] Mart. 3.85 (trans. D. R. Shackleton Bailey): *Quis tibi persuasit naris abscidere moecho? non hac peccatum est parte, marite, tibi. stulte, quid egisti? nihil hic tua perdidit uxor, cum sit salva tui mentula Deiphobi.* See Plaut. *Mil.* 1388–9 for a character who wishes to castrate an adulterer.

[38] Hermesianax, *Fragments* (*Leontion*) 2.4. [39] Ov. *Met.* 6.613–18. [40] *Dig.* 9.2.5.3.

[41] Gal. *Aff.Dig.* 4 5.17–18 K. [42] Diog. Laert. 5.9.

> flourished, because by so brave an end it validated the illustrious performance of what it professed and not only adorned Anaxarchus' life but rendered his death more renowned.[43]

Anaxarchus is able to turn the tables on his captor, both figuratively by refusing to be terrorised, and literally by spitting his severed tongue into Nicocreon's mouth. He is presented as martialling his oratorical skills one last time. Additionally, according to Philo, 'certain wise men' bit off their own tongues to prevent themselves from speaking when subjected to torture.[44] One example of this is the orator Antiphon who, in one version of his biography, was likewise captured by enemies, in his case Antipater of Corinth, and bit off his own tongue to prevent himself from revealing secrets about his city-state Athens.[45] Somewhat more positively, some individuals mutilated themselves as a way of honouring their dead.[46]

Seneca the Elder describes a variety of gruesome ways in which children might be mutilated in order to make them more effective beggars, with the mutilator choosing to inflict a particularly suitable mutilation on each child: 'this child has a ready tongue and sharp eyes: let them be torn out by the roots'.[47] Women might be mutilated by their husbands or fathers in order to make them less physically appealing; Petronius' *Satyricon* includes a character named Habbinas who states that if he had a daughter he would cut off her ears so as to prevent her from purchasing and wearing expensive earrings, although whether such a thing ever actually occurred is debatable.[48] Individuals might have their tongues cut out to prevent them from speaking inconvenient truths. Thus, Martial recounts an enslaver cutting out the tongue of an enslaved individual before crucifying him and ponders what the master was attempting to prevent the enslaved individual from saying, while Suetonius records that the emperor Caligula sentenced an equestrian to death by beasts in the arena then, when the man

[43] Val. Max. 3.4 (trans. D. R. Shackleton Bailey): *cum a tyranno Cypriorum Nicocreonte torqueretur, nec ulla vi inhiberi posset quo minus eum amarissimorum maledictorum verberibus invicem ipse torqueret, ad ultimum amputationem linguae minitanti 'non erit' inquit, 'effeminate adulescens, haec quoque pars corporis mei tuae dicionis,' protinusque dentibus abscisam et commanducatam linguam in os eius ira patens exspuit. multorum aures illa lingua et in primis Alexandri regis admiratione sui attonitas habuerat, dum terrae condicionem, habitum maris, siderum motus, totius denique mundi naturam prudentissime et facundissime expromit. paene tamen occidit gloriosius quam viguit, quia tam forti fine illustrem professionis actum comprobavit, Anaxarchique non vitam modo decoravit sed mortem reddidit clariorem*. See also Cic. *Tusc.* 2.52; Diog. Laert. 9.59.

[44] Philo, *That the Worse Is Wont to Attack the Better* 48 (trans. F. H. Colson and G. H. Whitaker): τινὰς τῶν σοφῶν.

[45] Plut. *Mor. Lives of the Ten Orators: Antiphon* 849B–D. [46] [Plut.] *Cons. Ad Apoll.* 22.

[47] Sen. *Controv.* 10.2 (trans. M. Winterbottom): *Huic lingua velox, oculi acuti: extirpentur radicitus.*

[48] Petron. *Sat.* 67.

protested his innocence, had him removed from the arena, had his tongue cut out, and then had him put back in.[49] This attempt to prevent the enslaved speaking inconvenient truths was not just done pre-emptively; Plautus presents the character Euclio vowing to cut off the tongue and tear out the eyes of an enslaved attendant who has revealed that he possesses a pot of gold.[50]

Barbarians of various types are frequently described as mutilating their enemies. The Germans cut out eyes and, on one memorable occasion, 'they sewed up the mouth of one of them after first cutting out his tongue, which one of the barbarians held in his hand, exclaiming, "At last, you viper, you have ceased to hiss"'.[51] According to Athenaeus, the Scythians cut off the noses of everyone whose territory they invaded, leading to these people afterwards being known collectively as the Rhincolauretai or 'Dock-noses'.[52] This does not seem to have been an isolated event; according to Strabo, the Aethiopians invaded Egypt to settle a dispute and cut off the noses of those that they perceived to be in the wrong. They then settled them all at a place called Rhinocolura, 'Docked-nose-ville', 'assuming that on account of their disgraceful faces they would no longer dare do people wrong'.[53]

Individuals could be mutilated in order to prevent them from taking on a role that required bodily integrity. Josephus records that Antigonus either cut off or bit off Hyrcanus' ears so that he would not be able to be king or high priest.[54]

Finally, as we have seen, Caesar ordered his soldiers to aim for their opponents' faces in combat, but in one-to-one altercations the face was a favourite target too. The gouging out of an individual's eye(s) features prominently in ancient literature.[55] It was a common threat made to the enslaved by their enslavers and is recorded as actually occurring on occasion; the emperor Hadrian stabbed an enslaved attendant in the eye with a stylus in a fit of rage.[56]

49 Mart. 2.82; Suet. *Calig.* 27.

50 Plaut. *Aul.* 188–9; this threat is repeated at 250.

51 Flor. 2.30 (trans. E. S. Forster): *uni os obsutunr, recisa prius lingua, quam in manu tenens barbarus 'tandem' ait 'vipera sibilare desisti'.* See also Tac. *Hist.* 3.84 for a German cutting off the ear of a tribune.

52 Ath. 12.524d; see also Strabo, *Geog.* 12.759.

53 Strabo, *Geog.* 16.31 (trans. H. L. Jones): ὡς οὐκ ἂν ἔτι τολμήσοντας κακουργεῖν διὰ τὴν αἰσχύνην τῆς ὄψεως.

54 Cut off: Joseph. *AJ* 14.10; bit off: Joseph. *BJ* 1.9; a rabbinic parallel, on the mutilation of a Sadducean high priest by biting his ear, is found in the Tosephta, *Parah* 3.8.

55 See Nutting, 1922 on *oculus effodere.*

56 For threats, see Plaut. *Aul.* 53, *Trin.* 463–5, *Pers.* 797. For Hadrian, see Galen 5.17–18 K.

Prosthetic Eyes

The loss of one or even both eyes is commonly attested in ancient Greek and Roman literary and documentary evidence. Despite the expertise of ancient Greek and Roman physicians in relation to some aspects of eye surgery – such as cataract couching, for example – the loss of an eye could not be treated medically or surgically. So how did people who were impaired in this way deal with their situation? There is some evidence that they appealed to the gods for assistance, but despite the claims of one of the supplicants at Epidauros that Asklepios poured a drug into his eye socket and his eye grew back and his sight was restored, it is unlikely that they were any more helpful than the physicians.[57] There is also some evidence that, like Thelyphron in Apuleius' *Metamorphosis* (discussed earlier), they resorted to attempting to disguise or at least to cover their missing eye with an eyepatch; Cleisophus, a flatterer of Philip II of Macedon, covered his eye with a bandage in imitation of the king, Plautus depicts a sailor and a soldier (or, at least, a man posing as a soldier) doing so, and an object that has been tentatively identified as a leather eyepatch has been recovered through archaeological excavation at the Roman fort of Vindolanda on Hadrian's Wall.[58] These would serve not only as a means of covering what could potentially be a gruesome injury, but also provide a degree of protection to the sensitive empty socket.

But what of ocular prostheses or artificial eyes? Ocular prostheses have a longer history than one might think – examples have been recovered during archaeological excavations of prehistoric sites in Spain and Iran – but is there any evidence to suggest that they were utilised in classical antiquity?[59] There are three roughly contemporaneous literary references (albeit from very different contexts) that could be seen to reference artificial eyes in the Roman imperial period. The first is one of Martial's epigrams, in which he excoriates a woman named Laelia: 'You use bought teeth and hair and are not ashamed of it. What will you do with your eye, Laelia? That's not to be bought.'[60] We

[57] *IG*² I, 121–122.9.

[58] Ath. 6.248f (Satyrus, *Life of Philip* fr. 3, *FHG* 3.161, fr. 24); Plaut. *Mil.* 1430; Plaut. *Cur.* 392–400; Birley, 1992. According to Vindolanda curator Barbara Birley, the leather object from Vindolanda has also been identified as a leather pouch for lead sling bullets.

[59] Spain: see Enoch, 2009 for an artificial eye made of ochre found with a man who died aged 40–45 dating to 7,000 years ago at Cingle del Mas Nou i Cava Fosca, Ares del Maestro, Castellón Province. Iran: see Enoch, 2007 and Moghadasi, 2014 for an artificial left eye made of bitumen, engraved to resemble a real human eye, with a pupil and with gold wires inset to resemble capillaries found with a woman who died aged 28–32 at Burnt City – it is worth noting that use of this caused an abscess in the socket.

[60] Mart. 12.25.

can read this either as a straightforward denial that ocular prostheses even existed in Ancient Rome (or, if they did, they were not known to Martial), unlike prosthetic hair and teeth, or we can perhaps be more flexible in our interpretation and consider Martial differentiating between prosthetic hair and teeth which, although artificial, restore a degree of functionality, and an ocular prosthesis, which cannot. The second reference is from one of Dio Chrysostom's discourses, and he makes the following point: 'About Pelops, too, the story ran that he had an ivory shoulder, as if there were any use in a man having a golden or ivory hand or eyes of diamond or malachite; but the kind of soul he had men did not notice.'[61] Once again, this is not so easy to interpret. Is it a straightforward statement that people were in the habit of utilising artificial eyes made of diamond or malachite, or is it hyperbole? The third reference is from Lucian's science fiction novel, *True Story*, in which he describes a race of beings called Arboreals who live on the moon: 'The eyes that they have are removable, and whenever they wish they take them out and put them away until they want to see: then they put them in and look. Many, on losing their own, borrow other people's to see with, and the rich folk keep a quantity stored up.'[62] While this is clearly make-believe (Lucian even has his narrator preface this account with the disclaimer 'I am reluctant to tell you what sort of eyes they have, for fear that you may think me lying on account of the incredibility of the story'), it does contain several points of interest for our purposes, points that were perhaps inspired by Lucian's observation of prosthesis-using contemporaries.[63] First, that prosthesis users might not wear their prostheses all the time, but choose to reserve them for particular occasions upon which they would be the most useful. Second, that people might lose their prostheses, something more likely to happen if the prostheses in question were small, such as eyes or teeth, and frequently being put on and taken off.[64] And third, that wealthy people might have more than one prosthesis.

[61] Dio Chrys. *Or.* 8.28 (trans. J. W. Cohoon): περὶ δὲ τοῦ Πέλοπος ἔλεγον ὅτι καὶ τὸν ὦμον ἐλεφάντινον ἔχοι, ὥσπερ τι ὄφελος ἀνθρώπου χρυσῆν χεῖρα ἢ ἐλεφαντίνην ἔχοντος ἢ ὀφθαλμοὺς ἀδάμαντος ἢ σμαράγδου· τὴν δὲ ψυχὴν οὐκ ἐγίγνωσκον αὐτοῦ ὁποίαν τινὰ εἶχεν.

[62] Luc. *Ver. hist.* 1.25 (trans. A. M. Harmon): τοὺς ὀφθαλμοὺς περιαιρετοὺς ἔχουσι, καὶ ὁ βουλόμενος ἐξελὼν τοὺς αὑτοῦ φυλάττει ἔστ᾽ ἂν δεηθῇ ἰδεῖν· οὕτω δὲ ἐνθέμενος ὁρᾷ· καὶ πολλοὶ τοὺς σφετέρους ἀπολέσαντες παρ᾽ ἄλλων χρησάμενοι ὁρῶσιν. εἰσὶ δ᾽ οἳ καὶ πολλοὺς ἀποθέτους ἔχουσιν, οἱ πλούσιοι. This was perhaps inspired by the Graiai of Greek mythology, two or three sea hags who shared a single detachable eye and tooth between themselves.

[63] Luc. *Ver. hist.* 1.25 (trans. A. M. Harmon): περὶ μέντοι τῶν ὀφθαλμῶν, οἵους ἔχουσιν, ὀκνῶ μὲν εἰπεῖν, μή τίς με νομίσῃ ψεύδεσθαι διὰ τὸ ἄπιστον τοῦ λόγου.

[64] See, for example, Palestinian Talmud, Shabbat 6.5 that discusses a woman being tempted to replace her gold tooth if it falls out of her mouth on the Sabbath due to its value, and not so tempted to replace her wooden tooth, as that is more easily replaced. For discussion of this, see Cohen and Stern, 1973, p. 103.

One further potential reference to them found in an epitaph is ambiguous. Is the *faber ocularius* attested in this epitaph a maker of prosthetic eyes for humans or a maker of artificial eyes for statues?[65] Or is it somewhere between the two: a maker of artificial eyes for humans to be worn post-mortem, such as those produced and utilised during mummification in Egypt?

There is some additional evidence from the Palestinian Talmud, but that too is problematic:

> "[Mishnah:] 'And thus it happened with one who vowed not to benefit from his sister's daughter. She was taken into R. Yishmael's house and they made her beautiful.' R. Yishmael asked him: Did you take a vow regarding her? He answered: No! Thus he [R. Yishmael] annulled the man's vow. In the same hour, R. Yishmael started weeping [...]. [Talmud/Gemara] Thus, he made her an [artificial] eye of gold and a tooth of gold and said to him [the man] as follows: 'benefit from what is upon her!'[66]

There are other versions of this teaching, but these simply refer to the gold tooth.[67]

While based on this evidence alone it cannot be stated definitively that ocular prostheses were known to the Romans and utilised by them, it is worth focusing on one aspect of these references and exploring it further. When Dio Chrysostom refers to prosthetic eyes, he makes a point of including two examples of materials used to make them: diamond and malachite. Why diamond and malachite, of all the precious and semi-precious stones known and utilised in classical antiquity? Is it because of their expense and concurrent prestige? Or is it for another reason, such as the qualities that those two types of stone were thought to have? As far as diamonds are concerned, according to Nonnos, they were 'the gem made stone in the showers of Zeus which protects against the stony glare of Medusa, that the baleful light of that destroying face may do him no harm'.[68] As far as malachite is concerned, according to Aristotle, malachite mined on the Chalcedonian island Demonesus was utilised as a medicament for eye conditions.[69] According to Vitruvius, wall paintings

[65] *CIL* VI 9402 (also *Inscr. Grut.* 645): *Dis Manibus / L(ucio) Licinio L(uci) f(ilio) Statoiria/ no L(ucius) Licinius L(uci) l(ibertus) Patroclus / faber oculariarius / frat(ri) cariss(imo) f(ecit).*

[66] Palestinian Talmud/Yerushalmi Nedarim 9,8 (41c) (Venice edition/print): קונם שאיני נושא את פלנית כעורה כו עשה לה עין של זהב שן של זהב בלשון הזה אמר לו זכה במה שעליה וכשמת רבי ישמעאל כו' כתיב בנות ישראל על שאול בכינה וגו'.

[67] Tractate Nedarim 9; 41c.

[68] Nonnus, *Dion.* 47.587–93 (trans. W. H. D Rouse): Διὸς πετρούμενον ὄμβρῳ λᾶαν, ἀλεξητῆρα λιθογλήνοιο Μεδούσης, ὄφρα φύγῃ σέλας ἐχθρὸν ἀθηήτοιο προσώπου.

[69] Aristotle, *On Marvellous Things Heard* 58/834b.

containing malachite 'affect the vision of the eyes with brilliance'.[70] Pliny the Elder provides considerably more information about the relationship between malachite and vision:

> Their special asset is their colour, which is limpid without being at all faint. On the contrary, it combines body and clarity, and, wherever one peers through the stones, reproduces the transparency of sea-water, the stones being in an equal degree translucent and brilliant. In other words, they dissipate their colour and also allow the sight to penetrate within. There is a story that in this island there stood on the burial-mound of a prince named Hermias, not far from the tunny-fisheries, the marble statue of a lion, into which had been inserted eyes made of 'smaragdus'; and these, it is said, blazed so brightly, even far below the surface of the sea, that the tunnies fled in terror, and the fishermen were long puzzled by this strange behaviour until finally they changed the gemstones in the eye-sockets.[71]

It is notable that the colour of malachite was green, and green was considered particularly beneficial to eyes and eye health during the Roman imperial period.[72] Other green stones, such as *smaragdus* (emerald), were also linked with vision.[73] Both diamond and malachite are associated with vision in ancient literature, and perhaps, if ocular prostheses did exist and they were made from diamond and/or malachite, this was the reasoning behind the choice of those materials.

As we have seen, inserting eyes into statues was common enough practice for at least one person to (potentially) make it their entire profession. Consequently, it would be surprising indeed if ocular prostheses, or at least the concept of ocular prostheses, whether worn inserted into the eye socket or outside of it, were completely unknown or never even occurred to the Greeks and Romans. But perhaps we need to bear in mind a statement of Aristotle that 'when seeing is removed the eye is no longer an eye, except in name – it is no more a real eye than the eye of a statue or of a painted figure'.[74] An ocular prosthesis, no matter how fine, could not, after all, restore one's sight, and, as we have seen, those who pretended to be in

[70] Vitr. *De arch.* 7.5.8 (trans. F. Granger): *fulgentes oculorum reddunt visus.*

[71] Plin. *HN* 37.66–7 (trans. D. E. Eichholz): *dos eorum est in colore liquido nec diluto, verum ex umido pingui quaque perspicitur imitante tralucidum maris, pariterque ut traluceat et niteat, hoc est ut colorem expellat, aciem recipiat. ferunt in ea insula tumulo reguli Hermiae iuxta cetarias marmoreo leoni fuisse inditos oculos e smaragdis ita radiantibus etiam in gurgitem ut territi thynni refugerent, diu mirantibus novitatem piscatoribus, donec mutavere oculis gemmas.*

[72] Vitr. *De arch.* 5.9.5; Sen. *Ira* 5.9.2; Gal. *Subf. Emp.* 6.54; for discussion, see Trinquier, 2002, pp. 114–27. Collyrium stamps seem to have been usually made of steatite, shale, or serpentine; for discussion, see Baker, 2011.

[73] Meadows, 1945; Plantzos, 1997.

[74] Arist. *De an.* 2.1, 472 B.

possession of body parts, such as hair and teeth, that they were not for reasons of vanity were the target of considerable criticism.

The extent to which any sort of aid to vision was utilised in antiquity is much debated.[75] Glass and rock crystal lenses and lens-like objects have been recovered during numerous archaeological excavations of sites dating back to the Bronze Age, and such objects were capable of magnification (tests have been done on them that prove this), but whether people actually utilised them for that specific purpose, as opposed to simply redirecting or reflecting light, is contentious. We should also consider the potential overlap between glass and rock crystal used for utilitarian reasons, such as heat, light, magnification, and for decorative purposes, such as furniture, jewellery, etc. Seneca the Younger discusses several means of magnification.[76] It would appear that the use of aids to augment and improve vision ranged from the rudimentary to the scientifically and technologically advanced – water, mirrors, glass, lenses. Some lens-like objects have been found in contexts that suggest they were being used with light reflection or magnification in mind, such as workshops in Tanis in Egypt and Pompeii in Italy.

Who was responsible for making such items? Perhaps glassworkers (considerable advancements were made in these technologies during the Roman imperial period, such as the invention of glassblowing) or lapidaries (considerable advancements were made in these technologies during the Hellenistic period), both of whom would have been well aware of the properties and capabilities of the materials they utilised on a daily basis. It has been suggested that craftsmen who manufactured articles requiring fine details, such as carving, engraving, and inscribing, utilised magnifying lenses in the service of their craft, and that producing such work without the aid of a magnifying lens would have been impossible.[77]

Perhaps we should consider an ocular prosthesis in a different light: since it could not restore vision and, if it were made from a substance such as diamond or malachite, was deliberately not life-like and so entirely obvious, intended to be noticed, should we consider a Roman ocular prosthesis as cosmetic and ornamental, an extreme form of conspicuous consumption, much like the Capua Limb? And perhaps we should also consider ancient ideas about the sense of sight. The ancient schools of thought about optics emphasise the tactile nature of sight, its ability to touch and even penetrate – vision involves a form of contact between the

[75] Sines and Sakellerakis, 1987; Enoch, 1996, 1998; Plantzos, 1997.
[76] Sen. *QNat.* 1.3.9 and 1.6.5–6. [77] Sines and Sakellarakis, 1987.

organ of sight and its object; depending upon the theory of vision, the eye is either an active or passive participant in the process of seeing.[78] The eye could project or deflect light, fire, even envy. But what if one's sense of sight was impaired in some way? To look upon something was to interact with it – if you could not see, you could not interact.[79] The loss of sight, the most severe and permanent form of which was the loss of an eye, was not just an impairment but a disability too, as it cut you off from appropriate social behaviour and custom. As a result, someone who could not see was at a considerable societal disadvantage, perhaps even fatally weakened and vulnerable.[80] This required treatment or at least mitigation, so perhaps this is the reason why when Dio Chrysostom described ocular prostheses, he specifically mentioned diamond and malachite, both materials particularly associated with the sense of sight.

The ancient evidence for ocular prostheses is sparse, but that which there is suggests that if they did exist, there was a certain amount of rationale behind their design, commission, and manufacture. An ocular prosthesis could not restore vision the way that a prosthetic toe, foot, or leg could restore mobility, but it could serve other purposes relating to the ancient understanding not only of the workings of the sense of sight, but also the maintenance of eye health, and, ultimately protection.

Prosthetic Noses

While, as we have seen, there is a considerable amount of literary and archaeological evidence for the use of prosthetic hair and teeth, and even some literary evidence for the use of prosthetic eyes in classical antiquity, the evidence for prosthetic noses is very slight indeed.

The Byzantine emperor Justinian II reigned from 668 to 695 CE before being overthrown. To prevent him from seeking to retake the throne, he was subjected to deliberate facial mutilation – common practice in the seventh century CE – and his nose was cut off.[81] Physical imperfection barred an imperial candidate from ascending to the throne, and this type of physical imperfection would have been highly visible and difficult to disguise.[82] However, he succeeded in retaking the throne in 705 CE, and reigned before being overthrown a second time and executed in 711 CE. According to

[78] Bartsch, 2006, p. 59. [79] Squire, 2016, p. 25.

[80] See Fredrick, 2002, p. 4; Barton, 2002, p. 219 on the perceived power of vision.

[81] Theophanes the Confessor, *Chronicle* 6187.

[82] See Leviticus 21.18 for the prohibition against imperfect men serving as priests; Skinner, 2014 suggests the removal of the nose could have been symbolic of castration and emasculation.

Agnellus, Justinian was able to bypass the usual ostracism that resulted from facial disfigurement by wearing a prosthetic nose made of gold.[83] Assuming that this uncorroborated story is true, the choice of gold was likely significant; not only was it the most precious of metals, it was also imperishable.[84] However, Christian Laes doubts its veracity and has suggested that it might have been inspired by an Hadith story about 'Arafajah, one of the followers of the Prophet Mohammed who, when his nose was cut off, used a prosthetic nose made of silver until the silver oxidised, leading to the Prophet ordering 'Arfajah bin As'ad to use a prosthetic nose made of gold instead.[85] Whatever the truth of Justinian's impairment, it is, however, notable that none of the coins from his second reign depict him as disfigured, although he was subsequently known as Justinian Rhinotmetos ('Slit-nosed'). There is also some scholarly debate over the likelihood that he subsequently underwent some sort of reconstructive surgery.[86] While other Byzantine emperors of the seventh century CE were subjected to facial mutilation, only Justinian II succeeded in regaining his throne and ruling despite having been mutilated and impaired in this way.

How might such a prosthetic have been worn? A mummy, unfortunately unprovenanced but thought to date from the Roman period in Egypt and currently housed in the Ungarischen Nationalmuseum in Budapest, has a truncated nose and this disfigurement is covered by a wooden prosthetic nose fixed to their face with straps.[87] The prosthesis was attached to the face after the deceased had undergone the mummification process, so this may simply have been a post-mortem body modification, or it may have been a prosthesis that the deceased wore in life and had restored to them after the mummification process was complete in preparation for their afterlife. Certainly, an ancient prosthetic nose would not have fixed itself to its user's face; some type of harness would have been necessary to ensure that it was securely fastened and not liable to fall off at an inopportune moment, thus mortifying its user.

[83] Agnellus of Ravenna, *Agnelli Liber Pontificalis Ecclesiae Ravennatis* c.137, MGH SSRLI 367 (trans. O. Holder-Egger): *et potitus imperio, nares sibi et aures ex obrizo fecit.*

[84] Skinner, 2014.

[85] Laes, 2019, p. 14. On 'Arfajah bin As'ad, see Ghaly, 2010, pp. 128–9. However, there is also the case of the Byzantine general Tatikios and his gold prosthetic nose, recorded by Guibert of Nogent in his account of the First Crusade, *Deeds of God through the Franks.*

[86] See Delbrueck, 1914 for the proposed identification of the 'Carmagnola' porphyry head as Justinian II, with the suggestion that he underwent a rhinoplasty undertaken by an Indian surgeon; see Heiburg, 1914 for refutation of this; see Remensnyder et al., 1979 for detailed discussion of ancient rhinoplasty; see Breckenridge, 1981 for a more recent summary of the debate.

[87] Merei and Nemeskeri, 1958; Selinger, 2012, p. 28.

Prosthetic Teeth

There is literary, documentary, archaeological, and bioarchaeological evidence for prosthetic teeth and other types of dental appliances in classical antiquity; after prosthetic hair, prosthetic teeth are the most frequently attested type of prosthesis in the classical era.

Despite claims that ancient Egypt was the source of dentistry, it is Etruria and the Etruscan civilisation that seems to have been responsible for the innovation of dental appliances and prosthetic teeth. A total of twenty-one Etruscan dental appliances, spanning a period of 400 years, from the mid-seventh century BCE to the fourth or third century BCE, are known.[88] Fourteen of these have been recovered from sites in Etruria proper, including Tarquinia, Orvieto/Bolsena, Chiusi, and Populonia, with others recovered from nearby territories, including Latium, Campania, and the *Ager faliscus*, and as far afield as Eretria in Greece and Sardis in Turkey. Etruscan dental appliances are distinctive in that they are all constructed from bands of gold and resemble the contemporary dental appliance known as a pontic or bridge. The precise configuration of the gold bands varies from device to device: thirteen take the form of bands wrapped around one or more teeth, eight take the form of bands made into individual rings attached in a linear series, and some include replacement teeth (human, animal, or gold).[89] Since Etruscan jewellery is frequently made from gold wire, it would appear that the choice of gold bands for the dental appliances was a deliberate choice; the gold bands are much wider and would have been much more visible.[90] They were entirely cosmetic in purpose; the pure gold utilised, much purer than that used in Etruscan jewellery, would never have tarnished.[91] They seem to have been worn by women only and positioned in the maxillary dentition, where teeth had either been lost or were deliberately removed – a process known as dental evulsion – to accommodate them.[92] In view of the small number of dental appliances that have been discovered to date, despite the excavation of numerous Etruscan cemeteries, Jean Mackintosh Turfa has raised the possibility that these appliances were not necessarily worn by Etruscan women but by non-Etruscan women who, having previously undergone dental evulsion, married into Etruscan families and then sought a remedy for what could have been viewed in Etruscan society as a type of facial disfigurement.[93]

88 For a catalogue, see Becker and Turfa, 2017; see also Turfa and Becker, 2019, pp. 94–8.
89 Becker and Turfa, 2017, p. 84. See, for example, Science Museum inv. A622194; Science Museum inv. A622195.
90 Becker and Turfa, 2017, p. 99.
91 Becker and Turfa, 2017, p. 101.
92 See Capasso, 1986, p. 55, for the initial suggestion, made without any supporting evidence.
93 Becker and Turfa, 2017, pp. 134–7.

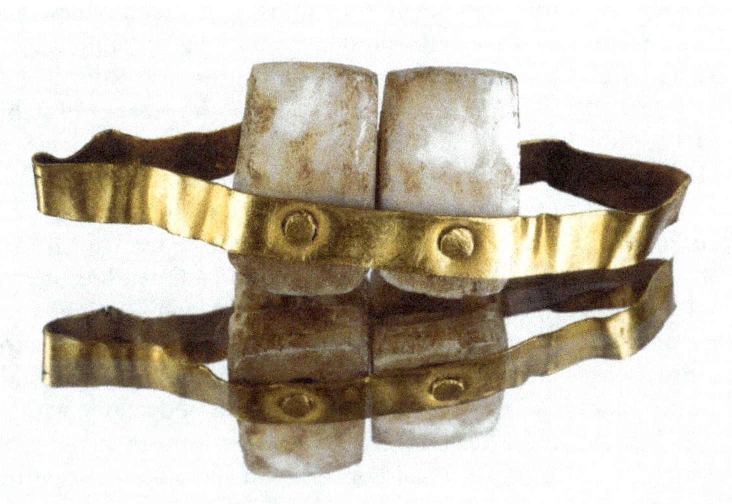

Figure 2.5 Etruscan dental appliance. Science Museum inv. A622194. Image courtesy of the Science Museum, London.

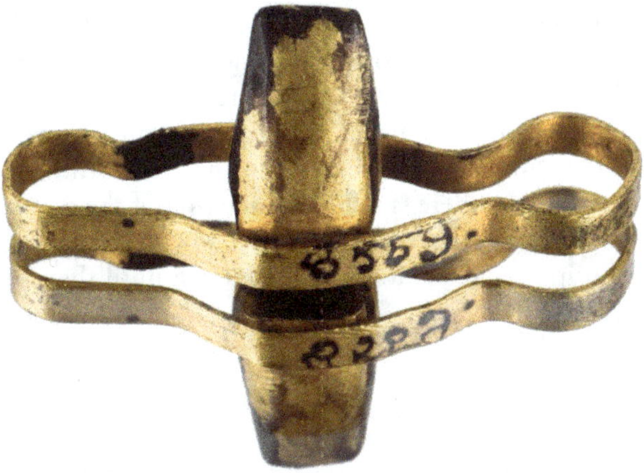

Figure 2.6 Etruscan dental appliance. Science Museum inv. A622195. Image courtesy of the Science Museum, London.

While the Etruscan phenomenon of utilising dental appliances and prosthetic teeth may have influenced neighbouring communities, the literary and archaeological evidence for Hellenistic and Roman dental appliances attests very different interpretations of the practice of stabilising loose teeth or replacing missing ones and considerable variety across the Mediterranean in the period from the fourth century BCE to the second century CE.[94] The earliest evidence is documentary, from extracts from the fifth century BCE Roman law codes known as the *Twelve Tables* that are likely older than this and compilations of earlier texts, although it is preserved in the writings of Marcus Tullius Cicero dating from the mid-first century BCE.[95] These laws, intended as a form of sumptuary legislation, state 'If a man's teeth are joined with gold, it shall be no violation of the law to bury or burn his body along with that gold.'[96] There is, however, no indication of what form this gold took – for example, whether it was a band or a wire or something else entirely. Medical treatises that mention gold as a means of treating loose teeth are equally uninformative. The Hippocratic treatise *On Joints*, dating to the mid-fifth century BCE, instructs 'If the teeth at the point of injury are displaced or loosened, when the bone is adjusted fasten them to one another, not merely the two, but several, preferably with gold, but failing that, with thread, till consolidation takes place.'[97] Similar instructions are found in Celsus' *On Medicine*, dating to the early first century CE: 'But if teeth become loosened by a blow, or any other accident, they are to be tied by gold to firmly fixed teeth, and repressants must be held in the mouth, such as wine in which some pomegranate rind has been cooked, or into which burning oak galls have been thrown.'[98] In both cases the context is medical, but there is also consideration of the cosmetic implications of missing teeth. These methods are, however, clearly temporary, designed to position and stabilise the loose teeth until they are loose no longer.

94 On teeth in ancient Greece and Rome, see Cootjans and Gourevitch, 1983.

95 *Laws of the Twelve Tables* 10.8–9, preserved in Cic. *Leg.* 2.24.60.

96 Cic. *Leg.* 2.24.60 (trans. C. W. Keyes): *At cui auro dentes iuncti escunt, ast im cum illo sepeliet uretve, se fraude esto.*

97 Hippoc. *Art.* 33.9–10 (trans. E. T. Withington, with minor adjustments): καὶ ἢν μὲν διεστραμμένοι ἔωσιν οἱ ὀδόντες οἱ κατὰ τὸ τρῶμα καὶ κεκινημένοι, ὁπόταν τὸ ὀστέον κατορθωθῇ, ζεῦξαι τοὺς ὀδόντας χρὴ πρὸς ἀλλήλους, μὴ μοῦνον τοὺς δύο, ἀλλὰ καὶ πλέονας,2 μάλιστα μὲν δὴ χρυσίῳ, ἔστ᾽ ἂν κρατυνθῇ τὸ ὀστέον, εἰ δὲ μή, λίνῳ.

98 Celsus, *Med.* 6.12 (trans. W. G. Spencer, with minor adjustments): *At si ex ictu vel alio casu aliquid labant dentes, auro cum iis, qui bene haerent, vinciendi sunt; continendaque ore reprimentia, ut vinum, in quo malicorium decoctum, aut in quo galla candens coniecta sit.*

Comedic writings such as satires and epigrams are more informative about prosthetic teeth and the individuals who apparently wore them.[99] The earliest such reference is found in one of Horace's satires, dating to between 35 and 30 BCE. He describes two elderly witches, Canidia and Sagana, visiting the Gardens of Maecenas on the Esquiline Hill for the purpose of digging up some of the pauper's corpses buried on the site in its previous life as a pauper's graveyard, and their encounter with a statue of the god Priapus.[100] The climax of the satire is Priapus farting and scaring the witches away, 'then amid great laughter and mirth you might see Canidia's teeth and Sagana's high wig come tumbling down, and from their arms the herbs and enchanted love-knots'.[101] Note that Horace uses the Latin word *dentes* here, clearly differentiating false teeth from any other sort of dental appliance such as a band or a wire. For the scene to be funny, the Roman audience had to have been familiar with prosthetic teeth, and not just the gold bands favoured by the Etruscans or the gold thread utilised by physicians for treating loose teeth. However, it also highlights one of the potential problems with utilising false teeth and that is the ever-present danger that they might fall out, always embarrassing but potentially more embarrassing in certain contexts such as dining. Lucillius, a writer of epigrams during the reign of the emperor Nero in the mid-first century CE (54–68 CE), offers an insight into the way that prosthetic teeth were viewed by the Romans when he refers to them in conjunction with prosthetic hair and cosmetics: 'You bought hair, rouge, honey, wax, and teeth. For the same outlay you might have bought a face.'[102]

Martial, likely influenced by Lucillius, and writing during the reign of the emperor Domitian in the late first century CE (81–96 CE), takes a similar approach in a number of his epigrams. In one early epigram, he links prosthetics and cosmetics, and he refers to several users of them by name:

> Fidentinus, do you take yourself for a poet on the strength of my verses and want it believed? Just so Aegle thinks she has teeth in virtue of purchased bones and Indian horn. Just so Lycoris, who is blacker than a falling

[99] Since the original purpose of the epigram was to commemorate remarkable individuals or events, it is rather fitting that much of the literary evidence for ancient prostheses comes in this form; see Taub, 2017, p. 30, for discussion.

[100] On Canidia, see Paule, 2017.

[101] Hor. *Sat.* 1.8.47–50 (trans. H. R. Fairclough): *Canidiae dentes, altum Saganae caliendrum excidere atque herbas atque incantata lacertis vincula cum magno risuque iocoque videres.*

[102] Lucillius, *Greek Anthology* 11.408 (trans. W. R. Paton): Ἠγόρασας πλοκάμους, φῦκος, μέλι, κηρόν, ὀδόντας· τῆς αὐτῆς δαπάνης ὄψιν ἂν ἠγόρασας.

> mulberry, fancies herself in white lead. You too by the reasoning that makes you a poet will have a head of hair when you are bald.[103]

This description of Aegle's prosthetic teeth as being made from bones and horn (that is, ivory) again makes it clear that this is a different sort of appliance from the Etruscan gold band, something akin to contemporary dentures, and this is also the case in another epigram where he contrasts the genuine black teeth of Thais with the false white teeth of Laecania.[104] His other references to prosthetic teeth are less informative about the appliances themselves, but do continue the practice of linking them with prosthetic hair and cosmetics. Thus, he describes Galla as using not only prosthetic teeth but also prosthetic hair and a prosthetic eyebrow, but also implies that she uses a considerable amount of cosmetics on her face as well, and Laelia as using prosthetic teeth and hair.[105]

Finally, Lucian, writing in the late second century CE, refers to a dental appliance akin to those described by Hippocrates and Celsus, and comprising some manner of gold for positioning and stabilising loose teeth. This one, however, is found in the mouth of a wealthy elderly woman rather than someone who has undergone some sort of trauma: 'I went to live with an old woman and for a time got my victuals from her by pretending to love a hag of seventy with only four teeth still left, and those four fastened in with gold!'[106]

There are several references to prosthetic teeth in the Talmud.[107] Rabbis agree that prosthetic teeth are permissible, whether they are made from gold, silver, or some other substance, perhaps ivory or wood.[108] Unlike the Roman authors, they view prosthetic teeth in a positive manner, believing them to increase the beauty of the woman wearing them.[109] However, they also come up in discussions regarding what people are permitted to do on the Sabbath, and whether women are permitted to go out wearing prosthetic teeth on the Sabbath, because if the prosthetic teeth fall out of their

103 Mart. 1.72 (trans. D. R. Shackleton Bailey): *Nostris versibus esse te poetam, Fidentine, putas cupisque credi? sic dentata sibi videtur Aegle emptis ossibus Indicoque cornu; sic, quae nigrior est cadente moro, cerussata sibi placet Lycoris. hac et tu ratione qua poeta es, calvus cum fueris, eris comatus.*

104 Mart. 5.43.

105 Galla: Mart. 9.38; Galla is also mentioned in many of Martial's other epigrams, see 2.34, 3.51, 3.54, 3.90, 4.38, 4.58, 5.84, 7.18, 7.58, 9.4, 9.78, 10.25, 11.19. Laelia: Mart. 12.23.

106 Luc. *Rhet.* 24 (trans. A. M. Harmon): ἔπειτα δὲ γραΐ συνοικήσας τὸ πρῶτον μὲν ἐγαστριζόμην πρὸς αὐτῆς ἐρᾶν προσποιούμενος γυναικὸς ἑβδομηκοντούτιδος τέτταρας ἔτι λοιποὺς ὀδόντας ἐχούσης, χρυσίῳ καὶ τούτους ἐνδεδεμένους.

107 For discussion, see Cohen and Stern, 1973.

108 Babylonian Talmud, Shabbat 65a.

109 Palestinian Talmud/Yerushalmi Nedarim 9.8 (41c); Babylonian Talmud Nedarim 66a–b.

mouths they may be tempted to put them back in, and this action would constitute labour.[110]

Archaeological evidence supports the descriptions of dental appliances found in at least some of these literary sources. Six gold or silver wire dental appliances have been recovered from sites across the eastern Mediterranean and the Levant, and a seventh has been recovered from Rome; these have been dated from the fourth or third centuries BCE to the first or second centuries CE. The last of these is particularly interesting as it corresponds to Lucian's contemporaneous description in that it was found in the mouth of a skeleton of a woman aged around fifty years old who was cremated and interred in a tomb in the Collatina necropolis and comprises a single gold wire wrapped around five teeth.[111] However, it also seems to have a space for two false teeth that replaced the central incisors. Unfortunately, only the right of these has survived, but it seems to have been the woman's own tooth, repurposed as its own replacement.[112] Four bronze 'crown-like prosthetic artefacts' thought to date from the second to fourth century CE and apparently found in the Judean mountains were acquired in an antiquity market in Jerusalem, and it has been suggested, based on the references to prosthetic teeth in the Talmud, that these were worn by women to cover their missing or damaged pre-molars.[113] Due to their shape, it is unlikely that these objects were functional; rather, it has been suggested that they were cosmetic and designed to look like jewellery, specifically a type of bead that was in widespread use during the Roman period.[114]

Conclusion

While the loss of facial features in classical antiquity seems to have been fairly common, facial prosthesis use, at least in respect of prosthetic eyes and noses, was clearly not. There are several possible explanations for this. First, if the loss of a facial feature is common, then, as with the loss of a limb or part of a limb, coping strategies are clear and the pressure to 'pass' is less. Literary, documentary, and bioarchaeological evidence tells us that the loss of one or both eyes, or simply just the loss of sight in one or both eyes, and the loss of teeth were very common, so individuals who experienced this were not unusual in classical antiquity, and since the members of their

[110] Palestinian Talmud, Shabbat 6.5.

[111] On this find, see Minozzi et al., 2007. It is discussed in greater detail in Becker and Turfa, 2017, pp. 283–99.

[112] Minozzi et al., 2007. [113] Rosenfeld et al., 2000, p. 641. [114] Rosenfeld et al., 2000, p. 643.

communities would have been well aware of their impairments, attempts to 'pass' would have been generally pointless. Added to this, facial prostheses such as prosthetic eyes and noses would have been somewhat problematic to use and could not necessarily be relied upon to stay attached to the individual's body. Perhaps wearing a patch of some sort that could be tied tightly around one's face and be relied upon to stay where it was put until it was removed was preferable to the alternative of one's false eye or nose falling off at an inopportune moment.[115] There is also the question of hygiene, particularly in relation to the use of a prosthetic eye or tooth that had to be physically inserted into and removed from the body.

One exception to this general rule, however, seems to be prosthetic teeth and other types of dental appliance. These do appear to have been relatively common, first among the Etruscans in the form of gold bands, and then among Roman and Jewish communities during the imperial period in the form of dentures. They also appear to have been replete with social and cultural significances relating to prestige, wealth, status, gender, and sexuality.

One additional point worth considering is that the facial prostheses that have survived from classical antiquity, like the extremity prostheses that have survived, have done so because they were included in the burials of their users, even if the vast majority of the examples that are contained in modern museum collections have now been separated from their users' bodies and little or no information survives about them and has to be tentatively reconstructed through examination by forensic dentists. In all cases, they seem to have been attached to their users' bodies in death as they would have been during life, rather than simply included alongside the individual as a grave good, even if they were not treated as such by excavators and collectors. Interring them in this manner supports the literary evidence and indicates that they were not forbidden by the sumptuary laws, unlike other luxury goods, so we can infer from this that they were seen as something beyond just jewellery, although they did in fact have a lot in common with jewellery and may have even been inspired by and designed to complement it.

This can perhaps reinforce the insight into the way that prostheses were viewed by their users, and, in turn, the way that prostheses and prosthesis users were viewed by their peers, that we have already been given by extremity prostheses. Like an extremity prosthesis, since an ancient facial

[115] There are literary references to people wearing adhesive patches (*splenia*) to cover up small facial disfigurements; see Mart. 2.29.9–10, 8.33.22; Plin. *Ep.* 6.2.2.

prosthesis was designed, commissioned, and manufactured specifically for an individual in order to meet their unique set of needs, it is highly unlikely that one could simply have been reused, such as, for example, an artisan's tools would have been, although one could potentially have been repurposed, particularly the more valuable materials such as metal, which could have been melted down and reused. So, the fact that this does not seem to have occurred, at least in the cases for which we have evidence, is certainly significant. It would appear that facial prostheses, like extremity prostheses, were viewed, both by their users and by others, as a true substitute for or replacement of the individual's missing body part.

CHAPTER 3

Hair Prostheses

Introduction

Ancient medical practitioners divided cosmetics into those which preserved beauty (*kosmetikon*) and those which unnaturally embellished it (*kommotikon*).[1] The former were considered acceptable, but the latter were not.[2] From the fifth century BCE onwards, treatises from a wide range of literary genres contain recipes for both types of cosmetics, yet, simultaneously, there is a long tradition of male Greek and Roman authors that excoriate women (and sometimes men) for seeking to augment and amplify their natural beauty with artificial substances.[3] Perhaps the most famous example of Classical Greek attitudes towards women using cosmetics can be found in Xenophon's *Estate Management*, where the character of Ischomachus chastises his wife for utilising them:

> I noticed that her face was made up: she had rubbed in a lot of white lead in order to look even whiter than she is, and alkanet juice to make her cheeks rosier than they truly were; and she was wearing boots with thick soles to appear taller than she naturally was. So I said to her, 'Tell me, wife, how should I appear more worthy of your love as a partner in our goods, by disclosing to you our belongings just as they are, without boasting of imaginary possessions or concealing any part of what we have, or by trying to trick you with an exaggerated account, showing you counterfeit money and wooden necklaces painted gold and describing clothes dyed purple that would fade? . . . Please assume, wife, that I do not prefer white paint and alkanet dye to your real colour; but just as the gods have made horses delight in horses, cattle in cattle, sheep in sheep, so human beings find the human body undisguised most delightful'.[4]

[1] Gal. *Comp. Loc.* 1.2. [2] Olson, 2009, p. 294.

[3] The Roman idea (and ideal) of female natural beauty is expressed most frequently in elegiac poetry; see, for example, Lilja, 1965, pp. 119–32; Richlin, 1992, pp. 44–6; Wyke, 2002, pp. 152–3; Olson, 2009, 2012, pp. 58–9.

[4] Xen. *Oec.* 10.2–3, 7 (trans. E. C. Marchant and O. J. Todd): "Ἐγὼ τοίνυν, ἔφη, ἰδών ποτε αὐτήν, ὦ Σώκρατες, ἐντετριμμένην πολλῷ μὲν ψιμυθίῳ, ὅπως λευκοτέρα ἔτι δοκοίη εἶναι ἢ ἦν, πολλῇ δ'

Yet, there is a considerable amount of archaeological evidence to suggest that in their daily lives women utilised cosmetics anyway, such as the *pyxides* shown in Figure 3.1, containing tablets made from white lead and alkanet, recovered from a fifth century BCE burial in the Kerameikos cemetery in Athens.[5] It is notable that Xenophon has Ischomachus include not just the white lead face powder and alkanet rouge that Ischomachus' wife uses to colour her face, but also the high-heeled shoes that she wears to increase her height; she is utilising artificial aids to augment not just her

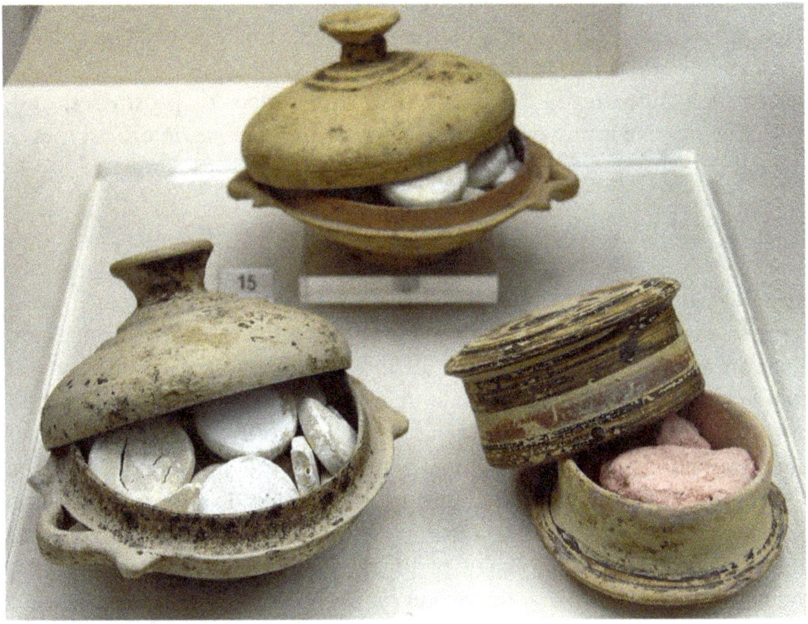

Figure 3.1 Corinthian *pyxides*, circa fifth century BCE. Kerameikos Archaeological Museum inv. 15598, 15539, and 15537. Image courtesy of Wikimedia Commons.

ἐγχούσῃ, ὅπως ἐρυθροτέρα φαίνοιτο τῆς ἀληθείας, ὑποδήματα δ' ἔχουσαν ὑψηλά, ὅπως μείζων δοκοίη εἶναι ἢ ἐπεφύκει, Εἰπέ μοι, ἔφην, ὦ γύναι, ποτέρως ἄν με κρίναις ἀξιοφίλητον μᾶλλον εἶναι χρημάτων κοινωνόν, εἴ σοι αὐτὰ τὰ ὄντα ἀποδεικνύοιμι καὶ μήτε κομπάζοιμι, ὡς πλείω ἔστι μοι τῶν ὄντων, μήτε ἀποκρυπτοίμην τι τῶν ὄντων μηδέν, ἢ εἰ πειρῴμην σε ἐξαπατᾶν λέγων τε, ὡς πλείω ἔστι μοι τῶν ὄντων, ἐπιδεικνύς τε ἀργύριον κίβδηλον καὶ ὅρμους ὑποξύλους καὶ πορφυρίδας ἐξιτήλους φαίην ἀληθινὰς εἶναι; . . . Καὶ ἐμὲ τοίνυν νόμιζε, εἰπεῖν ἔφη ὁ Ἰσχόμαχος, ὦ γύναι, μήτε ψιμυθίου μήτε ἐγχούσης χρώματι ἥδεσθαι μᾶλλον ἢ τῷ σῷ, ἀλλ' ὥσπερ οἱ θεοὶ ἐποίησαν ἵπποις μὲν ἵππους, βουσὶ δὲ βοῦς ἥδιστον, προβάτοις δὲ πρόβατα, οὕτω καὶ οἱ ἄνθρωποι ἀνθρώπου σῶμα καθαρὸν οἴονται ἥδιστον εἶναι"'. On Ischomachus' wife's use of cosmetics and its significance, see Glazebrook, 2009.

[5] Kerameikos Archaeological Museum inv. 15598, 15539, and 15537.

face but also her physique – so-called 'technologies of the body'. Likewise attested in the literary, documentary, and archaeological records as means of augmenting the body are 'false' teeth, as we saw in the previous chapter, and also 'false' or 'purchased' hair, in the form of both wigs and hair pieces or extensions.[6] In this chapter, I will examine the literary, documentary, archaeological, and bioarchaeological evidence for the use of prosthetic hair in classical antiquity.[7] It may come as a surprise but prosthetic hair is the most well-attested type of prosthesis utilised in classical antiquity, and consequently may have also been the most commonly utilised one. After all, one does not necessarily have to have experienced the traumatic loss of a body part to wear a wig or a hairpiece the way that one does in order to wear an extremity or facial prosthesis, wigs and hairpieces seem to have been much more readily available than other types of prostheses, and, consequently, we know much more about them than we do other types of ancient prosthesis.

Hair Loss in Classical Antiquity

Although an ancient individual did not need to lose all their hair to wear a wig or a hairpiece, this does seem to have been the most common reason given in ancient literary evidence for individuals doing so. This hair loss could occur in any number of ways in classical antiquity, both natural and unnaturally, and of the numerous ways in which hair could be lost unnaturally through cutting, shaving, plucking, etc., these ways could be voluntarily, with the individual in question cutting or plucking their hair or shaving their head of their own volition, or involuntarily, with the individual having their hair cut or plucked or their head shaved against their will. It is possible that the reason for losing one's hair was a significant factor in leading an individual to start using prosthetic hair.

Natural Hair Loss

Ancient medical authors set out different theories regarding the nature of hair and hair growth and this meant that their theories about the precise causes of hair loss varied.[8] The Hippocratic treatises *On the Nature of the Child* and *On Glands*, possibly produced by the same individual,

[6] On prosthetic hair, see Draycott, 2019c.
[7] This chapter contains some material first collated for Draycott, 2019c.
[8] For a general overview, see Matthews, 2019.

considered hair to be produced by moisture, with hair growing from the parts of the body that were the most porous, thus allowing the moisture to travel to where it was needed in order for the hair to grow.[9] The treatise *On Fleshes* agreed that moisture played a part but suggested that heat was also involved.[10] However, other treatises argued that too much heat was responsible for hair loss since it warmed up and burnt the roots of the hairs.[11] These ideas can be found circulating in other texts that have survived from the Classical period, with Aristotle attributing hair loss to the cooling of the head, connecting it with the production of semen, and proposing that this cooling of the head was caused by sexual intercourse, hence why – he thought – women, children, and eunuchs did not go bald.[12] These Classical ideas were a significant influence on Galen in relation to his thoughts on the causes of hair loss, which he attributed to a lack of moisture nourishing the hair.[13] The Late Antique physician Dysarius attributed hair loss to dryness, explaining that as the human body aged, its constitution changed, becoming cooler and drier, and this resulted in hair being lost as part of the natural ageing process.[14]

Since it was recognised that hair is lost as part of the natural ageing process, a bald head is one of the visual signifiers of old age, or at the very least a difference in generations between figures if more than one figure is depicted, in ancient art.[15] Thus, we see Geras, the Greek the personification of old age, and Senectus, the Roman personification of old age, depicted as bald.[16]

For some, however, hair loss as part of the natural ageing process could begin earlier than for others.[17] Today the most common type of hair loss is male pattern baldness, which starts in the late twenties or early thirties, with most men having experienced some degree of hair loss by their late thirties and around half of all men having experienced male pattern baldness by the age of fifty.[18] In classical antiquity, although it was recognised that nothing could prevent hair loss in old age, victims of early onset male pattern baldness were publicly mocked.[19] Not even powerful individuals such as dictators or emperors were immune from this sort of ribaldry,

[9] Craik, 2009, p. 118; see also Craik, 2014 for proposed dates and authorship of the Hippocratic treatises. Hippoc. *Nat. puer.* 9; Hippoc. *Gland.* 4.

[10] Hippoc. *Carn.* 14. [11] Hippoc. *Nat. puer.* 9. [12] Arist. *Gen. an.* 5.783b.

[13] See for example Gal. *MM* 14.8. [14] Macrob. *Sat.* 7.10. [15] Emery, 1999, p. 18.

[16] *LIMC* s.v. Geras, s.v. Senectus. [17] For discussion, see Draycott, 2018.

[18] www.nhs.uk/conditions/hair-loss/Pages/Introduction.aspx (accessed January 2021).

[19] For understanding of hair loss, see Celsus, *Med.* 6.1.1. For mockery, see Mart. 5.49. Conversely, see Mart. 12.82 for an account of the sycophant Menogenes complimenting a virtually bald man on his luxurious head of hair and resultant resemblance to Achilles.

although the ways in which they dealt with it varied considerably.[20] With regard to women, today female pattern baldness is far less common than male pattern baldness and normally starts after the menopause, although up to half of all women who give birth experience more hair loss than usual.[21] In classical antiquity, victims of female pattern baldness or other types of hair loss were mocked just as victims of male pattern baldness were, but they were also subjected to a degree of moralising regarding how their actions and their lifestyles had contributed to it.[22] Seneca blames female pattern baldness on women inappropriately acting like men and equates female victims of hair loss with male ones.[23] Hair seems to have been a crucial component of female beauty, and once women lost their hair they were considered to be much less sexually attractive than they had been previously.[24]

Since hair loss that occurred as part of the natural ageing process was understood as having occurred naturally, it was not considered to be a kind of mutilation the way that the loss of other types of body parts were.[25] It was, however, recognised that hair lost as part of the natural ageing process was unlikely to grow back. According to Aristotle, 'a man who has once become bald never after recovers his hair'.[26] Consequently, it is not surprising that there is some evidence for attempts to secure assistance with lost hair from a deity, with divine intervention perhaps considered the only means of arresting the process. At least one individual, Heraieos of Mytilene, sought the assistance of the god Asklepios to cure his baldness: his miraculous healing following the application of a drug to his head is recorded among the *iamata* from the sanctuary of Asklepios at Epidauros. Another, Tullia Superiana, sought the assistance of the goddess Minerva to help her regrow her hair.[27] Although they are not inscribed so we do not know who dedicated them or why they dedicated them, considering their forms, it is possible that these terracotta scalps are evidence of votive offerings made by individuals afflicted with male pattern baldness.[28] Considering the sheer volume of votive heads and half heads that have been recovered through archaeological excavations, it is certainly possible

[20] Suet. *Iul.* 45.1–2, 51.1; Suet. *Galb.* 21.1; Plut. *Vit. Galb.* 13.4; Suet. *Dom.* 18.1, 18.2.
[21] www.nhs.uk/conditions/hair-loss/Pages/Introduction.aspx (accessed January 2021).
[22] Ov. *Am.* 1.14. [23] Sen. *Ep.* 95.20–1.
[24] Ov. *Ars am* 3.242–250; Apul. *Met.* 2.8. On hair and female attractiveness, see Sensi, 1980–1.
[25] Arist. *Metaph.* 5.27.4.
[26] Arist. *Cat.* 10.13a (trans. H. P. Cooke and H. Tredennick): οὔτε φαλακρὸς ὢν πάλιν κομήτης ἐγένετο, οὔτε νωδὸς ὢν ὀδόντας ἔφυσεν.
[27] Epidaurian iamata A19 (*IG* IV^2, 1.19). *CIL* XI 1305 = *ILS* 3135.
[28] Wellcome Collection inv. A114891 and A634932.

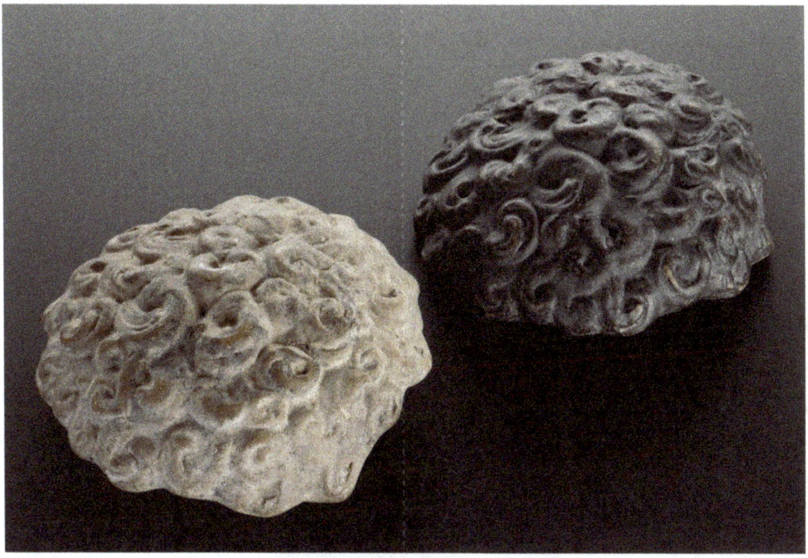

Figure 3.2 Terracotta ex votos. Wellcome Collection inv. A114891 and A634932. Image courtesy of the Wellcome Library.

that some of these were likewise dedicated for hair-related reasons. While hair loss was not as physically disabling as the loss of an extremity, it does seem to have been quite socially disabling, with responses to it ranging from rendering individuals objects of scorn and ridicule, or even objects of outright disgust, and it certainly impeded their ability to go about their usual business.

Hair Loss Due to Ill Health

Hair loss could occur if an individual suffered from a period of ill health, caused either by the illness or by the treatment prescribed for it. See, for example, the case of Stratonike, the wife of Seleucus, whose illness and subsequent hair loss seems to have been widely known, sympathised with, and humoured:

> Something similar and much more comical was done, she said, by Stratonice, the wife of Seleucus, who set a competition for the poets, with a talent as the prize, to see which of them could best praise her hair, in spite of the fact that she was bald and had not even a paltry few hairs of her own. Nevertheless, with her head in that pitiful state, when everybody knew that a long illness had affected her in that way, she listened to those rascally poets

> while they called her hair hyacinthine, and platted soft braids of it, and compared to wild parsley what did not even exist at all![29]

There could, however, be a moralising component present in discussions of hair loss, particularly if the individual's lifestyle was considered to have contributed to it. Plutarch attributes premature baldness in men to heavy drinking, while Seneca the Younger opines that women's lifestyle choices have caused them to start going bald and suffering from gout like men.[30]

For diseases of the head and the hair itself, such as alopecia, Galen reasoned that the moisture that produced and nourished the hair had gone bad in some way.[31] This marble head (Figure 3.3) is perhaps evidence of a votive offering

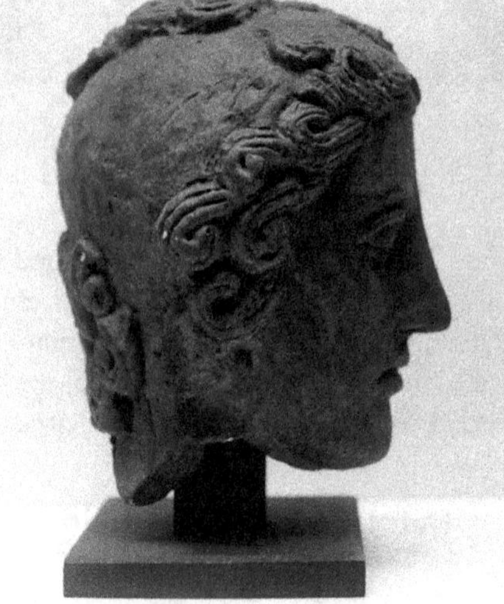

Figure 3.3 Terracotta ex voto, Temple of Minerva Medica, Rome, third or second century BCE. Antiquarium Comunale. Image courtesy of the Wellcome Library.

[29] Luc. *Imag.* 5 (trans. A. M. Harmon): Παραπλήσιον δὲ καὶ μακρῷ τούτου γελοιότερον Στρατονίκην ποιῆσαι τὴν Σελεύκου γυναῖκα. τοῖς γὰρ ποιηταῖς ἀγῶνα προθεῖναι αὐτὴν περὶ ταλάντου, ὅστις ἂν ἄμεινον ἐπαινέσαι αὐτῆς τὴν κόμην, καίτοι φαλακρὰ ἐτύγχανεν οὖσα καὶ οὐδὲ ὅσας ὀλίγας τὰς ἑαυτῆς τρίχας ἔχουσα. καὶ ὅμως οὕτω διακειμένη τὴν κεφαλήν, ἁπάντων εἰδότων ὅτι ἐκ νόσου μακρᾶς τὸ τοιοῦτον ἐπεπόνθει, ἤκουε τῶν καταράτων ποιητῶν ὑακινθίνας τὰς τρίχας αὐτῆς λεγόντων καὶ οὔλους τινὰς πλοκάμους ἀναπλεκόντων καὶ σελίνοις τοὺς μηδὲ ὅλως ὄντας εἰκαζόντων.

[30] Plut. *Mor.* 652f; Sen. *Ep.* 95.20–1. [31] Gal. *MM* 14.8.

made by an individual afflicted with a condition that caused partial hair loss, such as alopecia areata or ringworm.

However, frequently hair was considered an obstacle to medical treatment, leading to it being removed either by cutting the hair or shaving the head.[32] Rather unusually, one terracotta votive head from the Temple of Minerva Medica in Rome depicts a woman with a partially shaved head.[33] According to Celsus, invalids suffering from a variety of conditions ranging from insanity to epilepsy to ophthalmia should have their heads shaved as part of their medical treatment.[34] Caelius Aurelianus recommended cutting the hair for the relaxing and loosening effect that it had on the patient, and thought that it encouraged the pores to empty and fluid to evaporate.[35] Medicaments were frequently applied to the head, so in order for them to be efficacious they needed to be rubbed into the scalp, and other medical procedures, such as cupping and bloodletting, required likewise.

Hair Loss Due to Voluntary Body Modification

Hair could be deliberately or inadvertently removed in pursuit of a 'look' that was considered particularly desirable. Since grey or white hair was considered a sign of age, individuals could pluck their white hairs out. According to Macrobius, the emperor Augustus' daughter Julia had her enslaved attendants pluck out her white hairs:

> Julia was getting prematurely grey and took to plucking her grey hair in secret. One day her father surprised her hairdressers with his arrival, and they stopped their work. Pretending not to notice the grey hairs on their garments, Augustus chatted about some other topics for a while before steering the conversation around to the topic of age, then asked his daughter whether – some years hence – she would rather be bald or grey: when she replied, 'I, father, would prefer to be grey', he reproved her fib by saying, 'Then why are these women trying so hard to make you bald?'[36]

32 Matthews, 2019, p. 94.

33 Antiquarium Comunale inv. 5411, can be seen in Gatti Lo Guzzi, 1978, 134A.

34 Celsus, *Med.* 1.4.1, 3.18.8, 3.20.4, 3.23.7, 4.2.6, 4.2.9, 4.11.8, 6.2.2, 6.6.8 E, 6.6.15, 6.7.1 D, 6.7.4, 6.7.8 B, 7.7.15 D.

35 Caelius Aurelianus, *Chronic Diseases* 1.12, 3.131; in this, he was perhaps drawing on the teachings of Asclepiades of Bithynia; for discussion, see Matthews, 2019, p. 95.

36 Macrob. *Sat.* 2.7 (trans. R. A. Kaster, with minor alterations): *Eadem Iulia mature habere coeperat canos, quos legere secrete solebat. subitus interventus patris aliquando oppressit ornatrices. dissimulavit Augustus deprehensis super vestem earum canis, et aliis sermonibus tempore extracto induxit aetatis mentionem interrogavitque filiam utrum post aliquot annos cana esse mallet an calva; et cum illa respondisset, 'ego, pater, cana esse malo', sic illi mendacium obiecit: 'quid ergo istae te calvam tam cito faciunt?'*

An alternative scenario in which undesirable hair might be plucked out, and its consequences, is presented by Diodorus Siculus:

> There was, he said, a certain middle-aged man who took two wives. The younger, eager to have her husband resemble her, pulled out his grey hairs, while the old woman pulled out the black ones, until between them he was soon left quite bald. A similar fate, he said, would be in store for the people of Tucca; for as the Romans put to death those who were at odds with them and the Lusitanians did away with their enemies, the city would soon be left empty.[37]

A more drastic solution involved dying the entirety of one's hair, although, since ancient dyes were highly abrasive, this ran the risk of damaging the hair. According to Ovid, on one occasion his mistress dyed her hair and this caused most of her hair to fall out.[38] Another method of hair styling that might damage the hair and cause it to fall out was using hot tongs to create curls.

Hair could also be deliberately removed for specific religious ritual purposes. It has been suggested that in classical antiquity the ritual cutting of hair, or 'hair sacrifice', served as a substitute for human sacrifice on a *pars pro toto* basis, with hair considered appropriate for this purpose because the head is the seat of the soul, and its hair could stand for the whole person as a metonym.[39] With regard to the Roman period specifically, the Latin word for hair (*capillus*) is itself a diminutive of the word for head (*caput*), so it literally means 'little head', and the term 'caput' was also used in legal contexts to refer to citizenship, and consequently a change in an individual's status was referred to as 'lessening of the head' (*capitis deminutio*).[40] Those who voluntarily either shaved their heads or cut their hair beyond the norm for religious or ritual purposes included priests of the cult of Isis, sailors who had survived a shipwreck, men who had been acquitted of a capital crime, and formerly enslaved individuals. According to Plutarch, the reason why the priests of Isis shaved their heads and removed all other body hair was due to a concern for purity.[41] Their shaved heads are frequently depicted in ancient works of art. For sailors, to dream of having

[37] Diod. Sic. 33.7.6–7 (trans. C. H. Oldfather): ἔφη γάρ τινα μέσον ἤδη τὴν ἡλικίαν ὄντα γαμῆσαι δύο γυναῖκας, καὶ τὴν μὲν νεωτέραν ἐξομοιοῦν ἑαυτῇ φιλοτιμουμένην τὸν ἄνδρα ἐκ τῆς κεφαλῆς τὰς πολιὰς ἐκτίλλειν αὐτοῦ, τὴν δὲ γραῦν τὰς μελαίνας, καὶ πέρας ὑπ' ἀμφοτέρων αὐτὸν ἐκτιλλόμενον ταχὺ γενέσθαι φαλακρόν. τὸ παραπλήσιον δὲ καὶ τοῖς τὴν Τύκκην οἰκοῦσιν ἔσεσθαι· τῶν μὲν γὰρ Ῥωμαίων ἀποκτεινόντων τοὺς ἀλλοτρίως πρὸς αὐτοὺς ἔχοντας, τῶν δὲ Λυσιτανῶν ἀναιρούντων τοὺς αὐτῶν ἐχθρούς, ταχὺ τὴν πόλιν ἐρημωθήσεσθαι.

[38] Ov. *Am.* 1.14. [39] Hallpike, 1969, p. 149. [40] Levine, 1995, p. 85; Richlin, 1995, p. 206.

[41] Plut. *Mor. De Is. et Os.* 4.

a shaved head indicated a shipwreck was to come, as the reason that they shaved their heads or cut their hair was in order to make an offering of thanks to a deity, usually Poseidon, Isis, or the Dioscuri, for having escaped death, with the hair representing themselves and serving as a *pars pro toto* sacrifice.[42] This might also be connected to the fact that it was taboo for sailors to cut their hair or fingernails while at sea unless there was a terrible storm.[43] For men acquitted of a capital crime, the reasoning was similar.[44] Enslaved individuals who had recently been emancipated cut their hair at the temple of Feronia in order to make a hair sacrifice to signify dying as an enslaved person and being reborn as a Roman citizen.[45]

Hair Loss Due to Involuntary Body Modification

Someone's hair could be cut, or their head shaved, entirely against their will. Such an act would likely be undertaken quite violently, using some sort of method of restraint. Under such circumstances, the individual in question would likely view it as an act of assault and a type of physical mutilation, especially if they were part of a culture that placed a considerable emphasis on hair, and this sort of enforced head shaving has been described as being not only a violation of an individual's body-space and a form of violent assault, but also an act loaded with meaning in terms of power relations and transformation.[46] This transformation was unlikely to be viewed as a positive one by the individual in question. One situation in classical antiquity in which an individual's hair could be cut or their head shaved against their will was during the enslavement process, as individuals who were enslaved lost personal autonomy and became property, and their hair was cut or their head was shaved upon capture to indicate their servile position, with this style being subsequently maintained for the sake of ease.[47] Accordingly, many depictions of the enslaved

[42] Artem. *On.* 1.18: dreams of long flowing hair equate with profit; Artem. *On.* 1.22: dreams of hair loss equate with loss, unless the dreamer is in the habit of shaving his head, in which case the reverse is true. See Plaut. *Rud.* 5.2.16 and Juv. 12.81 for examples of sailors shaving their heads.

[43] Non. 1, *Hermotimus* 86. [44] Mart. 2.74; Plin. *Ep.* 7.27.

[45] Plaut. *Amph.* 1.1.306; Serv. 8.564; Livy 34.52.12, 45.44; Plut. *Vit. Flam.* 13.6; Juv. 5. See Fabre, 1981, pp. 19–20 on manumission ceremonies. See also King Prusias II of Bithynia in Polyb. 30.18, discussed in Arena, 2012, pp. 33–4.

[46] Aldhouse-Green, 2004a, p. 301. See also Artem. *On.* 1.30: 'If a man dreams that his beard has fallen off, or that it has been shaved off or forcibly ripped off by anyone, it signifies, in addition to loss of his blood relations, harm together with shame.'

[47] Petron. *Sat.* 110; Ach. Tat. 5.17, 8.5; Apul. *Met.* 9.12; Cyprian, *Letters* 77.3; Thompson, 2003, p. 241. See Aldhouse-Green, 2004a and b on captors' interaction with the enslaved and their hair as a sign of dominance.

in ancient literature and art present them as having short hair. As discussed earlier, a considerable amount of a woman's beauty and sexual attractiveness seems to have resided in her hair, so it is not surprising to see instances of women's hair being cut in classical antiquity as a means of policing or punishing female sexuality. Thus, a woman in an abusive relationship might experience this, as Lucian demonstrates through the character of Ampelis in his *Dialogues of the Courtesans*: 'If a man isn't jealous or angry, Chrysis, and never hits you, cuts your hair off, or tears your clothes, is he still in love with you?'[48] A woman accused of adultery might have her head shaved or her hair cut as a punishment, but also as a visible sign of her disgrace.[49] If an individual lost their hair under these sorts of circumstances, it may not have been possible or even permissible for them to cover themselves.

Literary Evidence for False Hair in Classical Antiquity

False hair is the most frequently mentioned type of prosthesis in ancient Greek and Latin literature. While the ancient Greeks do not seem to have utilised false hair outside of the theatre, there seem to have been several different types of false hair available to ancient Romans, and the literary evidence makes it clear that both women and men utilised them.[50] A full wig was known as a *capillamentum* or a *caliendrum*, while a hairpiece or hair extension used to supplement one's own hair was known as a *galerus* or a *galerum*. A full wig was significantly more time-consuming for a wig-maker to create than a hairpiece or a hair extension, so it would have been commensurately significantly more expensive to purchase.[51] This probably restricted use of full wigs – or at least high-quality full wigs – to the wealthier members of ancient Roman society. While nothing is known about the manufacture of wigs and hair pieces, according to Ovid and

[48] Luc. *Dial. meret.* 8 (trans. M. D. McLeod): "Οστις δέ, ὦ Χρυσί, μήτε ζηλοτυπεῖ μήτε ὀργίζεται μήτε ἐρράπισέ ποτε ἢ περιέκειρεν ἢ τὰ ἱμάτια περιέσχισεν, ἔτι ἐραστὴς ἐκεῖνός ἐστιν; See also Men. *Pk.* in which Polemon cuts off Glykera's hair in a fit of jealousy.

[49] Tac. *Germ.* 19; see also Paul, 1 *Corinthians* 11.4–8 for comparison, and the possibility that this was done in Jewish communities.

[50] See Lee, 2015, p. 70, for wigs not being common in Greece prior to the Hellenistic period; Xen. *Cyr.* 1.3.2 describes wigs as a Median fashion, while playwrights such as Arist. *Thesm.* 258 utilise them in scenes of male to female transvestitism.

[51] Fletcher and Salamone, 2016; experimental archaeological reconstruction of an ancient Egyptian wig (*circa* 1400 BCE) by a professional wig-maker resulted in the estimation that such a wig would have taken around 200 hours or one month to create – if an ancient Egyptian wig-maker could only produce a maximum of twelve wigs per year, he or she would have needed to charge enough for each wig to make this limitation on their professional activities worth their while; see also Cox, 1977.

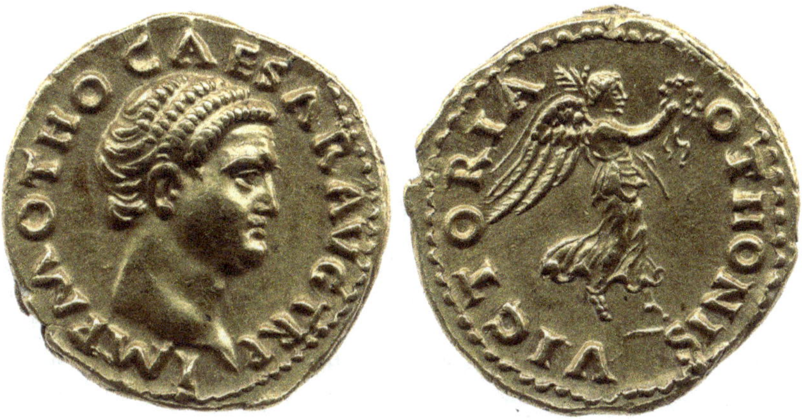

Figure 3.4 Gold aureus, Rome, 69 CE, British Museum inv. R.6333. Image courtesy of the British Museum.

Martial they could be purchased near the Porticus Philippi, in front of the temple of Hercules and the Muses.[52] According to Suetonius (circa 60–122 CE), the emperor Otho had thinning hair and wore a wig of such high quality that nobody could distinguish it from his natural hair; presumably such a wig was specially made by an artisan at the height of their powers.[53] It is worth noting, however, that portraits of Otho, whether on coins or carved in the round, do depict a peculiar hairstyle that might well be intended to demonstrate the difference between natural hair and prosthetic hair.[54] If this is indeed the case, it would appear that Otho suffered from something akin to what we know today as male pattern baldness.[55]

Tertullian, in his polemic *On the Apparel of Women*, gives us perhaps the fullest description of prosthetic hair in ancient literature:

> You affix I know not what enormities of subtle and textile perukes; now, after the manner of a helmet of undressed hide, as it were a sheath for the head and a covering for the crown; now, a mass drawn backward toward the neck. The wonder is that there is no open contending against the Lord's prescripts! It has been pronounced that no one can add to his own stature. You, however, do

[52] For wigs and hair pieces in the Porticus Philippi, see Ov. *Ars am* 3.167–8; Mart. 5.49.12–13; on this, see Dalby, 2000, p. 241. Toner, 2015, p. 95 states that barbers made wigs, but does not provide any evidence to support this claim.

[53] Suet. *Oth.* 12.

[54] British Museum inv. R6333; *RIC*I 13, p. 260; *RE*I 21, p. 367. www.britishmuseum.org/collection/term/BIB3158.

[55] On this, see Draycott, 2018.

> add to your weight some kind of rolls, or shield-bosses, to be piled upon your necks! If you feel no shame at the enormity, feel some at the pollution; for fear you may be fitting on a holy and Christian head the slough of someone else's head, unclean perchance, guilty perchance and destined to hell. Nay, rather banish quite away from your 'free' head all this slavery of ornamentation. In vain do you labour to seem adorned: in vain do you call in the aid of all the most skilful manufacturers of false hair. God bids you 'be veiled'. I believe he does so for fear the heads of some should be seen![56]

He believes that women who convert to Christianity should alter their physical appearance to reflect their new-found religiosity since modesty will ensure their salvation.[57] He differentiates between things worn (*cultus*) and things that beautify (*ornatus*), and includes false hair in the latter category.[58] Tertullian's contemporary Clement of Alexandria also criticised women for wearing wigs and hair pieces on numerous occasions in his writings. Like Tertullian, Clement describes prosthetic hair as inherently polluting:

> But additions of other people's hair are entirely to be rejected, and it is a most sacrilegious thing for spurious hair to shade the head, covering the skull with dead locks. For on whom does the presbyter lay his hand? Whom does he bless? Not the woman decked out, but another's hair, and through them another head. And if 'the man is head of the woman, and God of the man', how is it not impious that they should fall into double sins? For they deceive the men by the excessive quantity of their hair; and shame the Lord as far as in them lies, by adorning themselves meretriciously, in order to dissemble the truth. And they defame the head, which is truly beautiful.[59]

Tertullian's and Clement's rather specific objections were influenced by their adherence to Christianity.[60] Elsewhere in ancient literature, the wearing of

[56] Tert. 2.7.1–2 (trans. S. Thelwell): *Affigitis praeterea nescio quas enormitates sutilium atque textilium capillamentorum, nunc in galeri modum quasi uaginam capitis et operculum uerticis, nunc in ceruicum retro suggestum. Mirum quod non contra domini praecepta contenditur! Ad mensuram neminem sibi adicere posse pronuntiatum est. Vos sane adicitis ad pondus, collyridas quasdam uel scutorum umbilicos ceruicibus adstruendo. Si non pudet enormitatis, pudeat inquinamenti, ne exuuias alieni capitis forsitan immundi, forsan nocentis et gehennae destinati sancto et christiano capiti supparetis. Immo, omnem hanc ornatus seruitutem a libero capite propellite. Frustra laboratis ornatae uideri, frustra peritissimos quosque structores capillaturae adhibetis: Deus uos uelari iubet, credo ne quarumdam capita uideantur.*

[57] Raditsa, 1985, p. 306. [58] For discussion, see Lawler, 1929, p. 22.

[59] Clem. Al. 3.63.1–2 (trans. W. Wilson): Ἀλλοτρίων δὲ αἱ προσθέσεις τριχῶν τέλεον ἔκβλητοι, ὀθνείας τε ἐπισκευάζεσθαι τῇ κεφαλῇ τὰς κόμας ἀθεώτατον νεκροῖς ἐνδιδυσκούσας πλοκάμοις τὸ κρανίον· τίνι γὰρ ὁ πρεσβύτερος ἐπιθήσει χεῖρα; τίνα δὲ εὐλογήσει; Οὐ τὴν γυναῖκα τὴν κεκοσμημένην, ἀλλὰ τὰς ἀλλοτρίας τρίχας καὶ δι᾽ αὐτῶν ἄλλην κεφαλήν. Εἰ δὲ "κεφαλὴ γυναικὸς μὲν ἀνήρ, ἀνδρὸς δὲ ὁ Χριστός", πῶς οὐκ ἄθεον διττοῖς αὐτὰς περιπίπτειν ἁμαρτήμασιν; Τοὺς μὲν γὰρ ἀπατῶσι, τοὺς ἄνδρας, διὰ τὴν ὑποβολὴν τῆς κόμης, καταισχύνουσι δὲ τὸν κύριον τὸ ὅσον ἐπ᾽ αὐταῖς ἑταιρικῶς κοσμούμεναι εἰς ἀπάτην ἀληθείας καὶ τὴν ὄντως οὖσαν καλὴν βλασφημοῦσαι κεφαλήν.

[60] See Upson-Saia, 2011 for discussion of how early Christian women were expected to dress simply as a sign of their conversion to Christian ideals.

wigs and hair pieces is frequently strongly criticised in male-authored ancient literature due to the artifice that is perceived to be involved – criticisms that are likewise found in male-authored discourses about cosmetics.[61] A pagan contemporary of Tertullian and Clement, Philostratus the Elder, makes this clear in his discussion of feminine beauty:

> The woman who beautifies herself seeks to supply what is lacking; she fears the detection of her deficiency. The woman whose beauty is natural needs nothing adventitious, for she is self-sufficient to the point of utter perfection. Eyes underlined with kohl, false hair [κόμης προσθέσεις], painted cheeks, tinted lips, all the enhancements known to the beautifier's art, and all the deceptive bloom achieved by rouge have been invented for the correction of defects; the unadorned is the truly beautiful.[62]

False hair comes in for a considerable amount of criticism from Roman authors, particularly when it is being worn by elderly women attempting to disguise their baldness.[63] Ovid records an occasion in which his mistress, a fashionable young woman, having attempted to colour her hair and style it with a curling iron, has only succeeded in damaging it to the point where a considerable amount of it has fallen out, and he uses this as a reason to excoriate her for her vanity and frivolity, as well as taking the opportunity to say, essentially, 'I told you so':

> I said: 'Stop dyeing your hair!' Now you've no hair left to colour . . . Alas, what suffering [your hairs] had to bear! How they offered themselves patiently to the steel and fire, as their waves were twisted and tied in ringlets! I cried: 'That's wicked, wicked to scorch your hair! It's fine as it is: go carefully with the steel! Take the pressure away! No one ought to burn it: your hair itself teaches others how to pin theirs' . . . Why search your neat hair for what's vilely lost? Silly girl why hold the mirror sadly in your hand? It's no use contriving to stare at yourself: you need to forget about yourself, to please. No mistress of magic herbs has wounded you, no Thessalian witch soaked you in treacherous water: no illness's power has touched you – perish the thought! – No evil tongue has thinned your dense hair. Your hand did it and you're paying for your crime . . . Alas! She scarcely contains her tears and with her hand hides her delicate cheeks painted with blushes. She holds her former hair in her lap, and stares at it, ah

[61] See Olson, 2009; for expanded discussion on Roman cosmetics, see Olson, 2012, pp. 58–80.

[62] Philostr. *Ep.* 22 (trans. A. R. Benner): Ἡ καλλωπιζομένη γυνὴ θεραπεύει τὸ ἐλλιπὲς φοβουμένη φωραθῆναι ὃ οὐκ ἔχει· ἡ φύσει καλὴ οὐδενὸς δεῖται τῶν ἐπικτήτων ὡς προσαρκοῦσα ἑαυτῇ πρὸς πᾶν τὸ ὁλόκληρον. ὀφθαλμῶν δὲ ὑπογραφαὶ καὶ κόμης προσθέσεις καὶ ζωγραφίαι παρειῶν καὶ χειλέων βαφαὶ καὶ εἴ τι κομμωτικῆς φάρμακον καὶ εἴ τι ἐκ φυκίου δολερὸν ἄνθος, ἐπανόρθωσις τοῦ ἐνδεοῦς εὑρέθη· τὸ δὲ ἀκόσμητον ἀληθῶς καλόν.

[63] See, for example, Hor. *Sat.* 1.8.47–50; Mart. 1.72, 2.41, 5.43, 9.38, 12.23, 14.56; Luc. *Rhet.* 24; Lucillius, *Greek Anthology* 11.310; Macedonius, *Greek Anthology* 11.374.

> me, a tribute not fitting for that place! Calm yourself, doing your face! The harm's reparable. Shortly your natural hair will be seen again.[64]

Yet if Ovid is merely rather smug and snide about his poor mistress' experience of hair loss, Martial is overtly critical about the women of his acquaintance that experience the same and attempt to do something about it. He opines that Laelia should be ashamed of resorting to wearing a wig, and presumably Galla, who not only wears false hair but also false eyebrows, should feel twice as much shame as Laelia.[65]

People were thought to utilise wigs and hair pieces to deceive and pretend to be something they were not. This might be young and beautiful, but also, and potentially more significantly, in a state of good rather than poor health, as medical treatises make it clear that hair was an indicator of many things regarding an individual's constitution and underlying state of health.[66] Hair was considered an important component of female sexual attractiveness, and women were considered to be much less sexually attractive as a result of hair loss.[67] Roman writers such as Horace, Ovid, Martial, and Lucillius give examples of women who wear wigs to either appear much younger than they are or to hide signs of debilitating illness.[68] Lucian goes one further and

[64] Ov. *Am.* 1.14 (trans. A. S. Kline): *Dicebam 'medicare tuos desiste capillos!' Tingere quam possis, iam tibi nulla coma est ... Cum graciles essent tamen et lanuginis instar, heu, male vexatae quanta tulere comae! Quam se praebuerunt ferro patienter et igni, ut fieret torto nexilis orbe sinus! Clamabam: 'scelus est istos, scelus urere crines! Sponte decent; capiti, ferrea, parce tuo! Vim procul hinc remove! non est, qui debeat uri; erudit admotas ipse capillus acus' ... Quid male dispositos quereris periisse capillos? Quid speculum maesta ponis, inepta, manu? Non bene consuetis a te spectaris ocellis; ut placeas, debes inmemor esse tui ... Non te cantatae laeserunt paelicis herbae, non anus Haemonia perfida lavit aqua; nec tibi vis morbi nocuit – procul omen abesto! – Nec minuit densas invida lingua comas. Facta manu culpaque tua dispendia sentis; ipsa dabas capiti mixta venena tuo ... Me miserum! lacrimas male continet oraque dextra protegit ingenuas picta rubore genas. Sustinet antiquos gremio spectatque capillos, ei mihi, non illo munera digna loco! Collige cum vultu mentem! reparabile damnum est. Postmodo nativa conspiciere coma.* For discussion of this poem, see Zetzel, 1996; Papaioannou, 2006. Zetzel, 1996, pp. 74–7, has interpreted this as a reference to Propertius' work on a similar theme, in which he likewise warns his unnamed mistress against female adornment and vanity regarding her hair, clothing, and use of cosmetics.

[65] Mart. 12.23, 9.38.

[66] See for example Luc. *Dial. meret.* 39.11, in which a courtesan wears a wig over grey hair, presumably to allow her to continue working; and compare with 39.12, in which a courtesan whose hair was cut off while she is ill now wears a wig, likewise presumably to allow her to keep working.

[67] See Muson. 21 for discussion of the ways that women arrange their hair to appear more beautiful; Ov. *Ars am* 3.135–58 goes into considerable detail about which hairstyle a woman should choose depending upon the nature of her physical attributes. See Ov. *Ars am* 3.242–50 and Apul. *Met.* 2.8 for the loss of hair making women less attractive. On hair and female attractiveness, see Sensi, 1980–1. However, in the interests of fairness, it is also clear from ancient literary descriptions that bald men were likewise considered unattractive, it is simply that their hair is not ruminated on by ancient authors in precisely the same way that women's is.

[68] Hor. *Sat.* 1.8.47–50; Ov. *Am.* 1.14; Mart. 9.38, 12.23; Lucillius, *Greek Anthology* 11.68, 11.310.

presents the courtesan Philematium, who is not only aging and going grey, but has also been so ill that her hair has fallen out; her profession necessitates that men find her attractive, hair is necessary for sexual attractiveness, hence the wig.[69] This deception and pretence extended to the use of wigs and hair pieces as a means of disguising one's identity to facilitate misbehaviour. Thus, Juvenal claims that the empress Messalina wore a blonde wig to spend the night in a brothel competing with the prostitutes that worked there, and Cassius Dio tells a similar story of the emperor Elagabalus, while Suetonius claims that the emperors Gaius and Nero wore wigs to roam the streets and cause trouble at night.[70]

What is clear, however, is that wigs and hair pieces were risky. The prospect of someone's wig coming loose and either slipping or falling off entirely is frequently presented as a source of amusement.[71] Avienus tells a story of a horseman whose wig fell off during his routine and, when he was faced with public ridicule, turned the situation to his advantage through a display of wit: 'As the horseman saw that he was the laughing-stock of so many thousands, he shrewdly brought cunning to his aid and turned away the jest from himself. "Why be surprised," he remarked, "that my assumed locks have gone, when my natural hair deserted me first?"'[72] The spectacle of someone wearing a bad or unsuitable wig is also played for laughs.[73] Ovid tells of an occasion where he interrupted a woman dressing and she was in such a hurry that she put her wig on back to front.[74] While amused, he was also repulsed: 'Ugly is a bull without horns; ugly is a field without grass, a plant without leaves, or a head without hair.'[75]

Archaeological Evidence for False Hair in Classical Antiquity

Relatively few Roman wigs and hair pieces have survived in the archaeological record due to the very specific conditions necessary for the preservation of the organic materials that they were normally made from

69 Luc. *Dial. meret.* 11.4.

70 Juv. 6; Cass. Dio. 80.2; Suet. *Calig.* 11.1; Suet. *Ner.* 26.1. For discussion of Messalina's purported transgression, see Joshel, 1995, pp. 77–8.

71 See for example the witch Sagana in Hor. *Sat.* 1.8.47–50.

72 Avienus, *Fables* 11.7–12 (trans. J. W. Duff and A. M. Duff): *ille sagax, tantis quod risus milibus esset, distulit admota calliditate iocum, 'quid mirum' referens 'positos fugisse capillos, quem prius aequaevae deseruere comae?'*

73 See Petron. *Sat.* 110, where Petronius depicts two of his *Satyricon* characters covering up their shaven heads with women's wigs.

74 Ov. *Ars am* 3.244–7.

75 Ov. *Ars am* 3.249–50 (trans. J. H. Mozely): *Turpe pecus mutilum, turpis sine gramine campus, et sine fronde frutex, et sine crine caput.*

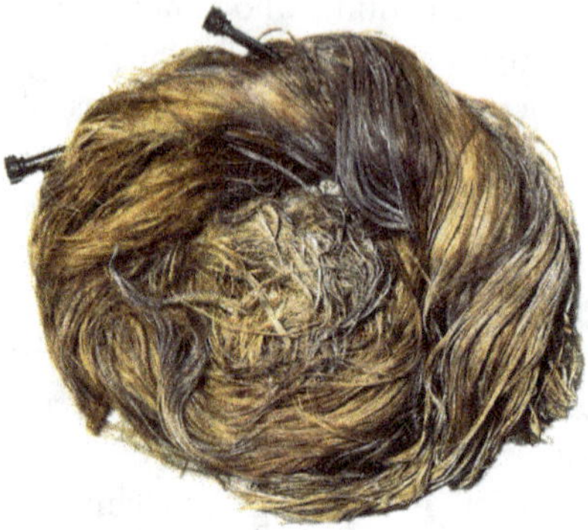

Figure 3.5 Roman wig, York, late-third to early-fifth century CE. Yorkshire Museum inv. YORYM:1998.695. Image courtesy of the Yorkshire Museum.

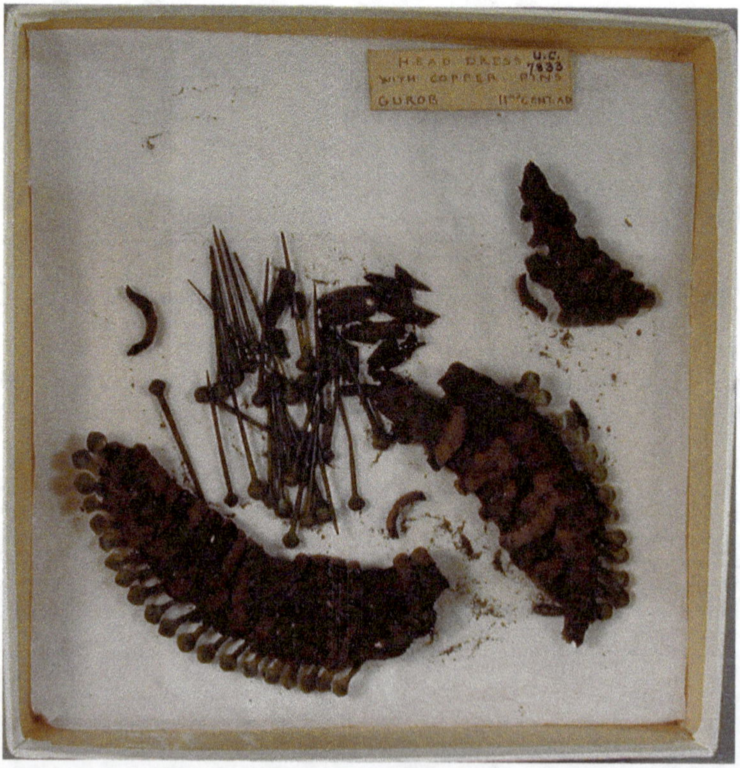

Figure 3.6 Roman hairpiece from Gurob in the Fayum, late first or early second century CE. Petrie Museum inv. UC7833. Image courtesy of The Petrie Museum of Egyptian Archaeology, UCL.

(hair, leather, plant fibres, etc.). However, examples of hair pieces made from human hair have been recovered from several locations around the Roman Empire. Three comprising dark brown and blonde sections of hair attached to pieces of leather and dating from the second century CE were recovered from burials excavated at Les Martres-de-Veyre in France.[76] One comprising a piece of plaited hair was found inside a cremation urn at Rainham Creek in Britain.[77] Another comprising a section of blonde hair in conjunction with two cantharus-headed jet pins which remain in situ threaded through the hair dating from the late third century to the early fifth century CE was found inside a lead sarcophagus at York in Britain.[78] Two more comprising hair attached to pieces of linen were found in tandem with the mummified bodies of their owners in the necropolis of Dush in the Kharga Oasis in Egypt.[79] One of the mummies was a woman of approximately twenty years old, the other was a child of approximately seven years old; both had very short and sparse growth of natural hair, and it has been suggested that this was a side-effect of typhoid, so the hair pieces served as a means of disguising this.[80] Another was found at Gurob in the Fayum and comprises a piece of plaited hair that would have been fixed to the wearer's head with sixty-two bronze pins in the 'orbis' hairstyle that dates from either the late first or the first half of the second century CE.[81] The length and styles of these hair pieces indicate that they were worn to supplement existing hair, although it is impossible to say for certain. The frequency with which the hair pieces are discovered braided and/or in conjunction with hair pins indicates that they were styled and arranged just as an individual's own hair would be.

However, one example of an entire wig made from auburn hair has been recovered from a tomb on the Via Latina in Rome, and, thanks to the preservation of the tomb's contents and the inscriptions on its marble sarcophagi, it is possible to state with certainty that this wig was worn by a wealthy woman named Aebutia Quarta, the daughter of Gaius Antestius

76 Audollent, 1921, p. 163; see also Audollent, 1923, pp. 311–12, pl. 8, nn. 3–6.

77 Wood, 1883, p. 108; Black, 1986, p. 225.

78 Yorkshire Museum inv. YORYM:1998.695. On the hair pins specifically, see Fletcher, 2016.

79 Fletcher, 1995, pp. 37–8. There was a tradition of wig-wearing in Egypt dating back to 3400 BCE, Fletcher, 2005, p. 3.

80 Woman: Mummy n.58.2.2.4, see Dunand et al., 1992, p. 142, pl. 33.3–4; Fletcher, 1995, Volume 1, pp. 37–38, p. 415; child: Mummy n.20.2.1.4, see Dunand and Lichtenberg, 1994, pp. 92–3 (with photographs); Dunand et al., 1992, pp. 51–2, pl. 24.1–4; Fletcher, 1995, Volume 1, p. 37, p. 415.

81 Petrie Museum inv. UC7833; Petrie, 1927, p. 5, pl. 4; Corson, 1965, p. 74; Allason-Jones, 2005, p. 135; Fletcher, 1995, Volume 1, p. 416; Volume 2, p. 947, pl. 819, pl. 820. On the hair pins specifically, see Fletcher, 2016.

Balbinus, in the late first and early second century CE.[82] Here, we could have an example of a woman who sought to follow fashion and amplify her natural beauty, or a woman whose own hair was for some reason lacking so she sought to disguise her deficiency by utilising the financial resources at her disposal, but either way her wealth enabled her to purchase and wear a wig of the highest possible quality in conjunction with her natural hair, and to hold it in place with a golden hairnet.[83]

As ancient writers such as Tertullian recounted, wigs and hair pieces could be made of substances other than human hair, although we have to wonder how convincing such items were, assuming they were intended as imitations of wigs and hair pieces made from human hair rather than as a distinct category of objects in their own right. A wig made from linen and tinted a shade of chestnut was reportedly recovered from the tomb of a Christian woman on the Via Ostiensis in the early eighteenth century; unfortunately, its current whereabouts, if it even still exists, are unknown.[84] A wig in the form of corkscrew curls on a plaited base with a plait hanging down at the back, made from grass fibres coated in beeswax, was recovered from a house at Harit in Egypt.[85] Another contemporaneous wig from Egypt resembles the one from Harit but is made from date palm fibres.[86] A hairpiece from Egypt made from string and linen was found attached to the mummy of a child.[87] Two other possible hair pieces made from plant fibres have been recovered from military sites in Britain: one from the Roman fort at Vindolanda in England and the other from the Roman fort at Newstead in Scotland.[88] However, there is some debate over whether they should be considered hair pieces at all, as opposed to hats or caps, or even baskets.[89]

82 For full details of the tomb, see Rossignani et al., 2005.

83 An Italian documentary about the excavation, *Carvilius, un enigna dall'antica Roma*, is available on Youtube: https://youtu.be/cwJ5nVvRNag (accessed January 2021). It contains a lengthy section on the wig and hairnet and uses an actress to demonstrate what Aebutia Quarta would have looked like with her hair arranged this way.

84 Bartman, 2001, p. 14, n. 69.

85 Cairo Archaeological Museum inv. JE.33434; Fletcher, 1995, Volume 1, p. 415; Volume 2, p. 945, pl. 815, pl. 816.

86 Cairo Archaeological Museum inv. Temp.Reg.18:1:26:26; Fletcher, 1995, Volume 1, p. 415; Volume 2, p. 946, pl. 817.

87 British Museum inv. EA.54051 (the hairpiece is not currently visible in the photograph of the mummy on the British Museum's website); Dawson and Gray, 1978, n. 78, n. 40, pl. 31a–b; Fletcher, 1995, Volume 1, p. 415; Volume 2, p. 946, pl. 818.

88 Vindolanda: Wild, 1993, pp. 61–8. Newstead: National Museum of Scotland inv. X.FRA 1183; Curle, 1911, p. 108, p. 358, pl. 15; Wild, 1993, p. 64, n. 7.

89 The Vindolanda Museum has labelled the Vindolanda example as a wig. The Newstead example was originally interpreted as a basket, see Curle, 1911, p. 108, pl. 15. However, today the National Museum of Scotland has it labelled as a hat.

Although we have no information about the manufacture of wigs and hair pieces in Ancient Rome, as we have seen, the ancient literary and archaeological evidence suggests that, for the most part, they comprised foundations made of leather or another type of material with human hair of varying lengths and colours attached. Where did this hair come from? One type of hair described as 'Indian hair' (*capelli Indici*) is known to have been imported from India because there is documentary evidence in the form of a record of customs dues being paid on it at Rome, and it was perhaps sought after because it was basic black in colour and so could be widely utilised.[90] Yet there is a considerable amount of literary evidence for another type of hair, known as 'captive hair' (*captivis comis*) because it was taken from German prisoners.[91] This type of hair seems to have been particularly popular during the reigns of Augustus and Domitian, perhaps because there was a considerable amount of military activity on the Rhine frontier at these times and thus a plentiful supply of German prisoners.[92] Why was German hair so popular? The Germans, particularly the Sicambrian and the Suebi tribes, were known for their long blonde or red hair (*flavus*; *rutilus*) tied up in the style known as the Suebian Knot (*nodus Suebicus*).[93] Their hair – not just its colour and texture, but also its chosen style – was one of the main differences between them and the Romans, and ultimately the transition from native hair style to Roman hairstyle was used as an indicator of the acquisition of *cultus*.

There was likely a practical benefit to the use of German hair for wigs and hair pieces as, unlike the Romans, both German men and women wore their hair long. Perhaps more important, however, is the fact that Germans were famous for their blonde (*flavus*) or red (*rutilus*) hair – colours that were not only unusual in Italy, but also replete with positive connotations such as divinity.[94] The fact that these hair colours were particularly associated with Germanic tribes is made clear from first Caligula's and later Domitian's attempts to falsify the origins of the 'prisoners' paraded in their sham triumphs by colouring the participants'

[90] *Dig.* 39.4.16.7. According to Arr. *Ind.* 6.9, Indian hair was dark like Ethiopian hair but not woolly.

[91] There is also evidence for hair dye consisting of 'German herbs'; see Ov. *Ars am* 3. 159–68. For discussion of Roman hair dye, see Bradley, 2009, pp. 170–4.

[92] Military activity such as Drusus' campaign against the Cherusci, Suebi and Sicambri in 11 BCE, recounted in Flor. 2.30.25. See also Ov. *Am.* 1.14.45–6, *Ars* 3.163–8, 3.242–50; Mart. 14.26 refers to 'Teutonic locks' (*teutonicos capillos*), Bartman, 1999, p. 39; Leary, 1996, p. 79. See also Mart. 5.37.8, 5.68, 14.26; Juv. 13.164–65; Claud. *Cons. Hon.* 4.446–7, Eutr. 1.383.

[93] For the Suebian Knot, see Tac. *Germ.* 38; Krierer, 2004, pp. 100–11.

[94] Sen. *Ira* 3.26.3; Sen. *Ep.* 124.22. See Barton, 1994, pp. 119–22 for the significance of colouring in ancient physiognomy.

hair these shades.[95] Petronius (circa 27–66 CE) portrays Encolpius as being especially pleased once his shaven head is covered with a wig: 'in fact, I was even more handsome than before, because my new hair was bright blond'.[96] It was also in all likelihood widely seen as symbolic, as ownership of German hair represented ownership of German people, and exotic and luxury goods were seen to represent the fruits of Roman imperialism.[97]

Conclusion

Hair loss seems to have been common in classical antiquity, with the potential to occur at all stages of life. This did not mean that hair loss was considered socially acceptable or passed without comment, however. For anyone that was not an elderly man, the social consequences of experiencing hair loss were considerable. One way of dealing with this hair loss was to utilise prosthetic hair, and, unlike extremity or facial prostheses, these seem to have been widely adopted both by individuals who had lost their hair and by individuals who had not but simply wished to supplement it.

Despite some literary and archaeological evidence for wigs and hair pieces made from other substances, most do seem to have been made from human hair. False hair is virtually unique among prostheses in that it can be made from a part of the human body, whether that body belongs to the intended user of the prosthesis or someone else entirely, and is thus perhaps seen as more authentic, more natural. In classical antiquity, the only other type of prosthesis where this was a possibility was the dental appliance, and, as far as we can tell from the available literary and archaeological evidence, neither the commissioners nor the makers of these items seem to have commonly capitalised upon this possibility in the way that the commissioners and makers of wigs and hair pieces did.

Hair was a fundamental physical feature for both men and women in classical antiquity, a means of expressing crucial information about gender, stage of life, social class, status, political affiliation, religious belief, and

95 For Caligula, see Suet. *Calig.* 47 and Pers. 6.46–7; Tac. *Agr.* 39 and Cass. Dio. 67.7.4. For discussion, see Beard, 2009, pp. 185–6.

96 Petron. *Sat.* 110 (trans. J. P. Sullivan): *immo commendatior vultus enituit, quia flavum conymbian erat.* Of course, this is a personal preference and entirely subjective; see Ov. *Am.* 2.4.37–44 for the poet's discussion of the type of women he finds attractive.

97 On Ovid and images of empire, see Habinek, 2002, pp. 46–9. On luxury and Roman imperialism generally, see Dalby, 2000.

even profession. Since hair was so significant and the possession of it so important, it is not surprising that those who were lacking sought to hide their deficiencies as far as they were able or permitted to do so, and false hair in the form of wigs and hair pieces was one way in which they could do this. The wearing of prosthetic hair provided a means of creating an alternative social and symbolic presentation of self that emphasised certain desirable qualities such as strength and vitality. It was not, however, without risk, as the wearing of wigs and hair pieces had negative connotations and often the hair utilised to make them did too; this is something that does not seem to have been the case with other types of ancient prostheses.

However, like other types of ancient prostheses, the prosthetic hair that has survived from classical antiquity has done so because it was included in the burials of its users, even if the vast majority of the examples that are contained in modern museum collections have now been separated from their users' bodies and little or no information survives about them. In cases of inhumation, they seem to have been attached to their users' bodies in death as they would have been during life, rather than simply included alongside the individual as a grave good, even if they were not treated as such by excavators and collectors. In cases of cremation, they appear to have been added to the urn in the latter stages of the process. This can perhaps reinforce the insight into the way that prostheses were viewed by their users and, in turn, the way that prostheses and prosthesis users were viewed by their peers that we have already been given by extremity prostheses.

Unlike extremity or facial prostheses, an ancient wig or hairpiece was not necessarily designed, commissioned, and manufactured specifically for an individual in order to meet their own unique set of needs, so such items could potentially have been reused. The fact that this does not seem to have occurred, at least in the cases for which we have evidence, is certainly significant. It appears that wigs and hair pieces were viewed, both by their users and by others, as a true substitute for or replacement of the individual's missing body part. If they were given away, it was into the perpetual keeping of a deity as a votive offering.[98]

[98] Myrinus, *Greek Anthology* 6.254.

CHAPTER 4

Design, Commission, and Manufacture of Prostheses

Introduction

In the twenty-first century, a prosthesis is universally recognised as a piece of medical technology. In the United Kingdom, the National Health Service houses regional Artificial Limb and Appliance Centres, where prosthetists design and manufacture prostheses by working in tandem with surgeons, physicians, physiotherapists, and – most importantly – the amputees themselves.[1] However, there are also increasing numbers of private companies, such as the Bespoke Prosthetics and Orthotics Company, that provide similar services for a fee.[2] Some of these companies, such as the Alternative Limb Project, offer not just what they describe as 'realistic' prostheses, but also 'alternative' ones.[3] Additionally, the advent of 3D printing has been a significant development in recent years, facilitating the efforts of companies that aim to create affordable prostheses for children, such as Limbitless Solutions, or organisations that seek to provide them for free, such as the University of Glasgow's student society Handprints e-NABLE Scotland.[4]

By contrast, however, in classical antiquity prostheses do not appear to have been perceived as a type of medical technology; they are not mentioned once in the surviving Greek or Latin medical literature, despite several lengthy discussions of amputation included therein, or in the surviving Greek or Latin technical literature that devotes space to assorted different types of medical apparatus. Thus, it is not a surprise that, to date, examinations of the use of technology for medical purposes in classical

[1] NHS: www.nhs.uk/Conditions/Amputation/Pages/Introduction.aspx#Prosthetics (accessed January 2021).

[2] Bespoke Prosthetics and Orthotics Ltd: www.bespoke-po.com/ (accessed August 2022).

[3] Alternative Limb Project: www.thealternativelimbproject.com/ (accessed January 2021).

[4] Limbitless Solutions: https://limbitless-solutions.org/ (accessed January 2021); Handprints e-NABLE Scotland: www.glasgowstudent.net/clubs/listings/handprints-enable-scotland/ (accessed January 2021).

antiquity have concentrated primarily on medical instruments; there have been some attempts to cover medical machines within discussions of the history of technology, but prostheses and other types of assistive technology have not featured.[5]

What about other types of evidence? Regarding documentary evidence, there are currently only two known references to individuals whose occupations could potentially have involved manufacturing prostheses. The first of these is found in an inscription that cannot be dated precisely but is thought to have been inscribed and set up along the Via Appia in Rome at some point between the first and third centuries CE. The inscription comprises an epitaph set up by Lucius Licinius Patroclus in memory of his brother:

> To the Spirits of the Departed; to Lucius Licinius Statorianus, son of Lucius; Lucius Licinius Patroclus, freedman of Lucius, maker of artificial eyes, set this up for his dearest brother.[6]

Patroclus gives his occupation as a 'maker of artificial eyes' (*faber ocular-iarius*). The term used here is unique, a *hapax legomenon*, and so it is unclear whether these artificial eyes were made for statues or for people, or perhaps even for both. The common assumption is the former.[7] Yet another inscription found in a grave near the Porta Capena states rather more definitively that an individual named Marcus Rapilius Serapio, presumably the individual whose grave the inscription was found in, 'inserted eyes into statues'.[8]

The second of these is found in a documentary papyrus dating to around 118 CE.[9] The papyrus is part of the Apollonios Archive and comprises a letter sent from a woman named Aline to her husband Apollonios, the *strategos* of the Hermopolite nome in Egypt during the period of the Jewish Revolt that lasted from 115 to 117 CE. In it, Aline updates Apollonios regarding her efforts to have a shrine built on their estate:

> Aline to Apollonios her brother, greetings. We give thanks to all the gods because of your safety … You wrote about your health … You are

[5] For studies on medical instruments, see the extensive work of Lawrence Bliquez, Ralph Jackson, Ernst Künzl, and Patricia Baker. For medical machines, see Drachmann, 1963, pp. 171–85; very briefly, Wilson, 2008, pp. 345–6.

[6] *CIL* VI 9402 = *Inscr. Grut.* 645 (trans. J. Draycott): *Dis Manibus / L(ucio) Licinio L(uci) f(ilius) Stato {i}ria/no L(ucius) Licinius L(uci) l(ibertus) Patroclus / faber oculariarius / frat(ri) cariss(imo) f(ecit).*

[7] See, for example, Holleran, 2012, p. 27.

[8] *CIL* VI 9403 = *ILS* 7713 (trans. J. Draycott): *M. Rapilius Serapio oculos reposuit statuis.*

[9] *P.Giss.* 20; also known as *W.Chr.* 94 and *P.Giss.Apoll.*11: http://papyri.info/ddbdp/p.giss.apoll;;11 (accessed January 2021). Translation and discussion of the papyrus in the context of it as an example of women's writing can be found in Bagnall and Cribiore, 2006.

> building . . . builders and carpenters . . . I am working at the wool as you wrote . . . tell me by letter which colour pleases you or send me a small sample of it. If you want your light, white garment to fall down, give heed to the purple. I was given a response by the Dioscuri of your estate, and a shrine has been built for them. **Areios the maker of artificial limbs provides the service for them; he was saying, 'If Apollonios writes to me about it, I will serve free of charge'. You really ought to write him a couple of lines, in order for him to come forward promptly in a manner worthy of you and the gods.** Your children are in good health and salute you. Write to us continuously about your health. Send what you have of Diskas . . . [Address on the verso] To Apollonios her brother.[10]

The term used to refer to Areios' occupation, *kōloplastēs* (*ὁ κωλοπλάστης*), is, like Lucius Licinius Patroclus' occupation *faber oculariarius*, a *hapax legomenon*, and has been translated as a 'manufacturer of artificial limbs'. Considering the context within which Areios is being discussed, it is possible that what he manufactures are votive offerings in the form of limbs.[11] However, the term that is normally used to indicate a manufacturer of votive offerings is *koroplastēs* (ὁ κοροπλάστης).

Additionally, in a discussion of artificial teeth found in the Talmud, the rabbis refer to them as being made by a *nagra* in response to a specific commission, and this Hebrew word can be translated as either 'carpenter' or, more generally, 'artisan'.[12] Another possible translation could be 'turner', if the artificial teeth were made from ivory.[13]

This demonstrates a fundamental difference between ancient and contemporary medical practice in relation to orthopaedic surgery, recovery, and rehabilitation: it was the individual's responsibility to prepare themselves for life with an impairment and equip themselves with the aids necessary to live this life, not their surgeon's nor their physician's nor

[10] *P.Giss.* 20 (trans. R. Bagnall, R. Cribiore and E. Ahtaridis, with adjustments; emphasis added): Ἀλινὴ Ἀπο[λλωνίῳ τῶι] ἀδελφῶ[ι . . . χαίρειν.] εὐχαριστοῦμεν πᾶ[σι τοῖς θεοῖς περὶ τῆς ὑγίας] σου ὅτι σε καὶ ἀπο[. . .] ἡ ἐπιστολή σου τὴν [. . .] που ἀπέστρεψεν [. . .] μων. ἡ δὲ προέλε[υσις . . .] ὥστε μηδὲν θεωρεῖσθα[ι . . .] ἀηδῶς ἔχειν διὰ τὸ διαστ[. . .] γενόμενον μετὰ κισσον[. . . ἔγρᾰ] ψας περὶ τῆς ὑγίας σο[υ . . . κ . . .] νοι εἰσίν. οἰκοδομ[εῖς . . .]ως[. . .] οἰκοδόμοις καὶ τέκτο[σι . . .]χο[. . .] γιον. ἐργά[σο]μαι τὰ ἔρια [καθὰ] ἔγρα[ψάς μοι ὁποῖ-] ον δέ σοι χρῶ[μ]α ἀρέσκει [δήλω]σον δι' ἐπ[ισ] τολῆς ἢ μεικρὸν ἔρ[γο]ν αὐτοῦ π[έμψο]ν. εἰ θέλεις ἀνᾰ βληθῆναί σ[ου τ]ὴν ἰσχνὴ[ν λε]υκὴν στολήν, φρόντισον τῆς πο̣[ρ]φύρας. ἐχρ[η]ματίσ[θ]ην ὑπὸ τῶν Διοσκούρων τῆς κτήσεως [σ]ου καὶ ᾠκοδόμηται αὐτῶν ὁ τόπος καὶ Ἄρειος [ὁ] κωλοπλάστης θεραπεύει αὐτοὺς καὶ ἔλεγ[ε]ν ὅτι, ἐὰ [ν] Ἀπολλώνιός μοι γράψῃ περὶ αὐτ[ῶ]ν̣, [θεραπεύ]σω προῖκα. ἀξιώσεις οὖν δίστιχον αὐτῶι γραφῆναι, ἵνα ἀξίως σου καὶ τῶν θεῶν ἀόκνως προσέλθῃ. τὰ παιδία σου ἔρρωται καὶ [ἀσπάζ] ε̣[τα]ί σε. σῦχ<ν>ῶς ἡμῖν γράφε περὶ τῆ[ς ὑγίας σου· πάντα ἃ] ἔχεις Δισκᾶτος πέμψον [. . .] [. . .]οι [. . .] Ἀπολλωνίωι ἀδελφῶι.

[11] For fuller discussion of Aline and Apollonios' healing shrine, see Draycott, 2014.

[12] Cohen and Stern, 1973, p. 103. [13] Cohen and Stern, 1973, p. 103.

any other type of healthcare practitioner's.[14] In the Hippocratic treatise *On Joints*, the author, who does not seem to subscribe to this rather narrow view of the ancient physician's remit, attempts to offer something of an explanation for this oversight before offering a justification for bothering to include information on how crutches can rehabilitate a patient in a medical treatise:

> One might say that such matters are outside the healing art. Why, forsooth, trouble one's mind further about cases which have become incurable? This is far from the right attitude. The investigation of these matters too belongs to the same science; it is impossible to separate them from one another. In curable cases we must contrive ways to prevent their becoming incurable, studying the best means for hindering their advance to incurability; while one must study incurable cases so as to avoid doing harm by useless efforts. Brilliant and effective forecasts are made by distinguishing the way, manner and time in which each case will end, whether it takes the turn to recovery or to incurability.[15]

Thus the author, having set out their stall regarding their view of rehabilitation and the importance of the physician's input into the patient's assistive technology, proceeds to recommend a variety of different types of crutch as, depending on the condition diagnosed and the treatment prescribed, the patient will require a particular type of crutch: one size does certainly not fit all.[16] It is clear that this physician, at least, viewed assistive technology as an integral part of the treatment they provided, even if his (or her) peers did not.

In accordance with this approach to rehabilitation, the literary and documentary accounts that we do have that mention prostheses indicate that they were highly individualised, and that individual prosthesis users went to a considerable amount of trouble to design, commission, and manufacture them, behaviour which met with varying responses from contemporaries. Surviving examples of prostheses, such as the Greville Chester Toe and the Cairo Toe, two roughly contemporary but very

[14] On rehabilitation in antiquity, see Horstmanshoff, 2012, although despite the title, this article does not actually discuss ancient rehabilitation in any kind of detail.

[15] Hippoc. *Art.* 58 (trans. E. T. Withington): γυμνάσια προσκρατύνει αὐτό. φαίη μὲν οὖν ἄν τις, ἔξω ἰητρικῆς τὰ τοιαῦτα εἶναι· τί γὰρ δῆθεν δεῖ περὶ τῶν ἤδη ἀνηκέστων γεγονότων ἔτι προσσυνιέναι; πολλοῦ δὲ δὲ οὕτως ἔχειν· τῆς γὰρ αὐτῆς γνώμης καὶ ταῦτα συνιέναι· οὐ γὰρ οἷόν τε ἀπαλλοτριωθῆναι ἀπ᾽ ἀλλήλων. δεῖ μὲν γὰρ ἐς τὰ ἀκεστὰ μηχανάασθαι, ὅπως μὴ ἀνήκεστα ἔσται, συνιέντα ὅπῃ ἂν μάλιστα κωλυτέα ἐς τὸ ἀνήκεστον ἐλθεῖν· δεῖ δὲ τὰ ἀνήκεστα συνιέναι, ὡς μὴ μάτην λυμαίνηται· τὰ δὲ προῤῥήματα λαμπρὰ καὶ ἀγωνιστικὰ ἀπὸ τοῦ διαγινώσκειν ὅπῃ ἕκαστον καὶ οἵως καὶ ὁπότε τελευτήσει, ἤν τε ἐς τὸ ἀκεστὸν τράπηται, ἤν τε ἐς τὸ ἀνήκεστον.

[16] Hippoc. *Art.* 58.

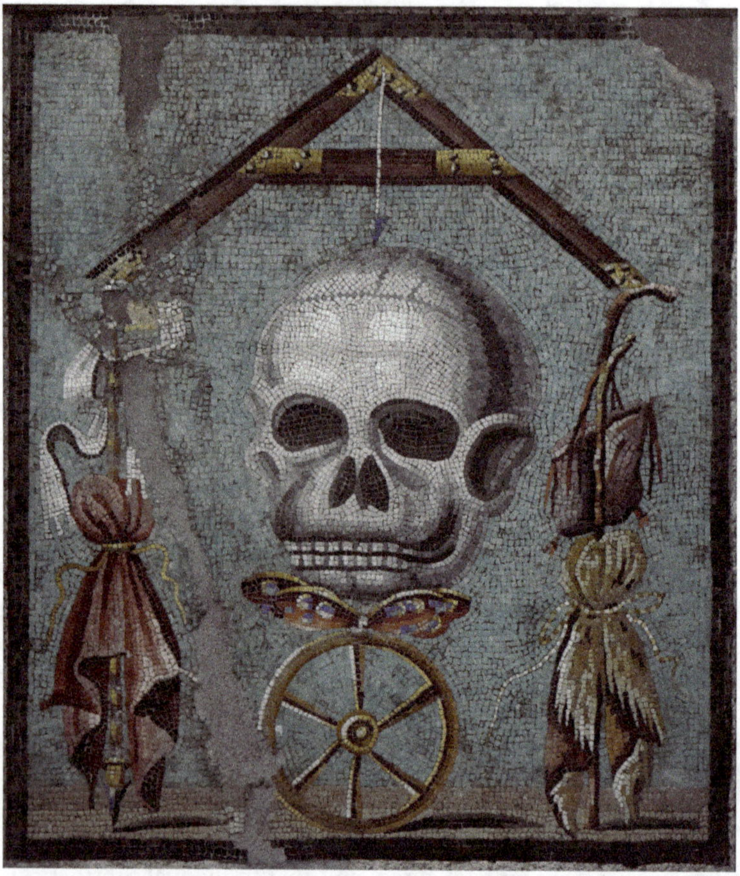

Figure 4.1 'Memento Mori' mosaic from the triclinium of the House/Workshop I.5.2, Pompeii, 30 BCE–14 CE. National Archaeological Museum of Naples inv. 109982. Image courtesy of Alamy.

different Egyptian prosthetic toes, support this. Even though these two prostheses served as replacements for the same lost body part (the big toe) and were utilised in the same way (fitted over the end of the foot and securely fastened with ties), they are very different objects. Artefacts such as these can provide an insight into the lived experience of impaired and disabled individuals in antiquity, a group that is often assumed to have been poor, pitiful, and entirely marginalised – in point of fact, a stick is one of the standard attributes of the beggar in ancient art. See, for example, the famous 'Momento Mori' mosaic recovered from the triclinium of a house turned workshop at Pompeii, dating to the period 30 BCE–14 CE, depicting death as the great leveller that cancels out all differences in class, status, and wealth. Here, the rich are represented by a purple robe and an elaborate sceptre on the left-hand side, while the poor are represented by a goatskin, a scrip, and a stick on the right-hand side.[17] These assumptions frequently carry over into later historical periods and even influence attitudes today. They can elucidate our understanding not only of the practical aspects of living with an impairment or disability (e.g. how did one achieve some semblance of, or any level of, physical mobility), but also of other aspects of the lives of the individuals that used them, such as their wealth and status; their access to knowledge, skill, and expertise in relation to the crafts of woodwork, metalwork, and leatherwork; their understanding of science and technology; and the extent to which its theoretical principles were applied to daily life, etc., thus enabling a much more developed understanding of this section of ancient society – one that has not yet been achieved despite a growing interest in impairment and disability in classical antiquity among scholars over the last two decades.

In this chapter, I will examine the literary, documentary, and archaeological evidence for the design, commission, and manufacture of prostheses in classical antiquity, and explore what it can tell us about prostheses, prosthesis use, and prosthesis users in classical antiquity.

Artisans

The earliest reference to a prosthesis in classical literature that can be viewed as historical rather than mythological is found in Herodotus' *Histories* and its date can be pinpointed to 479 BCE.[18] This account is also reasonably detailed, both with regard to the process by which the limb was lost, and with regard to the process by which it was replaced. According to Herodotus, Hegesistratus of Elis, a diviner for the Persians, after amputating part of his own foot to extricate himself from shackles and in doing so facilitate his escape from Spartan captivity, 'made himself a foot of wood'.[19] The Greek verb used, προσποιέω, literally means 'make over, add, or attach', and so it is possible that Hegesistratus did, in fact, make the

[17] National Archaeological Museum of Naples inv. 109982.

[18] This is not, however, the earliest reference to prostheses in world literature. This is found in the *Rigveda*, which was produced in India in the period *circa* 1500–1200 BCE, and it comprises an account of Vishpala, a female warrior with an iron leg.

[19] Hdt. 9.36–7 (trans. A. D. Godley): προσποιησάμενος ξύλινον πόδα.

extremity prosthesis himself, whittling or carving it from a suitable piece of wood. According to Gregory of Tours, a cleric from Poitiers, who lost the use of one of his feet after what he claimed was an assault by a demon, did just that:

> He cut a staff to the height of his knee, put a piece of leather on top of it, bent his foot back, and [attached] the staff to his knee; with the assistance of this peg leg he regained his mobility when he tried to move on foot.[20]

Yet it is also possible that Hegesistratus' prosthesis was made for him by one or more artisans, such as a carpenter, or a carpenter collaborating with a leather-worker, if this prosthesis was similar to the two prosthetic toes that have survived from first millennium BCE Egypt, which, although one was made of wood and the other made of cartonnage, were both tied on to the foot with leather laces.[21] This episode is contemporaneous with the surgical treatises included in the Hippocratic Corpus, and while none of these treatises mention extremity prostheses, they do discuss in detail the use of aids such as walking sticks, crutches, and corrective footwear, and so it may be possible to extrapolate something of the process of creating a prosthesis from the process of creating other types of assistive technology.

The use of mobility aids – staffs, walking sticks, canes, crutches – in classical antiquity has not been comprehensively studied.[22] However, even a cursory glance at the scattered ancient literary and material evidence for them indicates that these were deceptively complicated objects with a wealth of overt and covert significances.[23] The ways in which these items are depicted in material culture vary significantly. While they are frequently depicted in use by the elderly or otherwise infirm, this is not always the case; see, for example, Figure 4.2: this statuette from the third or second century BCE, which depicts a beautiful young woman posing in the manner of the goddess Aphrodite removing her sandal while simultaneously using a crutch to support herself. While they were certainly used for the practical purpose of walking, whether the user was afflicted with some sort of mobility impairment or not, they were also utilised for the symbolic purpose of indicating particular states such as positions of authority, leisure, and old age.[24] Consequently, considerable thought could go into, and considerable resources could be expended on,

[20] Gregory of Tours, *VM* 3.9 (trans. R. Van Dam): *Qui inciso fuste ad mensuram geniculi, et pelle superposita ad ipsum geniculum, extenso retrorsum vestigio, gressum, quem pede nitebatur agere, fuste adminiculante perficiebat.*

[21] See Finch, 2019 for details.

[22] Loebl and Nunn, 1997, p. 450. However, see now Draycott, in press b.

[23] Draycott, in press b.

[24] Loebl and Nunn, 1997; Draycott, in press b.

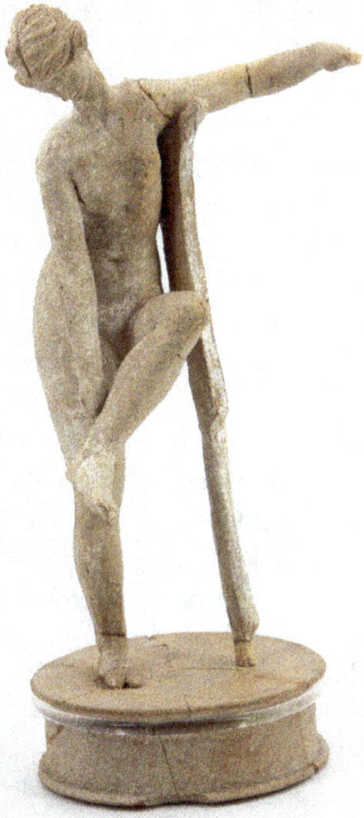

Figure 4.2 Italian statuette, third century or second century BCE. Museo Archeologico Nazionale di Taranto inv. 106495. Image courtesy of Museo Archeologico Nazionale di Taranto.

the creation of one. This started with the materials from which one was made: Theophrastus, in his botanical writing, recommended mallow (*Malva sylvestris*) for the creation of walking sticks because it grew to great heights quickly and was strong, and recommended bay (*Laurus nobilis*) specifically for the creation of walking sticks for the elderly because it was lightweight, although olive wood was frequently as well, presumably partly because its nature made it particularly suitable for tools but also because of its ubiquity in the ancient Mediterranean.[25] As discussed earlier, the author of the Hippocratic treatise *On Joints* described a variety of different types of crutch that could be used by

[25] Theophr. *Hist. pl.* 1.3.2, 5.7.7.

those suffering from mobility impairments, the type of crutch recommended depending very much upon the precise nature of the impairment.[26] For untreated dislocations that had occurred *in utero* or in early childhood, he (or she) advised either one or two crutches.[27] For dislocations that occurred in adulthood and were not successfully reduced, leading to one leg being significantly shorter than the other, he (or she) advised using a long crutch if the patient was capable of walking erect but either could not or did not want to place their foot on the ground, or a shorter crutch if they could or wanted to place their foot on the ground.[28] The author of *Instruments of Reduction* likewise made recommendations regarding the use of mobility aids, similar but not identical to those of the author of *On Joints*, and advised that a crutch should be short rather than long since if it were long the user would not use the impaired foot.[29]

There is some bioarchaeological evidence for the use of assistive technology in the form of staffs, sticks, canes, and crutches, the purposes of which seem to have been assistance with support and mobility by the physically impaired, and this shows the considerable variety of applications of this type of assistive technology. A skeleton from the Roman necropolis of Casalecchio di Reno in Bologna, dating to the second or third century CE, shows pathological changes in the upper body, particularly on the right hand side of the upper body, that is consistent with the use of one or perhaps even two pieces of assistive technology.[30] The deceased, an elderly male, suffered from considerable degeneration of the right hip, to the extent that his right foot would have been unable to touch the ground, which led him to need to utilise at least one and probably two pieces of assistive technology to enable locomotion, in line with the advice given by the author of *On Joints*.[31] These may have consisted of a crutch under his arm on the right hand side and a walking stick in his hand on the left hand side.[32] A skeleton from the Le Colombier cemetery in Vaison-la-Romaine, which dates to the fifth or sixth century CE, attests pathological changes on the right scapula that are consistent with crutch use.[33] The deceased, a male aged around 50–60 years old who has been tentatively identified as an enslaved individual based on the location of his burial in the cemetery, exhibited a stress fracture on his right scapula, indicating that he utilised a crutch on the right-hand side of his body, perhaps due to osteoarthritis in his right hip. Finally, a skeleton from the Shurafa cemetery near

[26] Hippoc. *Art.* 58. [27] Hippoc. *Art.* 53. [28] Hippoc. *Art.* 58. [29] Hippoc. *Mochl.* 23.

[30] Belcastro and Mariotti, 2000, p. 532; another individual from the same cemetery shows evidence for crutch use, but this is not as clear.

[31] Belcastro and Mariotti, 2000, pp. 530–1. [32] Belcastro and Mariotti, 2000, p. 538.

[33] Darton, 2010.

Helouan, of a man aged at least thirty years old who suffered from hydrocephalus which resulted in hemiplegia (partial paralysis) of the left-hand side of his body which necessitated the use of some sort of assistive technology in order to facilitate physical mobility, and the use of a long staff, held in both hands across the body as a means of supporting the weaker left-hand side, has been proposed as a solution to this individual's particular set of needs.[34]

Likewise, it is clear that considerable thought went into, and considerable resources were expended on, the creation of the corrective footwear recommended for the treatment of congenital conditions that affected the feet and, as a result, affected physical mobility, such as club-foot (*Talipes equinovarus*).[35] The author of *On Joints* advised treatment as early as possible, dressing and bandaging the foot in a very particular way, and then adding a sole made from a firm substance such as stiff leather or lead.[36] It is recognised that there will be variations in the condition and that the dressings and bandages should be likewise varied.[37] If the manual adjustment, dressing, and bandaging are not sufficient, one can go a step further and utilise corrective footwear. Something akin to a Chian or Cretan boot is advised because they were apparently unyielding.[38] In line with this advice, there are several ancient literary references to individuals with impaired feet utilising corrective footwear, although in both cases they unfortunately lost one or both of their shoes. The first is a music master named Damonidas, who lost a pair of boots that were specially made for his impaired feet, and, depending upon how you interpret his response, either rather generously or rather snidely prayed that they might fit the feet of the thief.[39] The second is a musician named Dorion, who lost his specially made shoe at a party, which led him to curse the thief that the shoe might come to fit him or, potentially, her.[40]

There is some archaeological evidence for the production and use of corrective footwear in antiquity. More than 4,000 shoes dating from the period of the first to the fourth centuries CE have been excavated at the

[34] Derry, 1913, pp. 455–6.

[35] On congenital deformities of the legs and feet, see Roberts and Manchester, 2010, pp. 57–9; for an example of clubfoot that was left untreated from a Romano-British cemetery, see Roberts et al., 2004. The modern incidence of *Talipes equinovarus* is 1 in 800–1,000 births, and it is more common in males and runs in families. See, for example, Hippoc. *Morb. sacr.* 3; Arist. *Hist. an.* 585b, 586a; Plin. *HN* 7.11.50 for ancient understandings regarding impairment and disability being heritable conditions. For depictions in ancient art, see Grmek and Gourevitch, 1998, pp. 151–2, pp. 282–7; Ziskowski, 2012. For discussion of the condition, see Horstmanshoff, 2013.

[36] Hippoc. *Art.* 62. For commentary, see Michler, 1963.

[37] Hippoc. *Art.* 62; see also Hippoc. *Mochl.* 32.

[38] Hippoc. *Art.* 62.

[39] Plut. *Mor.* 18d.

[40] Ath. 8.338a.

Roman fort of Vindolanda on Hadrian's Wall. Some of these shoes attest evidence of a certain amount of podiatric knowledge on the part of the individuals who made them, as they appear to have been altered at the initial point of production to mitigate the effects of over-supinated or over-pronated gait.[41] These shoes have metal bars fitted to the side of the heels on the outside of the shoes in order to provide extra support to the part of the foot that was turning either inward or outward.[42] More minor adjustments comprising clusters of hobnails inserted into particular parts of the soles can also be found on some shoes.[43] This is particularly common on the arch of the foot and the heel of the foot.[44] Unlike the metal bars that were most likely added by the shoemaker, the hobnails could have been added to the soles of the shoes at a subsequent point in time and not necessarily by a professional shoemaker. And, while not strictly corrective, there is literary evidence that suggests that shoes were altered to accommodate the requirements of individuals who suffered from gout, and this was accomplished by stuffing them with dog fur, presumably to soften the impact of leather on tender skin.[45]

Who would have made these pieces of assistive technology? In the case of staffs, sticks, walking sticks, canes, and crutches, perhaps a carpenter. In the case of corrective footwear, probably a shoemaker. According to Xenophon, shoemaking could be a highly specialised profession:

> In large cities, on the other hand, inasmuch as many people have demands to make upon each branch of industry, one trade alone, and very often even less than a whole trade, is enough to support a man: one man, for instance, makes shoes for men, and another for women; and there are places even where one man earns a living by only stitching shoes, another by cutting them out, another by sewing the uppers together, while there is another who performs none of these operations but only assembles the parts. It follows, therefore, as a matter of course, that he who devotes himself to a very highly specialized line of work is bound to do it in the best possible manner.[46]

Thus, some types of shoemakers might have been more suited to the production of corrective footwear than others. Shoemakers are frequently depicted in material culture in conjunction with the tools of their trade and

[41] Greene, 2019, p. 310. [42] See Vindolanda L–1992–3745 for an example.

[43] See Vindolanda L–1988–2118 for an example. [44] Greene, 2019, p. 319.

[45] Scribonius Largus, *Compositiones medicamentorum* 161.

[46] Xen. *Cyr.* 8.2.5 (trans. W. Miller): ἐν δὲ ταῖς μεγάλαις πόλεσι διὰ τὸ πολλοὺς ἑκάστου δεῖσθαι ἀρκεῖ καὶ μία ἑκάστῳ τέχνη εἰς τὸ τρέφεσθαι· πολλάκις δὲ οὐδ᾽ ὅλη μία· ἀλλ᾽ ὑποδήματα ποιεῖ ὁ μὲν ἀνδρεῖα, ὁ δὲ γυναικεῖα· ἔστι δὲ ἔνθα καὶ ὑποδήματα ὁ μὲν νευρορραφῶν μόνον τρέφεται, ὁ δὲ σχίζων, ὁ δὲ χιτῶνας μόνον συντέμνων, ὁ δέ γε τούτων οὐδὲν ποιῶν ἀλλὰ συντιθεὶς ταῦτα. ἀνάγκη οὖν τὸν ἐν βραχυτάτῳ διατρίβοντα ἔργῳ τοῦτον καὶ ἄριστα δὴ ἠναγκάσθαι τοῦτο ποιεῖν.

the products that they produced, and there does appear to be some variety in these depictions: see, for example, the funerary monument of Xanthippos, dating from around 420 BCE, in which he sits in a high-backed chair and presents his shoemaker's last.[47] Both the carpenter and the shoemaker, however, would in all likelihood have been working in conjunction with a physician who could supervise, instruct, and advise them during the manufacturing process. Would they have also made prostheses? A specialist artisan such as a shoemaker did not necessarily only produce footwear. One of Herodas' poems depicts two women, Coritto and Metro, discussing Coritto's newly acquired scarlet leather dildo, which Metro covets.[48] When Metro asks how Coritto came to have it, she replies that she was referred to the shoemaker Cerdon.[49] In the following poem, Herodas depicts Metro patronising the shoemaker in order to acquire a similar dildo for herself.[50] Cerdon presents a range of items to Metro and, while they are presented as women's shoes, it is thought that this catalogue of shoes is a carefully curated series of puns and sexual innuendos.[51] If shoemakers were in the habit of producing dildos and – presumably – the phalluses used in theatrical performances, it is not beyond the realms of possibility that they might also have produced other leather body parts, such as fingers, hands, toes, or feet, if commissioned to do so. After all, the mid-second century Alexandrian grammarian Dionysius was known as Dionysius Skytobrachion in an attempt to differentiate him from the many other ancient authors with the same name, the sobriquet translating to 'of the leather arm'. Although this has been interpreted as a reference to his prolific literary output (essentially, him having written so much that his arm must have been like leather), it could potentially be a reference to a prosthetic arm made from leather.[52] In the poems, Coritto is referred to Cerdon by the tanner Candas' acquaintance Artemis, and then she in turn refers Metro to Cerdon, so we can see how an amputee might have come to find an artisan willing or able to accommodate them.

[47] British Museum inventory 1805.0703.183; the object that he is holding has also been interpreted as an anatomical votive, perhaps indicating that Xanthippos suffered from some sort of physical impairment, and as a prosthetic foot, perhaps indicating that Xanthippos had undergone an amputation.

[48] Herod. 6. For a clear link being made between a foot and a phallus, see a cup housed in the Ashmolean Museum on which the foot is replaced by a phallus, inv. 1974.344, Beazley Archive 396. For dildos in classical antiquity, see Nelson, 2002.

[49] Herod. 6.87.88. [50] Herod. 7; for discussion of this poem, see Anagnostou-Laoutides, 2015.

[51] Herod. 7.56–64; for discussion of this aspect of the catalogue of shoes, see Sumler, 2010.

[52] Bliquez, 1996, pp. 2662–3, f. 33.

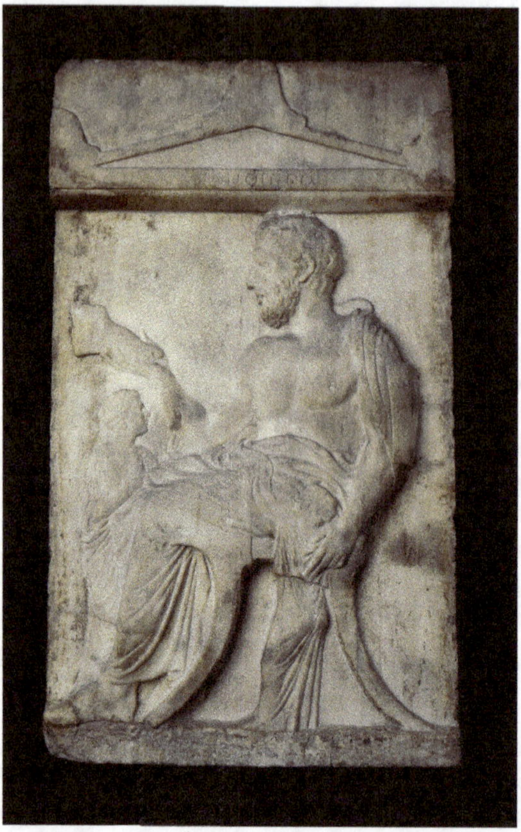

Figure 4.3 Funerary monument of Xanthippos, circa 420 BCE. British Museum inv. 1805, 0703.183. Image courtesy of the British Museum.

It is possible that individuals without much in the way of technical expertise or training could have manufactured rudimentary extremity prostheses such as peg-legs themselves, just as they apparently did walking sticks, as basic carpentry skills were easy to acquire and could be undertaken in one's home with minimal equipment, although we have to question how comfortable and, consequently, how wearable such objects would have been.[53] However, more elaborate objects comprising wood, organic materials, and even metals would have required the services of multiple types of artisan working in collaboration over a potentially

[53] See Arist. *Sph.* 31 for walking sticks; see Acton, 2014, p. 200, for carpentry at home.

extended period of time.[54] While a carpenter could have carved a wooden foot or leg, and potentially even a stick, staff, cane, or crutch to use in conjunction with it, a wooden hand or arm, or even a wooden facial prosthesis such as a nose or set of teeth, at the very least the services of a leather-worker would have been required to produce padding to cushion the socket of the extremity prosthesis, to ensure the user's comfort and prevent or at least minimise chafing, and potentially also as a means of attaching the prosthesis to the body of the user as securely as possible. Close examination of the original Capua Limb did not offer any indication of how it would have been attached to its user, leading to suppositions that some sort of leather or fabric belt would have been worn around the waist and the limb would have been attached to that.[55] Yet, close examination of the remains of the 'Hemmaberg Limb' has revealed that the prosthesis took the form of a cup padded with an organic material such as leather or another kind sort of textile.[56] If some sort of metal were involved – as in the case of the Capua Limb, which was plated with bronze, and of the 'Hemmaberg Limb', which included an iron ring around the socket – the services of one or more metal-workers would have been required too. For facial prostheses comprising luxury materials such as gold, silver, and ivory, the specialist expertise of a goldsmith, a silversmith, and an ivory worker would have been necessary, and epigraphic evidence attests that specialist artisans such as these clustered in cities like Athens and Rome, where it was worth their while to ply their trades.[57]

Although no treatises on the subjects of woodworking, metalworking, leatherworking, or bone and ivory carving written by artisans survive, depictions of artisans undertaking their crafts found in material culture such as frescoes, mosaics, and reliefs can be informative about certain aspects of their trades. Two reliefs of cutlers' workshops dating to the second century CE and on display in the Museo della Civilta Romana show the wares that the cutlers were capable of producing, and among the implements are surgeon's scalpels, indicating that artisans could be called upon to make pieces of medical technology. An interesting snippet of information about the possibilities of collaboration between physicians and artisans can be found in Galen's treatise *On Avoiding Distress*, where he details how he would design his own medical and

[54] During the Medieval period, there is firmer evidence of artisans such as blacksmiths working in collaboration with medical practitioners, at least in the production of herniary belts. See Brozzi, 1993; DeMarchi, 2006; Carbonelli, 1908. Thanks to Ileana Micarelli for bringing this to my attention.

[55] Bliquez, 1996, pp. 2669–70. [56] Eitler and Binder, 2019; Binder et al., 2016.

[57] See Joshel, 1992 for occupational inscriptions from the city of Rome.

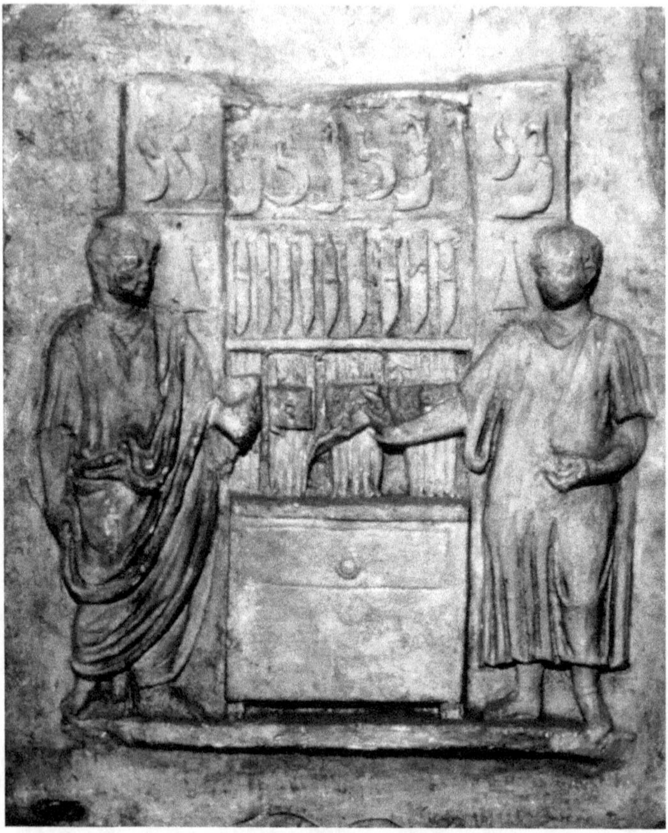

Figure 4.4 Roman relief, second century CE. Image courtesy of Alamy.

surgical instruments, create wax models of them, and then give these models to artisans so that they could create them for him.[58]

Inspiration

Where did individuals get the idea to replace their lost body parts with prostheses? Potentially here the myth of Pelops played a significant role, supplemented by well-known historical exemplars such as Hegesistratus of

[58] Gal. *Ind.* 4–5, 10. For archaeological evidence of the manufacture, or at least the repair, of medical instruments, see a shop from Pompeii in Italy, and another from Dion in Greece; discussion of the manufacture of medical instruments can be found in Bliquez, 2014, pp. 14–16.

Elis and his wooden foot or Marcus Sergius Silus and his iron hand. However, while one might be aware of the possibility of prostheses in theory, how did one go about putting that theory into practice and acquiring one?

In Classical and Hellenistic Greece, individuals were responsible for equipping themselves with their panoply, and while those of modest means might have had to do with hand-me-downs, those of considerable means could afford specially made, highly personalised ones.[59] An example of this has been recovered from one of the Macedonian tombs at Vergina; one of the sets of bones recovered from the tomb is that of a woman aged around thirty years old who has been identified as Philip II's seventh wife, the daughter of the Scythian king Atheas.[60] Bioarchaeological examination of her remains has determined that she had Schmorl's nodes, indicative of horse-riding from an early age, and had suffered a Schatzker type IV fracture of the left tibia, leading to leg shortening, atrophy, knee disfiguration, and mobility impairment.[61] Alongside her remains were a gold-plated quiver, seventy-four arrowheads, spearheads, and a suit of ceremonial armour. The armour includes a pair of gilded bronze greaves that do not match because they were made for a pair of legs where one was shorter and thinner than the other, the result of a poorly healed fracture; the left greave is 39 cm high and its maximum diameter is 30 cm, while the right greave is 41.6 cm high and its maximum diameter is 33.5 cm; thus, the left greave is significantly smaller than the right greave.[62] Here is evidence of an artisan paying attention to the specific medical requirements of their patron, as well as, potentially, the individual in question continuing to go about their business despite their impairment, or even having this business facilitated by their specially commissioned equipment.

Did armour, with its focus on the physical body of the warrior and their specific requirements, inspire prostheses? And were armourers responsible for producing extremity prostheses, whether for soldiers on active duty or veterans, in the first instance? As discussed earlier, it has been suggested that the Capua Limb was inspired by greaves.[63] Since it was recovered from a tomb in Capua that has been dated to around 300 BCE, contemporaneous to the Second Samnite War (327–304 BCE), it has been suggested that

[59] Acton, 2014, p. 137.

[60] See Hdt. 4.71.2 for the Scythian custom of sacrificing one of the king's concubines upon his death and burying her beside him; Antikas and Wynn-Antikas, 2016, p. 682, identify this woman as the first case of a royal woman with a documented disability in ancient Greece.

[61] Antikas and Wynn-Antikas, 2016, p. 689.

[62] Antikas and Wynn-Antikas, 2016, p. 687.

[63] Bliquez, 1996, p. 2672.

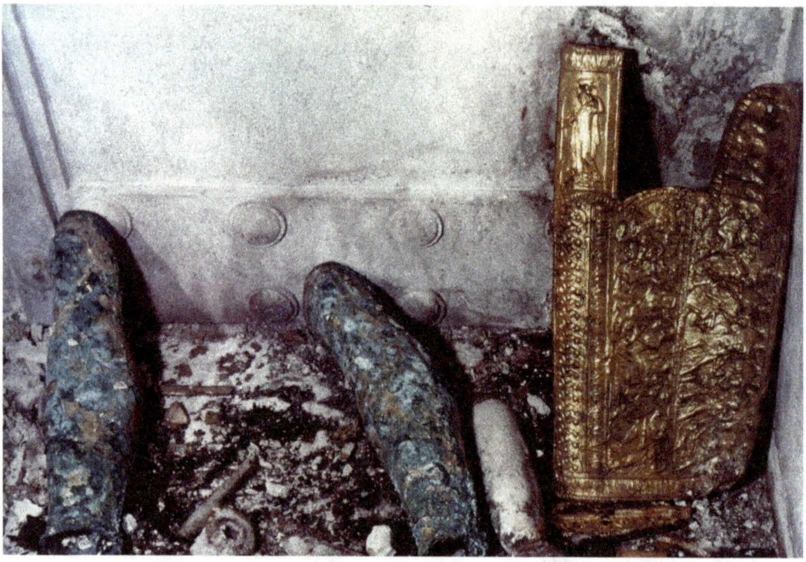

Figure 4.5 Macedonian greaves, from the tomb of Philip II of Macedonia, Amphipolis. Image courtesy of Alamy.

it was made for either a soldier or a gladiator who lost his leg in combat.[64] Since Capua was the chief centre for copper and bronze production in antiquity, it makes sense that an extremity prosthesis created there would utilise both the material and the creativity and skill of the artisans that made their livings working it.[65] Slightly later in date, the iron hand of Marcus Sergius Silus seems to have been designed with military application in mind, since he used it as a means of holding his shield. Since he lost his right hand fighting in the Second Punic War (218–201 BCE) yet wished to continue as a soldier, it makes sense that his prosthesis would have been designed, commissioned, and manufactured with that aim uppermost in mind. Since Roman soldiers of this period did not wear gauntlets, that piece of military equipment cannot have inspired Silus' hand the way that greaves apparently inspired the Capua Limb, and, if we consider the function of this hand, it seems to have been intended primarily as a way of holding a shield rather than anything else.[66] If Silus' prosthetic hand was intended to simply support his shield, we might imagine a simple cap

[64] Bliquez, 1996, p. 2671. [65] Plin. *HN* 34.95.

[66] In a manner of speaking, shields can provide an introduction to thinking about the logistics of prostheses since both need to be worn, carried, and handled by their users, both need to be tough yet

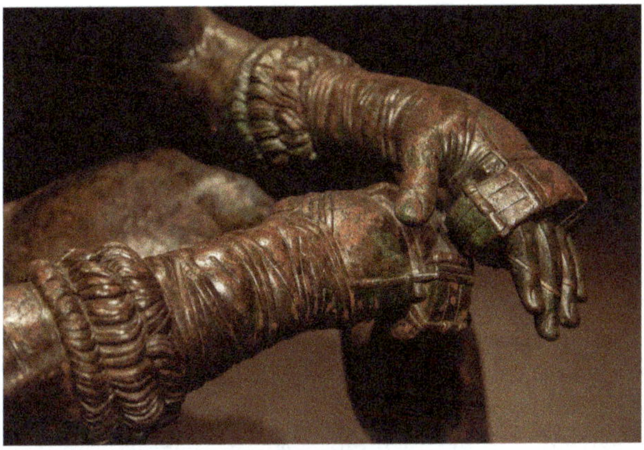

Figure 4.6 Detail of the Thermae Boxer, Baths of Constantine, Rome, third–second century BCE. Palazzo Massimo alle Terme inv. 1055. Image courtesy of Alamy.

placed over the stump to hold the shield in place used in conjunction with one or more leather straps attaching the shield to Silus' arm and torso. But Pliny does say 'iron hand' specifically, so potentially we need to envisage something more like a gauntlet or a boxing glove.[67] While Greek and Roman soldiers did not wear gauntlets, athletes who engaged in sports such as boxing and wrestling did, so it is possible that we should look to those for both inspiration for Silus' hand and an understanding of how it might have been possible to use it to bear a shield. Additionally, it is worth considering that the right hand, as the sword hand, was particularly vulnerable to attack and there are numerous literary accounts of soldiers losing theirs during combat, so it seems unlikely that Silus would have been the only one in this position, particularly since his story seems to have been so well known and so inspirational during the Roman Republic and Empire. While it is true that to date no archaeological examples of prosthetic hands or arms dating to the Graeco-Roman period have been found, there are references in ancient literature to prosthetic hands made from gold and ivory.[68]

The surviving examples indicate that extremity prostheses were extremely personal: they were designed, commissioned, and manufactured

pliable, and both are made from multiple different materials working in conjunction with each other. For discussion of how a shield could be shaped by the body of its user, see Noel, 2019.

67 Palazzo Massimo alle Terme inv. 1055.

68 Stat. *Theb.* 94–7; Dio Chrys. *Or.* 8.28. See also an improvised prosthetic hand comprising a knife strapped to the wrist from Longobard Italy; Micarelli et al., 2018.

according to an individual's specific preferences or requirements. Due to the technical knowledge, skill, and expertise required, not just in relation to the trade itself but also in relation to the capabilities of the human body, it is likely that the same artisans that produced personalised armour and weapons for ancient soldiers produced personalised prostheses for wounded soldiers and veterans.[69] Considering the ancient association of the impaired and disabled with crafts such as metalwork, epitomised by the Greek god Hephaistos and his Roman counterpart Vulcan, it is even possible that ancient artisans drew on their own experiences of impairment to inspire their innovative creations.[70] In one of Lucilius' epigrams, he mentions a blacksmith who, in addition to having a wife named Aphrodite and a son named Eros, had an impaired leg, making his similarity to Hephaistos extreme.[71] Thus, veterans such as Hegesistratus, the anonymous Capuan, and Marcus Sergius Silus would have been able to defy their societies' expectations and continue to play noteworthy roles in it at moments of historical significance, in which case their prostheses may then have inspired those of others.

Yet what of other types of prostheses – facial prostheses such as dental appliances and dentures, and wigs and hair pieces? These potentially had a very different trajectory, in keeping with the ways in which they are described in ancient literature as personal ornamentation and cosmetics. It is more appropriate to equate Etruscan dental appliances with jewellery and other types of personal ornamentation, and since they did not seem to have had a physical function but rather a symbolic one, we should perhaps speak of them having 'wearers' rather than 'users'. The gold bands replaced teeth but were not intended as a means of restoring the functionality of the lost teeth and assisting the wearer with tasks requiring use of the mouth and the teeth, such as speech and eating. They were, however, designed to be noticed as soon as the wearer opened her mouth, and serve as an indicator of her wealth, status, and prestige, and presumably a woman who wore gold in her mouth also wore gold elsewhere in the form of

[69] For discussion of the relationship between impairment and disability, and crafts, see Draycott, in press a.

[70] There seems to have been a consistent connection between physical impairment and crafts in classical antiquity, and this connection was expressed in a number of different ways. We see impaired individuals resorting to crafting to make a living and contribute to their communities (e.g. Hippoc. *Art.* 53), impaired individuals using their knowledge of crafting to create assistive technology for themselves and others (e.g. Hom. *Il.* 18.418–21), and individuals who craft for a living becoming impaired as a result of their crafting (e.g. Xen. *Oec.* 6.2; Arist. *Oec.* 1.2.3; Arist. *Pol.* 1.4.3–4, 8.2.1; Luc. *Somn.* 6–13).

[71] Lucilius, *Greek Anthology* 11.307.

earrings, necklaces, rings, hair ornaments, etc.: all these pieces of personal ornamentation worked in conjunction with each other to create a striking visual effect. Perhaps Etruscan gold jewellery inspired the creation of the dental appliances in the first place; there are certainly similarities in the gold-working techniques used to make Etruscan jewellery and Etruscan dental appliances, indicating that the same goldsmiths were responsible for both.[72] It has been proposed that the dental appliances were created as a means of obscuring the unsightly signs of tooth evulsion that women of neighbouring Italic tribes had undergone before joining Etruscan society through marriage.[73] In this way, something perceived as a flaw could be repurposed as an opportunity to emphasise one's more socially acceptable and desirable qualities. While later in date and different in form, it would appear that Roman and Jewish dental appliances and dentures were produced with similar aims in mind, as when they are mentioned in ancient literature they are generally done so in connection with women, their physical appearances, and other types of enhancement.

As for wigs and hair pieces, these had long been used as part of costumes in theatrical performances, a means of changing one's appearance to communicate certain information to onlookers, and this aspect of wigs and hair pieces was also taken advantage of by individuals who wished to disguise themselves, such as Hannibal Barca during the Punic Wars:

> During this winter he also adopted a truly Punic artifice. Fearing the treachery of the Celts and possible attempts on his life, owing to his establishment of the friendly relations with them being so very recent, he had a number of wigs made, dyed to suit the appearance of persons differing widely in age, and kept constantly changing them, at the same time also dressing in a style that suited the wig, so that not only those who had seen him but for a moment, but even his familiars found difficulty in recognizing him.[74]

This designation of wig-wearing as something that is done by 'others' is common in ancient Greek and Latin literature; wigs and hair pieces are initially something foreign – a Punic, a Median, or an Egyptian practice.

[72] Turfa and Becker, 2019, pp. 56–7. [73] Becker and Turfa, 2017, pp. 136–7.

[74] Polyb. 3.78 (trans. W. R. Paton, F. W. Walbank and C. Habicht): Ἐχρήσατο δέ τινι καὶ Φοινικικῷ στρατηγήματι 2τοιούτῳ κατὰ τὴν παραχειμασίαν. ἀγωνιῶν γὰρ τὴν ἀθεσίαν τῶν Κελτῶν καὶ τὰς ἐπιβουλὰς τὰς περὶ τὸ σῶμα διὰ τὸ πρόσφατον τῆς πρὸς αὐτοὺς συστάσεως, κατεσκευάσατο περιθετὰς τρίχας, ἁρμοζούσας ταῖς κατὰ τὰς ὁλοσχερεῖς διαφορὰς τῶν ἡλικιῶν ἐπιπρεπείαις, καὶ ταύταις ἐχρῆτο συνεχῶς μετατιθέμενος· ὁμοίως δὲ καὶ τὰς ἐσθῆτας μετελάμβανε τὰς καθηκούσας ἀεὶ ταῖς περιθεταῖς. δι᾽ ὧν οὐ μόνον τοῖς αἰφνιδίως ἰδοῦσι δύσγνωστος ἦν ἀλλὰ καὶ τοῖς ἐν συνηθείᾳ γεγονόσι.

Even once they become a regular part of Roman society, they are still referred to as something that undesirable individuals such as courtesans and prostitutes wear, even though it is clear that wigs were utilised much more widely, both as a means of disguising one's loss of hair and as a means of supplementing one's existing hair.

It is also worth bearing in mind that in the absence of the modern understanding of health and safety, or even basic principles of hygiene, the ancient workplace was always extremely hazardous. Its dangerous conditions caused health problems ranging from calluses and scars to permanent deformities or other, less immediately visible, issues such as breathing problems, so it is understandable that those who worked in it recognised this and sought to try and protect themselves. They attempted to do this using a variety of different types of protective equipment, ranging in complexity and ingenuity from the rudimentary to the advanced. So, just as warriors, whether soldiers or gladiators, wore armour to protect themselves from injury and death during combat, so too did other, less high-profile types of ancient workers use personal protective equipment as a matter of course in their daily lives. At the most basic level, agricultural workers, spending long hours in high temperatures, sought to prevent themselves from suffering the effects of too much sun by donning headgear. Calpurnius Siculus describes them wearing close-fitting leather caps, while the archaeologist Sir William Flinders Petrie recovered a Panama-style straw hat during his 1901–2 excavation season in Egypt which has been radiocarbon dated to between 420 and 568 CE, making it the oldest such hat in the world, which may have served a similar purpose.[75] According to Theophrastus, they also attempted to avoid potentially deadly bites and stings by wearing sturdy hand and foot coverings when venturing into dense undergrowth.[76] This makes sense when read against Erycius' poem about a man named Mindon who was bitten on the foot by a spider while cutting down a tree, the result of which was that the bite became infected, turned gangrenous, and his leg had to be amputated.[77] Additionally, it was common knowledge that specific plants had powerful properties, both positive and negative, that could affect those tasked with gathering them; Plutarch records that those who harvested the opium poppy were warned to be on their guard against the plant's soporific fumes and cover their noses and mouths with something, perhaps a mask made from leather or cloth, to prevent inhalation.[78] Breathing apparatus was also found in other

[75] Calp. *Ecl.* 1.7; Petrie Museum inv. 1902.31.22. [76] Theophr. *Hist. pl.* 9.5.2.
[77] Erycius, *Greek Anthology* 9.233. [78] Plut. *Mor.* 647f–648a.

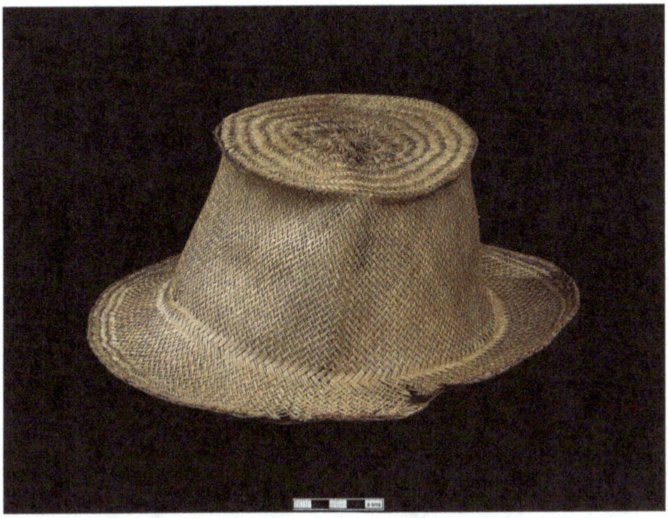

Figure 4.7 Egyptian straw hat, circa 420–568 CE. Pitt Rivers Museum inv. 1902.31.22. Image courtesy of the Pitt Rivers Museum, University of Oxford.

hostile environments. Pliny the Elder, who spent a considerable amount of time at the silver mines in Spain during his military service and described their workings in detail, recounted that those responsible for processing the minerals that were mined there tied masks made from animal bladders around the lower halves of their faces to cover their noses and mouths to prevent them from inhaling the dust and damaging their lungs while leaving their eyes unobstructed so they were able to see what they were doing, and his account was supported by Dioscorides.[79] Aristotle speculated as to why divers on the lookout for sponges, pearls, snails required to manufacture purple dye, or even salvage from shipwrecks would routinely bind sponges around their ears, and concluded that it was to protect their ear canals and ear drums, while Lycophron included information in his only surviving poem that indicates that, on occasion, they would don rudimentary leather wetsuits to inure themselves to the freezing temperature of the water they were required to submerge themselves in for extended periods of time.[80] While much ancient diving seems to have

[79] Plin. *HN* 33.40; see also Diosc. 5.94. For discussion of the dangers of lead mining in antiquity, see Nriagu, 1983.

[80] Arist. [*Pr.*] 32.3, 32.5; Lycoph. *Alex.* 72–80. For diving in antiquity, see Ioannidou, 2015; for sponges, see Rodríguez-Álvarez, (2018); Voultsiadou, 2007.

taken the form of what we know today as freediving, Aristotle's repeated musings on the subject make it clear that breathing apparatus akin to the contemporary snorkel was sometimes used, and it seems some divers went even further than that in their efforts to circumvent the inhospitable environment of the seabed, fashioning rudimentary diving bells out of cauldrons since these retained a certain amount of air even while submerged.[81] Since measures such as these were not only aimed at protecting the frail human body but were also aimed at augmenting it to provide a functional advantage in an inhospitable environment, somewhere that humans would not or could not normally go, it is not beyond the realms of possibility that this idea of augmentation may have been applied in a slightly different way and may also have inspired prostheses and assistive technology.

Materials

Both literary and archaeological evidence indicate that a variety of materials were used in the creation of prostheses in classical antiquity. These materials were likely used for both practical and impractical reasons.

The most basic and easily accessible material for an extremity prosthesis would have been wood. A wide range of different types of wood were available in major cities and towns in the classical world, whether grown locally or imported from elsewhere.[82] Ancient authors that discuss wood as a natural resource make clear that certain types were preferred for specific purposes; according to Theophrastus, mallow, holly, Judas-tree, and bay were commonly used for walking sticks, so it is possible that these were also utilised in the creation of extremity prostheses.[83] In an epigram about a farmer who loses his leg after a spider bite turns gangrenous, Mardonius specifies that his prosthesis is 'the branch of a tall olive'.[84] Wood would have been a good choice for extremity prostheses in classical antiquity due to its accessibility, affordability, and malleability, and it would have been relatively lightweight while simultaneously strong enough to bear the potentially considerable weight of the user.[85] However, certain types of wood could also have been used to make a statement: the Cairo Toe is made from elm, which is not native to

[81] Arist. *Part. An.* 2.16.659a9. [82] Meiggs, 1982. [83] Theophr. *Hist. pl.* 1.3.2, 5.7.7.
[84] Mardonius the Consul, *Greek Anthology* 11.374.
[85] For wooden extremity prostheses in which the type of wood utilised is not specified, see Hdt. 9.36–7; Plut. *Mor. De frat. amor.* 3.1; Mart. 10.100; Luc. *Ind.* 6.

Egypt and so is found only very rarely in archaeological contexts there.[86] When it was used, it seems to have been utilised specifically for its strength under compression, in chariot hubs.[87] Thus, this imported wood could have been specially selected for this purpose due to a combination of factors both practical and impractical, physical and symbolic.

An extremity prosthesis made entirely from metal seems unlikely; such an object would have been both heavy and unyielding. However, the Capua Limb attests bronze sheeting used to cover a wooden section with a central core of iron, while the 'Hemmaberg Limb' attests iron fittings in conjunction with wood and leather. If Marcus Sergius Silus' iron hand allowed him to bear his shield on his right arm instead of his left, as attested in the images of him depicted on his coinage, it seems more probably that it was wood covered with iron sheeting.[88] There is evidence for a wide range of metal-workers operating in the cities and towns of the classical world, both large and small establishments, and specialisation increased over the centuries, particularly in locations such as Athens and Rome, where specialist metal-workers are attested not only in the literary but also the epigraphic record.[89]

Gold seems to have been consistently utilised for dental appliances, likely in part because of its malleability but also because it was recognised not to be toxic. There is literary evidence ranging in date from the fifth century BCE through to the third century CE. The Laws of the Twelve Tables refer to 'teeth bound with gold', indicating the use of gold as a dental appliance by the Romans at least as early as the fifth century BCE, and gold wire is advised as a means of stabilising loose teeth in the Hippocratic treatise *On Joints*, dating to the fifth century BCE, and then again in Celsus' *On Medicine*, dating to the early first century CE, while Lucian describes a woman doing so in the second century CE, and the Hebrew Bible details the case of a woman with a gold tooth in the third century CE.[90] While the evidence for goldsmiths operating in Classical Athens is minimal, there is a considerable amount of evidence for them operating in Rome, during which time large quantities of unworked gold were imported to the capital from the provinces, notably Spain, Britain, Gaul, Dalmatia, and Dacia.[91] There are hundreds of inscriptions attesting different types of individuals who made their living from working

[86] Finch, 2019, p. 44. [87] Gale et al., 2000, p. 346. [88] Plin. *HN* 7.29.

[89] For specialist metalwork in Classical Athens, see Dem. 27.9; Xen. *Mem.* 3.10.9; Arist. *Pax* 1209–64.

[90] *Laws of the Twelve Tables* 10.8–9; Hippoc. *Art.* 33.9–10; Celsus, *Med.* 6.12; Palestinian Talmud tractate Nedarim 9.41c; Babylonian Talmud tractate Nedarim 66b.

[91] Plin. *HN* 33.78; Stat. *Silv.* 3.3.89.

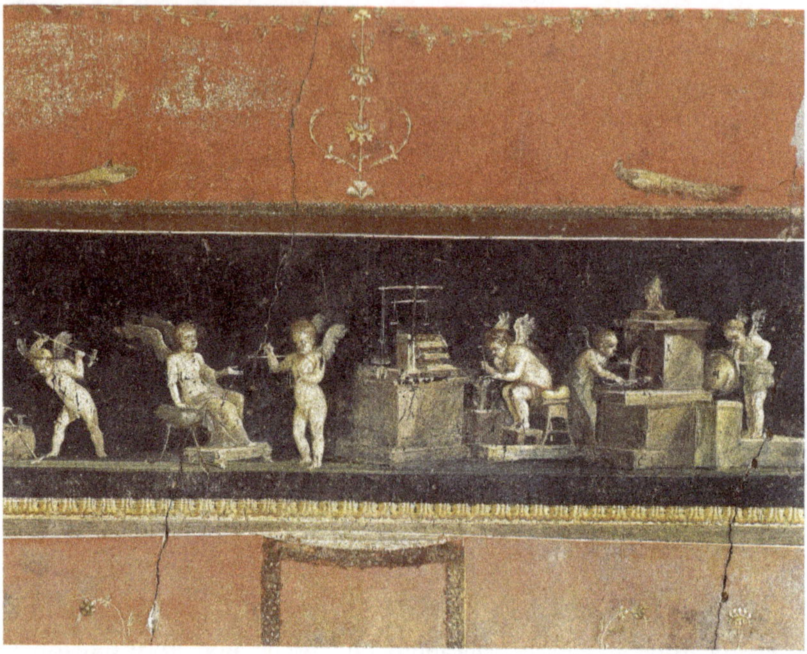

Figure 4.8 'Cupids as Goldsmiths' fresco from the House of the Vettii, Pompeii, 62–79 CE. Image courtesy of Alamy.

gold: *aurifices, brattiarii, inauratores, auri nextrices, barbaricarii*.[92] There is also epigraphic evidence of guilds of goldsmiths.[93] Goldsmiths could own their material, or have it provided by their patron or customer.[94] While this fresco (Figure 4.8) from the House of the Vettii in Pompeii, dating from the first century CE, shows cupids in the guise of gold workers, it is an authentic depiction of the trade.

There are a few examples of silver dental appliances surviving in the archaeological record. Silver was imported to Rome from the provinces, primarily Spain, and a considerable amount of silverware was produced in Campania. Epigraphic evidence attests to a considerable variety of individuals making their living from silver: *argentarii, celators, tritores argentarii, toreuticensis, flatuarii*, as well as an individual who added touches of gold to silver, an *inaurator*.

[92] Most of these individuals are male; however, there are some female metal-workers attested in the following inscriptions: *CIL* III 2117, V 7044, VI 6939, 2911.

[93] *CIL* VI 9202, 95. [94] See for example *CIL* VI 9222.

There are also literary references to false teeth made from bone and ivory.[95] During the Roman imperial period, ivory was initially imported from North Africa, although the eventual failure of North African ivory led to attempts to import it from Ethiopia and India.[96] The Sabrathenses maintained a trading station in the Piazza of the Corporations at Ostia and used it to import ivory, and more than 675 cubic feet of the substance (around 2,500 tusks) was recovered from the Horrea Galbana.[97] Seven inscriptions attesting ivory carvers (*eborarius* or *faber eborarius* in Latin) have been discovered in Rome, dating from the period of the first century BCE to the first century CE.[98] Five of the seven are associated with the area between the Porta Salaria and the Porta Pinciana, which is suggestive of there being a particular association between the trade and that area: perhaps it was recognised as an 'ivory quarter'.[99] An inscription also attests to a collegium of ivory and citrus wood workers (*eborarii et citrarii*) in Trastevere during the reign of Hadrian.[100] Ivory was used for chryselephantine statues of gods and other significant figures, in part because of the qualities of the material that caused ancient authors to liken it to beautiful skin, and in part because of its inherent prestige as an exotic imported material.[101] While ivory life-size human hands and feet have been recovered in the archaeological record, these have been interpreted as fragments of freestanding statuary or perhaps components of furniture rather than prostheses, but since there are literary references to ivory prostheses, it is possible that some individuals sported them in real life.[102] Yet, while ivory might have been appealing and considered a suitable material for an extremity prosthesis such as a hand or arm for a member of the social elite due to its resemblance to human skin and its luxurious and prestigious associations, it would probably not have withstood the stresses and strains of such usage for very long. Bone, due to its superior bending strength and elasticity, and its resistance to stress fractures, would have been a better choice.[103] In any case, it is clear that ivory and bone carvers worked closely with woodworkers and metal-workers to produce a range of products, and

[95] Mart. 1.72. [96] Plin. *HN* 8.7; Suet. *Ner.* 31.

[97] *CIL* XIV Suppl. P. 662 n. 14; Lanciani, 1898 p. 250.

[98] *CIL* VI 37374, 37793, 7885, 9375, 9397, 33423, 7655. While the individuals named in these inscriptions are all men, Plin. *HN* 35.40.147–8 mentions a renowned female ivory carver, Iaia of Cyzicus.

[99] St Clair, 2003, p. 11. [100] *CIL* VI 9528. [101] Lapatin, 2001, p. 6.

[102] Lapatin, 2001, p. 5. See, for example, the 'Corinth Arm', at Lapatin, 2001, p. 129: a well-carved, life-size forearm carved from elephant ivory that dates prior to 146 BCE, but there is no literary record of a chryselephantine statue in Corinth.

[103] St Clair, 2003, pp. 1–2.

literary, documentary, and archaeological evidence strongly suggests that prostheses were among these products.[104]

Wigs and hair pieces seem to have been primarily made from human hair, and there were several ways in which this hair could have been sourced. If an individual was having their hair cut or head shaved as a prelude to medical treatment, they might endeavour to keep the hair and commission a wig to be made from it. However, there was also a thriving trade in hair from both inside and outside the Roman empire. Hair was gleaned from newly captured prisoners who were to be sold as enslaved individuals; this type was referred to as 'captive hair' (*captivis comis*).[105] Hair was also imported from India; this type was referred to as 'Indian hair' (*capelli Indici*).[106] There is also literary and archaeological evidence for the use of materials such as leather, linen, and plant fibres. Perhaps the responsibility for making the wig depended upon the materials involved.

Meanings

While it is likely that practical considerations such as accessibility, cost, malleability, weight, etc., were taken into account when an individual selected the material for his or her prosthesis, the possibility that materials were selected for other reasons that are harder to pin down is a possibility. Since it is probable that each prosthesis created in classical antiquity was entirely original, an object that was designed, commissioned, and manufactured according to the specific needs of that one particular amputee, it is likely that additional concerns were catered to: if a simple peg-leg would have been sufficient for practical purposes such as mobility, why did the owner of the Capua Limb go to all the trouble of encasing his (or her) prosthesis in bronze? Would an ancient amputee enlist their prosthesis as a means of expressing their wealth, status, taste, or fashion sensibility? Could an ancient prosthesis offer a unique opportunity for conspicuous consumption? Dio Chrysostom commented on the myth of the hero Pelops in a way that was less than favourable: 'as if there were any use in a man having a golden or ivory hand or eyes of diamond or malachite; but the kind of soul he had men did not notice'.[107] Materials such as ivory, gold, and precious stones were frequently the target of accusations

[104] St Clair, 2003, p. 23. [105] Mart. 14.26. [106] *Dig.* 39.4.16.7.

[107] Dio Chrys. *Or.* 8.28 (trans. J. W. Cohoon): ὅτι καὶ τὸν ὦμον ἐλεφάντινον ἔχοι, ὥσπερ τι ὄφελος ἀνθρώπου χρυσῆν χεῖρα ἢ ἐλεφαντίνην ἔχοντος ἢ ὀφθαλμοὺς ἀδάμαντος ἢ σμαράγδου· τὴν δὲ ψυχὴν οὐκ ἐγίγνωσκον αὐτοῦ ὁποίαν τινὰ εἶχεν.

regarding *luxuria*, so potentially individuals who sought to utilise them in their prostheses would have been viewed negatively. One indication of this is presented by Lucian:

> Not long ago there was a rich man in Asia, both of whose feet had been amputated in consequence of an accident; they were frozen, I gather, when he had to make a journey through snow. Well, this of course was pitiable, and to remedy the mischance he had had wooden feet made for him, which he used to lace on, and in that way made shift to walk, leaning upon his servants as he did so. But he did one thing that was ridiculous: he used always to buy very handsome sandals of the latest cut and went to the utmost trouble in regard to them, in order that his timber toes might be adorned with the most beautiful footwear! Now are not you doing just the same thing? Is it not true that although you have a crippled, fig-wood understanding, you are buying gilt buskins which even a normal man could hardly get about in?[108]

The possibility that prosthesis users did not, in fact, display their prostheses but sought to cover them up with clothing or footwear is interesting in itself – were they, in fact, trying to pass their prosthesis off as the extremity that it had replaced? Or were they attempting to emphasise their prosthesis through combining it with eye-catching clothing or footwear, and making it even more impactful?

On several occasions, the fact that prostheses could be made from different materials according to the requirements of their users/wearers is mentioned specifically. In their discussion of artificial teeth in the Talmud, the rabbis and sages state that some women wear gold teeth, others wear silver, and still others wear 'artificial' ones, perhaps referring to ivory or even wooden ones.[109] The difference in the value of these materials is acknowledged, as a woman who wears a gold or silver false tooth is thought more likely to want to break the restrictions of the Shabbat to replace the tooth in her mouth if it falls out due to the cost of getting a replacement, while a woman who wears an 'artificial' false tooth, presumably a wooden one, is less likely to break the restrictions of the Shabbat to replace the

[108] Luc. *Ind.* 6 (trans. A. M. Harmon): Καὶ ἐγένετό τις οὐ πρὸ πολλοῦ ἐν Ἀσίᾳ πλούσιος ἀνὴρ ἐκ συμφορᾶς ἀποτμηθεὶς τοὺς πόδας ἀμφοτέρους, ἀπὸ κρύους, οἶμαι, ἀποσαπέντας ἐπειδή ποτε διὰ χιόνος ὁδοιπορῆσαι συνέβη αὐτῷ. οὗτος τοίνυν τοῦτο μὲν ἐλεεινὸν ἐπεπόνθει, καὶ θεραπεύων τὴν δυστυχίαν ξυλίνους πόδας πεποίητο, καὶ τούτους ὑποδούμενος ἐβάδιζεν ἐπιστηριζόμενος ἅμα τοῖς οἰκέταις. ἐκεῖνο δὲ γελοῖον ἐποίει, κρηπῖδας γὰρ καλλίστας ἐωνεῖτο νεοτμήτους ἀεί, καὶ τὴν πλείστην πραγματείαν περὶ ταύτας εἶχεν, ὡς καλλίστοις ὑποδήμασι κεκοσμημένα εἴη αὐτῷ τὰ ξύλα. οὐ ταὐτὰ οὖν καὶ σὺ ποιεῖς χωλὴν μὲν ἔχων καὶ συκίνην τὴν γνώμην, ὠνούμενος δὲ χρυσοῦς ἐμβάτας, οἷς μόλις ἄν τις καὶ ἀρτίπους ἐμπεριπατήσειεν.

[109] Palestinian Talmud, Shabbat 6.5; Babylonian Talmud, Shabbat 65a.

tooth in her mouth if it falls out because she can more easily obtain a replacement. Finally, Lucian, in his science fiction novel *True Story*, describes his fictional race, the Arboreals, as using artificial phalluses, with the wealthy Arboreals using ivory ones while the poor Arboreals use wooden ones.[110] While this is obviously a fictitious scenario, and there is no other evidence for the use of prosthetic genitalia in classical antiquity, Lucian may have been drawing on his observations of other types of prostheses in use, and noted differences in the materials used for prostheses according to the wealth and status of the individuals using them.[111]

Conclusion

The loss of body parts was common in classical antiquity, but it does not necessarily follow that prostheses and prosthesis use were. Based upon the frequency (or infrequency) with which prostheses are mentioned in ancient literature, it could be that prostheses were so common as to be unremarkable, or so uncommon as to be worth commenting on. However, it is necessary to consider the context in which these references occur, and why they include the information that they do.

Were prostheses considered necessary in classical antiquity? Modern studies have shown that prosthesis users are understandably much more likely to utilise prostheses that make their lives easier than those that make their lives harder, so it is possible that ancient prostheses were utilised as long as they did likewise. It is possible that there were a number of more viable alternatives available to an amputee in the form of sticks, staffs, crutches, wheeled conveyances, animals, and even humans.

How we interpret the ways in which prostheses, prosthesis use, and prosthesis users were viewed in ancient society depends very much on how we approach them. Were prostheses equated with clothing and dress? Were they equated with weapons and armour? Were they equated with scientific gadgets and instruments? Or were they equated with all three depending upon the circumstances? It is the latter scenario that seems the most likely: just as prostheses were highly individualised and personalised, so were the responses that people had to them. While one observer might admire an

[110] Luc. *Ver. hist.* 1.22.

[111] While there are literary references to women using dildos (e.g. Herod. 6.57–73, 6.87–8, 7.56–64) and numerous depictions of the practice on Greek painted pottery, I do not consider these to be prostheses because the women are not using them to replace body parts that they themselves have lost. I would, however, consider a literary reference to a eunuch using a dildo to be a prosthesis, but I am not aware of any such references.

individual's prosthesis as an exquisite piece of craftsmanship, an object of taste and refinement, and an indication that its user had overcome a significant personal setback in an ingenious way, another might think that same prosthesis an ostentatious and grotesque display of self-indulgent *luxuria* and even hubris, and a more or less successful attempt to deceive others regarding their corporeal integrity. A fellow amputee might be envious, particularly if they were themselves were unable to utilise a prosthesis and had to make do with a more rudimentary piece of assistive technology. Or they might be inspired and seek to acquire one themselves.

Since no comprehensive and detailed discussions of prostheses survive from classical antiquity (assuming that any ever existed in the first place), it is necessary to infer much about their design, commission, and manufacture from references to (somewhat) comparable objects such as clothing and jewellery, weapons and armour, medical instruments, and scientific gadgets.

CHAPTER 5

Living Prostheses

Introduction

> [Hephaistos] spoke and rose from the anvil, a huge, panting bulk, limping along, but beneath him his slender legs moved nimbly. The bellows he set away from the fire, and gathered all the tools with which he worked into a silver chest; and with a sponge he wiped his face and both his hands, and his mighty neck and shaggy breast, and put on a tunic, and grasped a stout staff, and went out limping; and **there moved swiftly to support their lord handmaids made of gold in the semblance of living girls. In them is understanding in their minds, and in them speech and strength, and they know cunning handiwork by gift of the immortal gods. They busily moved to support their lord.**[1]

The use of other entities as a type of assistive technology in classical antiquity was attested as early as the eighth century BCE, in Homer's *Iliad* and other mythological cycles that were circulating contemporaneously: the Greek god Hephaistos requisitioned the bodies of other humans and animals to compensate for his own deficiencies and even went so far as to create automata to act as his assistants in his forge.[2] These automata took the form of at least two golden handmaids.[3] Scholars have suggested that there is a specific reason why this assistive technology was

[1] Hom. *Il.* 18.410–18 (trans. A. T. Murray, revised by W. F. Wyatt; emphasis added): Ἦ, καὶ ἀπ' ἀκμοθέτοιο πέλωρ αἴητον ἀνέστη/ χωλεύων· ὑπὸ δὲ κνῆμαι ῥώοντο ἀραιαί./ φύσας μέν ῥ' ἀπάνευθε τίθει πυρός, ὅπλα τε πάντα/ λάρνακ' ἐς ἀργυρέην συλλέξατο, τοῖς ἐπονεῖτο·/ σπόγγῳ δ' ἀμφὶ πρόσωπα καὶ ἄμφω χεῖρ' ἀπομόργνυ/ αὐχένα τε στιβαρὸν καὶ στήθεα λαχνήεντα,/ δῦ δὲ χιτῶν', ἕλε δὲ σκῆπτρον παχύ, βῆ δὲ θύραζε/ χωλεύων· ὑπὸ δ' ἀμφίπολοι ῥώοντο ἄνακτι/ χρύσειαι, ζωῇσι νεήνισιν εἰοικυῖαι.

[2] The golden handmaids were also referred to by Philostr. *VA* 6.11.18–19. For further discussion of Hephaistos' use of assistive technologies, see Draycott, in press a.

[3] Interestingly, it does not appear that any ancient depictions of the golden handmaids have survived from classical antiquity, if they ever existed in the first place. This print (Figure 5.1) is entitled 'Thetis bittet Hephaistos, für ihren Sohn Achilleus eine Rüstung zu schmieden' and was engraved by Johann Heinrich Füssli in 1803.

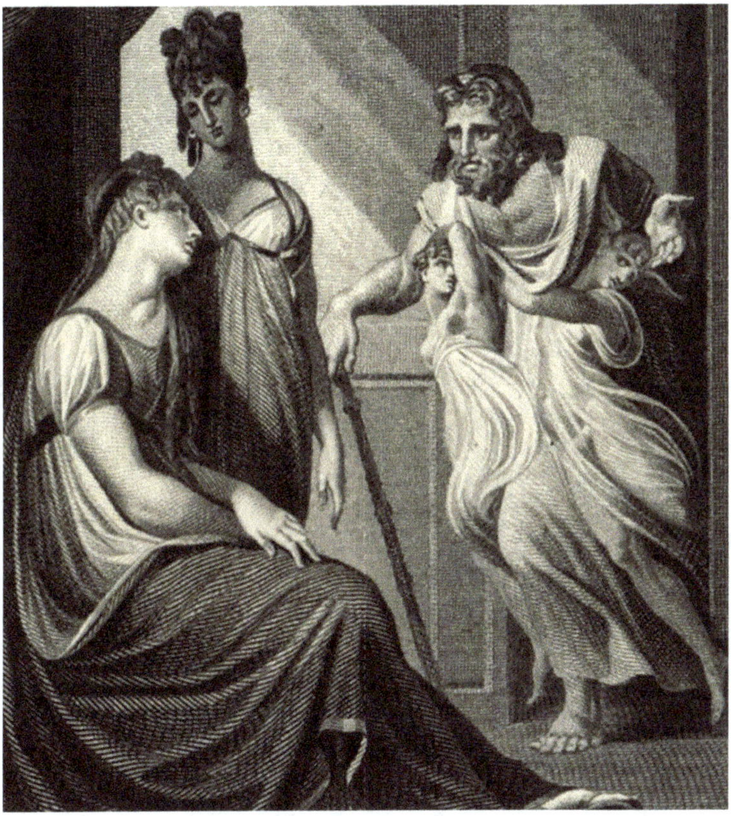

Figure 5.1 'Thetis bittet Hephaistos, für ihren Sohn Achilleus eine Rüstung zu schmieden' by Johann Heinrich Füssli. Image courtesy of Wikimedia Commons.

envisaged in human form rather than in the form of any of Hephaistos' other creations. According to Paipetis, 'the greater diversity of jobs is required from a robot, the more its form tends to become human, for a simple reason: The human body, through its age-long adaptive evolution within terrestrial environments, is the perfect "universal tool", therefore, if robots are to substitute for humans in their activities, they must assume their form.'[4] Additionally, according to Kalligeropoulos and Vasileiadou, 'two mythical robots, two self-moving manlike machines, having sense, speech and strength. Innovative technological visions: The strength, i.e. the feature that transforms low-power

[4] Paipetis, 2010, p. 108.

commands into powerful mechanical movements, the speech, i.e. the construction of machines producing sounds to communicate, and the sense, i.e. the particular inner structure that results in skilful, learning machines.'[5] All three of these have a resonance in relation to the requirements of assistive technology for an impaired individual: strength is necessary for the practical side of providing physical assistance; speech for interaction, understanding, and companionship; and sense for anticipation of needs and empathy. Whether or not the poet and the audience *believed* that Hephaistos had created automata/robots/androids to assist him is not the point; the point is that it seemed to be a reasonable supposition that someone with his sort of physical impairments would benefit from such assistive technology, and so they would look for achievable counterparts, namely humans and, potentially, some types of animals.

Yet, to date this is not an aspect of impairment and disability in classical antiquity that has been investigated in detail by scholars.[6] This chapter will examine the ways in which physically impaired individuals in classical antiquity utilised humans (whether family members, friends or acquaintances, or enslaved individuals) and, on occasion, animals as 'living prostheses', supplementing their own bodies and body parts with those of others.[7] It will also explore how impaired and disabled individuals viewed these 'living prostheses' and whether or not they were preferred to inanimate forms of assistive technology, such as the prostheses we have encountered so far.

Using Humans as Prostheses

It is extremely likely that, in the first instance, physically impaired individuals sought the assistance of their family, friends and household staff (whether freeborn, formerly enslaved, or enslaved) in their day to day lives; there is a degree of literary, documentary, and archaeological evidence to this effect, although, like many of the practical aspects of impairment and disability in classical antiquity, it is not foregrounded. This link between assistive technology and human assistance can be made explicitly as the individuals rendering this assistance are described in those very terms, even as

5 Kalligeropoulos and Vasileiadou, 2008, p. 79.

6 See van Schaik, 2019 for a very recent discussion of the crucial role that human caregivers played in the lives of the physically impaired and immobile in classical antiquity. For archaeological evidence of the existence of care and caregiving in past societies on an individual-by-individual basis, see Tilley, 2012; Tilley, 2015; Tilley and Schrenk, 2016.

7 I have taken the term 'living prostheses' from van Schaik, 2019.

assistive technology personified.[8] In some cases, this use is figurative, simply serving as a simile or a metaphor. For example, in Euripides' *Phoenician Women*, Antigone describes her mother Jocasta as having been Oedipus' staff: 'your wife, who toiled in caring for you and like a staff tended your blind footsteps'.[9] Similarly, in his *Hecuba*, the former queen of Troy addresses those left of her former subjects and describes them as her staff, 'leaning upon the crook of your arm as my staff, I shall hasten my limbs' slow-foot advance', and later in the play begs Odysseus for the life of her youngest daughter Polyxena, attempting to describe how much she needs her by likewise referring to her as her staff.[10] This practice of equating children (or substitute children) with staffs to support a parent in their old age seems to have been fairly common.[11] However, in other cases, this use is, or becomes, rather more literal: according to Macrobius, the reason that the Cornelii Scipiones bore that particular cognomen was that one of their family members 'used to guide his blind homonymous father, in place of a cane'.[12]

Even if impaired individuals were able to use assistive technology such as staffs, sticks, crutches, or extremity prostheses, they might still require differing degrees of physical assistance in conjunction with them. Marcus Sergius Silus wore an iron prosthetic hand but still required a single enslaved attendant to assist him in battle in a manner that is not specified.[13] Lucian's anonymous rich man wore two wooden feet but still required enslaved attendants to carry him around.[14] Considering how labour intensive the use of assistive technology can be and the physical toll that it can take on the body, causing chafing, blisters, aches, and pains even for a contemporary individual with state of the art apparatus, it is

[8] See for example Soph. *OC* 867; Eur. *Hec.* 65, 261.

[9] Eur. *Phoen.* 1548–9 (trans. D. Kovacs): ἄλοχος, παραβάκτροις ἃ πόδα σὸν τυφλόπουν θεραπεύμασιν αἰὲν ἐμόχθει.

[10] Eur. *Hec.* 65–7 (trans. D. Kovacs): κἀγὼ σκολιῷ σκίπωνι χερὸςδιερειδομένη σπεύσω βραδύπουνἤλυσιν ἄρθρων προτιθεῖσα; Euripides, *Hecuba* 281.

[11] See also Quint. Smyrn. 3.479, 5.446–7; John Damascene, *Baarlam and Ioasaph* 207. This is not the only way in which children were envisaged physically supporting their parents in their dotage: see, for example, the many literary and artistic depictions of the breastfeeding of parents by their nursing adult female children as a sign of *pietas*, discussed in Mulder, 2017.

[12] Macrob. *Sat.* 1.26 (trans. R. A. Kaster): *qui cognominem patrem luminibus carentem pro baculo regebat.*

[13] Plin. *HN* 7.29. It is notable that the enslaved individual is not named in Pliny's account and his (one assumes, considering the martial context, that the enslaved individual was male) presence is minimised as this does not fit the story that Pliny is telling and his promotion of Silus as an example to follow. See Laes, 2011; Schultze, 2011; Beagon, 2002.

[14] Luc. *Ind.* 6.

likely that an ancient individual was similarly afflicted and required support in the form of regular first aid.[15]

Some impaired individuals might require still more assistance, or a sustained level of assistance. Physically impaired individuals who were not capable of locomoting independently with the aid of one or two mobility aids, or the help of someone's strong arm, could still be mobile, albeit by being carried around, at least for journeys of short duration. A sedan chair or a litter (φορεῖον, κλίνη, or κλινίδιον in Greek; *sella* or *lectica* in Latin) allowed someone to be carried from place to place in either a seated position or a reclining position. Such modes of transport seem to have been used by the Persians with little fanfare, but as far as the Greeks were concerned they were fit only for invalids or for women, and if you were neither of those things they were a trapping of luxury and you were censured for being effeminate.[16] Roman generals used them while on military campaigns when ill or injured, but only invalids or women used them within the city.[17] It is notable that the physically impaired emperor Claudius' use of a covered conveyance in the city of Rome is emphasised, despite the fact that his predecessors had likewise used conveyances.[18] They are mentioned frequently in miraculous healing accounts, a key feature of which is the previously immobilised individual suddenly restored to health and able to get up from their sedan chair or litter and move independently.[19]

But what of those who were physically impaired but did not have access to such a comprehensive network of human assistance? A series of epigrams from the *Greek Anthology* takes the subject of a blind man and a mobility-impaired man working together to overcome their respective impairments:

> One man was maimed in his legs, while another had lost his eyesight, but each contributed to the other that of which mischance had deprived him. For the blind man, taking the lame man on his shoulders, kept a straight course by listening to the other's orders. It was bitter, all-daring necessity which taught them all this, instructing them how, by dividing their imperfections between them, to make a perfect whole.[20]

[15] For domestic medical practice, see Draycott, 2019d.

[16] Persians: Hdt. 3.146.3. Invalids: Dem. 54.20; Plut. *Vit. Per.* 27; Plut. *Vit. Eum.* 14.3; Andocides, *On the Mysteries* 62; Lys. 4.9, although this person is faking his injuries. Criticism: Din. 1.36. For discussion, see Casson, 1994, p. 67.

[17] Generals: Livy 24.42; Val. Max. 1.7, 2.8; Suet. *Aug.* 91. Invalids and women: Cass. Dio. 57.17.

[18] Cass. Dio. 60.2.3.

[19] *Epidaurian iamata* B17, B18, C14, C21; Luke 5.17–26; Matthew 9.1–8; Mark 1.1–12. For a comparison of these miraculous healing accounts, see Horn, 2013. For discussion of the presence of ramps at the entrances to healing sanctuaries, see Sneed, 2020.

[20] Philippus or Isodorus, *Greek Anthology* 9.11 (trans. W. R. Paton): Πηρὸς ὁ μὲν γυίοις, ὁ δ' ἄρ' ὄμμασιν· ἀμφότεροι δὲ/ εἰς αύτοὺς τὸ τύχης ἐνδεὲς ἠράνισαν./ τυφλὸς γὰρ λιπόγυιον ἐπωμάδιον

> The blind beggar supported the lame one on his feet, and gained in return the help of the other's eyes. Thus the two incomplete beings fitted into each other to form one complete being, each supplying what the other lacked.[21]

> A blind man carried a lame man on his back, lending him his feet and borrowing from him his eyes.[22]

> Both are maimed and strolling beggars; but the one has lost the use of his eyes, the other the support of his legs. Each serves the other; for the blind man, taking the lame one on his back, walks gingerly by the aid of eyes not his own. One nature supplied the needs of both; for each contributed to the other his deficiency to form a whole.[23]

This premise seems to have been a popular one in classical antiquity, as variations on it are also found in contemporary Jewish literature.[24] Considering this seemingly widespread appeal, then, perhaps it is not surprising that it continued to be popular after antiquity and has been used as a parable on mutual assistance and cooperation well into the twentieth century. The story was featured not just in works of literature but also works of art in a range of media; see, for example, Figure 5.2: this fresco from St Archangel Michael's Church in the Byzantine Lesnovo Monastery in north-eastern Macedonia, which dates to around 1347 CE. Interestingly, unlike the situations described earlier in which one individual is served by another or several others, in this scenario the two men are equals rather than a superior and their inferior. As a result, they have a symbiotic relationship.

Using Animals as Prostheses

While humans were likely the first choice for assistants to the physically impaired and disabled in classical antiquity, it is possible that on occasion animals were utilised for similar purposes. Visually impaired individuals

βάρος αἴρων/ ταῖς κείνου φωναῖς ἀτραπὸν ὠρθοβάτει·/ πάντα δὲ ταῦτ᾽ ἐδίδαξε πικρὴ πάντολμος ἀνάγκη,/ ἀλλήλοις μερίσαι τοὐλλιπὲς εἰς τέλεον.

21 Leonidas of Alexandria, *Greek Anthology* 9.12 (trans. W. R. Paton): Τυφλὸς ἀλητεύων χωλὸν πόδας ἠέρταζεν,/ ὄμμασιν ἀλλοτρίοις ἀντερανιζόμενος./ ἄμφω δ᾽ ἡμιτελεῖς πρὸς ἑνὸς φύσιν ἡρμόσθησαν/ τοὐλλιπὲς ἀλλήλοις ἀντιπαρασχόμενοι.

22 Plato the Younger, *Greek Anthology* 9.13 (trans. W. R. Paton): Ἀνέρα τις λιπόγυιον ὑπὲρ νώτοιο λιπαυγὴς/ ἦρε, πόδας χρήσας, ὄμματα χρησάμενος.

23 Antiphilus of Byzantium, *Greek Anthology* 9.13B (trans. W. R. Paton): Ἄμφω μὲν πηροὶ καὶ ἀλήμονες, ἀλλ᾽ ὁ μὲν ὄψεις,/ ὃς δὲ βάσεις· ἄλλου δ᾽ ἄλλος ὑπηρεσίῃ·/ τυφλὸς γὰρ χωλοῖο κατωμάδιον βάρος αἴρων/ ἀτραπὸν ὀθνείοις ὄμμασιν ἀκροβάτει./ ἡ μία δ᾽ ἀμφοτέροις ἤρκει φύσις· ἐν γὰρ ἑκάστῳ/ τοὐλλιπὲς ἀλλήλοις εἰς ὅλον ἠράνισαν.

24 Epiph. *Adv. haeres.* 64.70.5–17 (*Apocryphon of Ezekiel* fr. 1); Talmud Sanhedrin 91a–b; Lev Rabbah 4.5; Mekilta on Exodus 15:1. For discussion of these parables in the Jewish tradition, see Evans, 2000, pp. 64–5.

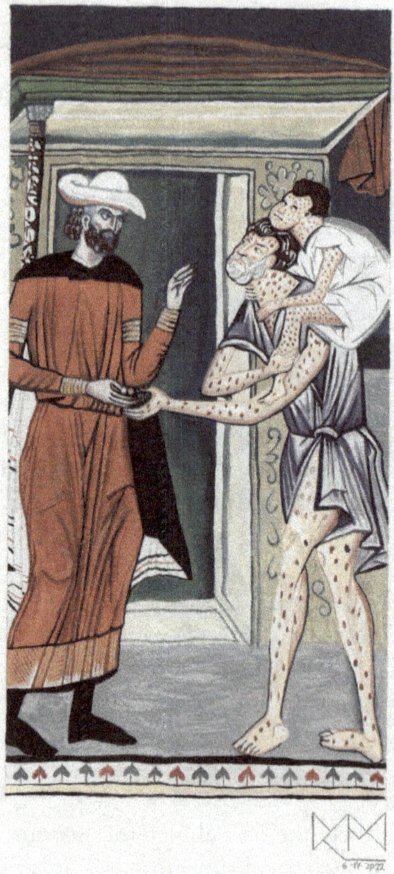

Figure 5.2 Fresco from St Archangel Michael's Church, the Lesnovo Monastery, Macedonia, 1347 CE. Image courtesy of Richard Marshall.

are often described in ancient literature as using their staffs as substitutes for their eyes (in fact, a degree of synaesthesia is apparent as these individuals are described as using their staffs as supplementary hands as they 'feel' their way), but it is possible that some utilised dogs just as a contemporary visually impaired individual might.[25] In this vein, it has

25 For the visually impaired using their staffs as guides, see for example Eur. *Phoen.* 1546; Prudent. 2.145–8. On synaesthesia in antiquity, see Butler and Purves, 2013. On seeing eye dogs, see Laes, 2018, p. 100 for discussion. See also Esser, 1959 and De Libero, 2002, p. 86.

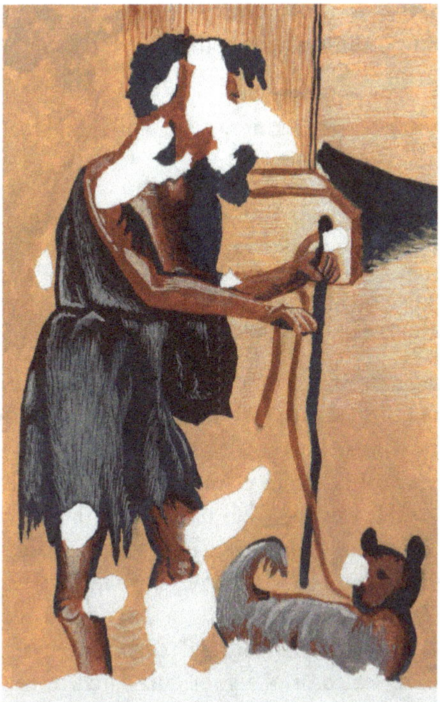

Figure 5.3 Section from the 'Forum Frieze' fresco from the atrium of the Praedia of Julia Felix, Pompeii, 62–79 CE. Naples National Archaeological Museum inv. 9059. Image courtesy of Richard Marshall.

been suggested that the so-called 'Forum Frieze' from the atrium of the Praedia of Julia Felix at Pompeii (II.4.3–12) depicts a blind man using a dog as a guide, and, if this suggestion is correct, this would be the earliest known depiction of a visually impaired individual using a guide or seeing eye dog (see Figure 5.3).[26] Unfortunately, the fresco is in a very poor condition so it is difficult to make out precisely what it depicts, but it appears to show a man holding a walking stick in his left hand, perhaps even leaning on it, and a lead in his right hand, which is attached to the collar of a dog, in conversation or perhaps begging with a woman and her companion.[27]

[26] Naples National Archaeological Museum inv. 9059.

[27] For discussion of the history of seeing-eye dogs, see Fishman, 2003, p. 452.

Another alternative is the monkey. There are references in ancient literature to monkeys imitating human behaviour, such as this anecdote recorded by Aelian:

> A monkey observed from a distance a nurse washing a baby in a tub, observed how first of all she took off its swaddling clothes and then after the bath wrapped it up; it marked where she laid it to rest, and when it saw the place unguarded, sprang in through an open window, from which it had a view of everything; took the baby from its cot; stripped it as it had chanced to see the nurse do; brought the tub out, and (there was water heating on some embers) poured boiling water over the wretched baby and even caused it to die most miserably.[28]

Granted, this is not a positive outcome for the baby (and certainly not for the nurse), and the point of the story is to prove Aelian's designation of the monkey as 'the most mischievous of animals' true, but it does make the point that monkeys could imitate human actions.[29] Numerous ancient literary sources from as early as Plautus in the third century BCE record Romans keeping monkeys as domestic pets and they are often depicted in Roman art; zooarchaeological evidence has proved the veracity of this (for example, the bones of a Barbary macaque have been recovered from the Sarno Baths in Pompeii).[30] An animal cemetery recently excavated at Berenike on the Red Sea coast of Egypt and dated to the first and second centuries BCE has revealed the skeletal remains of sixteen resus macaques that had been laid to rest with a considerable amount of care, arranged like sleeping babies or children and accompanied by grave goods including shells, a woollen blanket, amphoras, and piglet and kitten bones.[31] Perhaps monkeys such as these could have been trained to render assistance to individuals with physical impairments and limited mobility, and could

[28] Ael. *NA* 7.21 (trans. A. F. Scholfield): αὐτίκα γοῦν ἰδὼν ἐξ ἀπόπτου τροφὸν λούουσαν παιδίον ἐυ σκάφῃ, καὶ πρῶτον μὲν ὑπολύουσαν τὰ σπάργανα, εἶται ἐκ τοῦ λουτροῦ κατειλοῦσαν αὐτό, παραφυλάξας ἔνθα ἀνέπαυσε τὸ βρέφος, ὡς εἶδεν ἐρημίαν, ἐσέθορε διά τινος ἀνεῳγμένης θυρίδος, ἐξ ἧς οἱ πάντα2 σύνοπτα ἦν, καὶ ἄρας ἐκ τῆς εὐνῆς τὸ παιδίον, καὶ γυμνώσας ὡς ἔτυχεν ἰδών, καὶ κομίσας ἐς μέσον τὴν σκάφην, ζέον ὕδωρ (καὶ γὰρ ἦν ἐπί τινων ἀνθράκων θερμαινόμενον) τοῦ δυστυχοῦς παιδίου κατέχεε, καὶ μέντοι καὶ ἀπέκτεινεν αὐτὸ οἴκτιστα. Thanks to Christian Laes for bringing this passage to my attention.

[29] Ael. *NA* 7.21 (trans. A. F. Scholfield): Κακοηθέστατον δὲ ἄρα τῶν ζῴων ὁ πίθηκος ἦν. For a similar example of a monkey being trained to imitate human behaviour with similarly unsuccessful, albeit far less severe consequences, see Luc. *De Merc. cond.* 5. This monkey had been trained to dance in perfect time with the music made by singers and flautists but was easily distracted by treats such as figs and almonds, which would lead him to pull off his mask and tear it up. For other references to ancient performing monkeys, see Toynbee, 1973, reissued 2013, pp. 57–8. For ancient monkeys more generally, see Vespa, 2020.

[30] Bailey et al., 1999.

[31] Fox, 2020. The full publication of the site is hopefully forthcoming.

perhaps have been trusted with relatively simple, low-risk tasks such as fetching and carrying.

While, as discussed, humans could carry physically impaired individuals over short distances, animals were preferred for longer ones, usually equids such as donkeys or mules. The impaired individual who argues that he should be permitted to receive a pension on the grounds of his disability in Lysias' twenty-fourth speech discusses his use of equids to transport himself. While his accuser has suggested that his ability to use a horse means that he is not, in fact, disabled, the speaker argues that, on the contrary, he is only using a horse to get around because he is, in fact, disabled.[32] He equates the equids that he occasionally borrows from friends with the two sticks that he uses, as he 'use[s] both aids for the same reason'.[33]

Impairment, Disability, and Enslavement

How did the impaired and disabled individuals who utilised the bodies and body parts of other human beings and, on occasion, animals view this process of requisition? Did they attempt to rationalise or justify it? Or did they simply take it for granted? Seneca the Younger writes to Lucilius of a wealthy man of his acquaintance named Calvisius Sabinus:

> He had the bank-account and the brains of a freedman. I never saw a man whose good fortune was a greater offence against propriety. **His memory was so faulty that he would sometimes forget the name of Ulysses, or Achilles, or Priam, names which we know as well as we know those of our own attendants**. No major-domo in his dotage, who cannot give men their right names, but is compelled to invent names for them, no such man, I say, calls off the names of his master's tribesmen so atrociously as Sabinus used to call off the Trojan and Achaean heroes. **But none the less did he desire to appear learned. So he devised this short cut to learning: he paid fabulous prices for slaves, one to know Homer by heart and another to know Hesiod; he also delegated a special slave to each of the nine lyric poets. You need not wonder that he paid high prices for these slaves; if he did not find them ready to hand he had them made to order**. After collecting this retinue, he began to make life miserable for his guests; he would keep these fellows at the foot of his couch, and ask them from time to time for verses which he might repeat, and then frequently break down in the middle of a word. Satellius Quadratus, a feeder, and consequently a fawner, upon addle-pated millionaires, and also (for this quality goes with the other two) a flouter of them, suggested to Sabinus that he should have philologists to

[32] Lys. 24.11.

[33] Lys. 24.12 (trans. W. R. M. Lamb): ἐγὼ διὰ τὴν αὐτὴν αἰτίαν ἀμφοτέροις χρῶμαι.

> gather up the bits. Sabinus remarked that each slave cost him one hundred thousand sesterces; Satellius replied: 'You might have bought as many bookcases for a smaller sum'. But **Sabinus held to the opinion that what any member of his household knew, he himself knew also**. This same Satellius began to advise Sabinus to take wrestling lessons, sickly, pale, and thin as he was. Sabinus answered: 'How can I? I can scarcely stay alive now'. 'Don't say that, I implore you', replied the other, 'consider how many perfectly healthy slaves you have!' **No man is able to borrow or buy a sound mind**; in fact, as it seems to me, even though sound minds were for sale, they would not find buyers. Depraved minds, however, are bought and sold every day.[34]

While it is debatable by modern standards as to whether Calvisius Sabinus suffered from a mental impairment, his poor memory would certainly have been viewed as such by his elite Roman peers, and one of its consequences would have been a degree of social disability; Seneca's low opinion of his acquaintance's mental acuity is made explicit in the quoted passage. However, for our purposes this passage offers a fascinating insight into how an impaired individual with financial resources might go about acquiring specialist caregivers. Calvisius Sabinus seems to have either sought out enslaved individuals with the specific skill sets that he required, or, where none existed, invested money in having them trained up to his precise specifications.

A similar approach to dealing with an intellectual impairment and its ramifications is attested by Philostratus in relation to the orator Herodes Atticus and his son Atticus Bradua:

> [Atticus Bradua] had been misrepresented to [Herodes Atticus] as foolish, bad at his letters, and of a dull memory. At any rate, when [Bradua] could not master his alphabet, the idea occurred to Herodes to bring up with him

[34] Sen. *Ep.* 27.5–8 (trans. R. M. Gummere, with minor adjustments; emphasis added): *Calvisius Sabinus memoria nostra fuit dives. Et patrimonium habebat libertini et ingenium; numquam vidi hominem beatum indecentius. Huic memoria tam mala erat, ut illi nomen modo Vlixis excideret, modo Achillis, modo Priami, quos tam bene quam paedagogos nostros novimus. Nemo vetulus nomenclator, qui nomina non reddit, sed inponit, tam perperam tribus quam ille Troianos et Achivos persalutabat. Nihilominus eruditus volebat videri. Hanc itaque conpendiariam excogitavit: magna summa emit servos, unum, qui Homerum teneret, alterum, qui Hesiodum; novem praeterea lyricis singulos adsignavit. Magno emisse illum non est quod mireris; non invenerat, faciendos locavit. Postquam haec familia illi conparata est, coepit convivas suos inquietare. Habebat ad pedes hos, a quibus subinde cum peteret versus, quos referret, saepe in medio verbo excidebat. Suasit illi Satellius Quadratus, stultorum divitum adrosor, et quod sequitur, adrisor, et quod duobus his adiunctum est, derisor, ut grammaticos haberet analectas. Cum dixisset Sabinus centenis milibus sibi constare singulos servos; 'Minoris', inquit, 'totidem scrinia emisses'. Ille tamen in ea opinione erat, ut putaret se scire, quod quisquam in domo sua sciret. Idem Satellius illum hortari coepit, ut luctaretur, hominem aegrum, pallidum, gracilem. Cum Sabinus respondisset: 'Et quomodo possum? Vix vivo', 'Noli, obsecro te', inquit, 'istuc dicere; non vides, quam multos servos valentissimos habeas?' Bona mens nec commodatur nec emitur. Et puto, si venalis esset, non haberet emptorem. At mala cotidie emitur.*

> twenty-four boys of the same age named after the letters of the alphabet, so that he would be obliged to learn his letters at the same time as the names of the boys.[35]

Like Calvisius Sabinus' poor memory, Atticus Bradua's poor memory would not necessarily be considered an impairment today, but for the son of a Roman consul who would have been expected to follow in his father's footsteps, and of an internationally famous orator, it was a potentially extremely serious social disability. However, this ingenious means of alleviating it seems to have been successful; Bradua was himself appointed consul in 185 CE, and no further mention of his purported intellectual deficiencies is made.[36]

It is clear from the epigraphic evidence found in the columbaria owned by senatorial families dating to the early imperial period that have been excavated around the city of Rome that elite Roman households comprised many members with very specific job titles and narrow remits; the wealthier a household, the more enslaved individuals it had, and the more specialised their duties were. So, in a wealthy household it would not be surprising to find individuals whose sole duties were to assist those members of the household with tasks that, due to their impairments, they were physically unable to perform. Thus, for example, an *ornatrix* charged with dressing and adorning her mistress might find her duties extending to care of her mistress' prosthetic teeth or hair, while someone *a cubiculo* charged with managing the bedroom might find his or her duties extending to helping their master or mistress in and out of bed.

As Seneca makes explicit by reporting Calvisius Sabinus' speech, as far as the latter was concerned, the knowledge, skills, and experience that his enslaved attendants possessed were his knowledge, skills, and experience because he owned them and thus owned their talents too. Since an enslaved individual's primary function was to be of physical service to his or her enslaver, in providing this physical service, the enslaved individual became part of the enslaver's physical nature.[37] This belief in the enslaved individual as a constituent part of the enslaver had a long history.[38] So, just as Carvilius Sabinus requisitioned his enslaved attendants' memories, so might another

[35] Philostr. *VS* 2.1.588 (trans. W. C. Wright): διεβέβλητο δὲ πρὸς αὐτὸν ὡς ἠλιθιώδη καὶ δυσγράμματον καὶ παχὺν τὴν μνήμην· τὰ γοῦν πρῶτα γράμματα παραλαβεῖν μὴ δυνηθέντος ἦλθεν ἐς ἐπίνοιαν τῷ Ἡρώδῃ ξυντρέφειν αὐτῷ τέτταρας παῖδας καὶ εἴκοσιν ἰσήλικας ὠνομασμένους ἀπὸ τῶν γραμμάτων, ἵνα ἐν τοῖς τῶν παίδων ὀνόμασι τὰ γράμματα ἐξ ἀνάγκης αὐτῷ μελετῷτο.

[36] For discussion of learning difficulties in classical antiquity, see Laes, 2018, p. 57.

[37] Wrenhaven, 2011, p. 99. See also Blake, 2013.

[38] See for example Aristotle's discussion of enslavement at *Pol.* 1.1254a.

enslaver requisition their eyes, ears, voices, hands, arms, feet, or legs. In a manner of speaking, since most of the human hair that was used for the creation of wigs and hair pieces seems to have been harvested from prisoners of war, a wig or hairpiece owner was requisitioning another enslaved individual's hair, just not their own enslaved individual's.[39]

The fact that the impaired and disabled of classical antiquity utilised the bodies of others as supplements or even replacements for their own should not come as a surprise considering the reliance of ancient societies on enslavement. One of the words used to refer to enslaved individuals in classical antiquity was ἀνδράποδον (literally, a 'man-footed thing'), reminiscent of the word used to refer to cattle, τετραπόδης (literally, a 'four-footed thing').[40] Another was σῶμα, 'body', and the enslaved seem to have been perceived as proxy or surrogate bodies for their enslavers: according to Artemidorus, if you dreamed of your enslaved, you were really dreaming of yourself, and on certain occasions the enslaved literally stood as proxy or surrogate bodies for their enslavers, submitting to punishments or even death sentences on their behalves.[41]

In ancient Greece and Rome, slaves were conceptualised as tools and were parts of their master or mistress, entirely subsumed to their will: for example, Aristotle referred to the enslaved as 'living tools', while Varro described them as 'articulate tools' – in both cases, the emphasis is placed squarely on their functionality.[42] Yet there is an inherent contradiction here: while the enslaver might think that they want their enslaved attendants to be nothing more than automata, mere extensions of their own will, in order to serve their enslaver effectively an enslaved attendant needs to possess and display a degree of independent thought and initiative.[43] Their purpose was to provide 'bodily service for the necessities of life', although how their enslavers interpreted that could vary considerably according to their specific set of needs.[44] The fact that the very definition of freedom in classical antiquity was considered to be not living for the benefit of another does raise the question as to whether individuals who were not enslaved would, out of choice, proffer assistance to the impaired and disabled for fear of impugning their own dignity as free individuals.[45] According to Pseudo-Quintilian, Roman law decreed that if someone was responsible for blinding someone else, their punishment was literally 'an eye for an eye': either they themselves had to submit to being blinded, or they had

[39] For further discussion, see Draycott, 2019c. [40] Wrenhaven, 2011, p. 104.
[41] Artem. *On*. 4.30. For the enslaved sacrificing themselves, see Val. Max. 6.6.
[42] Arist. *Eth. Nic*. 1162b4; Varro, *Rust*. 1.17. [43] Fitzgerald, 2000, p. 27.
[44] Arist. *Pol*. 1254b25–7 (trans. H. Rackham): ἡ γὰρ πρὸς14 τἀναγκαῖα τῷ σώματι βοήθεια.
[45] Arist. *Rhet*. 1367a32–3.

to make amends in some way, such as 'giving' their eyes to the person they had blinded and serving as their guide.[46] In the hypothetical scenario proposed, a soldier blinds his prostitute lover and she, rather than choosing for him to be blinded, requests that he guide her; the soldier refuses and requests to be blinded, on the grounds that 'it would not do for a hero to give his hand to a prostitute for to show her the way'.[47] He is very clear about his reasoning: 'it's shameful for a hero to take on such an office'.[48] Is it shameful that a military hero should have to be seen publicly with a prostitute, or is it shameful that a free man should have to lower himself to waiting on someone else and performing a role normally taken by an enslaved person?

That is not to say that impaired and disabled individuals simply took this assistance for granted and never ruminated on what it signified. According to Pliny the Younger, one of his acquaintances, Domitius Tullus, was an invalid and was highly vocal about the indignities that he perceived his condition to have inflicted upon him:

> Crippled and deformed in every limb, he could only enjoy his vast wealth by contemplating it, and could not even turn in bed without assistance. He also had to have his teeth cleaned and brushed for him – a squalid and pitiful detail – and when complaining about the humiliations of his infirmity was often heard to say that every day he licked the fingers of his slaves.[49]

This gives us something of an insight into the degree of assistance that it was considered normal and appropriate for the enslaved to render their enslaver, and how those individuals who required more than was usual may have felt about it.

Finally, it is notable that in the series of epigrams from the *Greek Anthology* discussed earlier, the visually impaired man and the mobility-impaired man are described as beggars. This explains why they are reduced to helping each other rather than relying on assistance from members of their households. Likewise, part of the argument that Lysias' impaired individual makes regarding his eligibility for a pension is that he is in such straightened financial circumstances that he cannot even afford one enslaved attendant to assist him.[50]

[46] Quint. 297.

[47] Quint. 297.4 (trans. D. R. Shackleton Bailey): *Negat fas esse ut vir fortis manum meretrici praestet, ut iter demonstret.*

[48] Quint. 297.13 (trans. D. R. Shackleton Bailey): *Enim forti viro turpe est hoc officium subire.*

[49] Plin. *Ep.* 18.9–10 (trans. B. Radice): *Quippe omnibus membris extortus et fractus, tantas opes solis oculis obibat, ac ne in lectulo quidem nisi ab aliis movebatur; quin etiam (foedum miserandumque dictu) dentes lavandos fricandosque praebebat. Auditum frequenter ex ipso, cum quereretur de contumeliis debilitatis suae, digitos se servorum suorum cotidie lingere.*

[50] Lys. 24.7.

Conclusion

It has been argued that the presence of the enslaved in ancient Greece and Rome led to what has been described as the 'stagnation' of ancient technologies. While this argument has been refuted, it is worth considering in relation to assistive technology, if not other types of technology, in classical antiquity. The institution of enslavement and the use of the enslaved in classical antiquity is relevant to how we view prostheses and assistive technology in classical antiquity. In the contemporary world, an individual who acquires a physical impairment such as the loss of a limb must undergo an extensive period of rehabilitation, relearning how to do everything that they previously did with two limbs with one limb and a prosthesis instead, while an individual who develops a sensory impairment such as blindness or deafness may acquire and train with an assistance dog. This enables them to live independently, or as independently as possible. However, in classical antiquity most people, whether impaired or not, did not live independently. Rather, they lived with the enslaved and relied upon them for a wide range of daily activities, including those that a contemporary individual usually accomplishes without assistance. This raises perhaps the most fundamental question of this monograph: did an impaired individual in the classical world ever actually need a functional prosthesis? Should we even be attempting to evaluate ancient prostheses based on our contemporary assessments of their functionality or lack thereof, and judging them accordingly? Or should we perhaps be using entirely different criteria and viewing them as having a different sort of functionality, and being more akin to clothing or jewellery?

It is possible that the prostheses and other types of assistive technology that were used in classical antiquity were used precisely because they served purposes that other people could not easily serve. For example, in the case of the Egyptian individuals that lost their great toes, they would still have been able to walk unassisted, unlike someone who lost part or all of one leg, but their balance would have been negatively affected. So, prosthetic great toes would have served to improve their balance in a way that the assistance of another person or animal could not, hence examples of this type of prosthetic – the Greville Chester Toe and the Cairo Toe – having survived from classical antiquity.

Conclusion

The eleventh main instalment (the twentieth overall) in the *Assassin's Creed* action-adventure stealth video game franchise, *Assassin's Creed Odyssey*, was released in the autumn of 2018. The game, set in Greece in the year 431 BCE, during a fictionalised version of the Peloponnesian Wars, allows the player to explore an open-world version of ancient Greece, choosing whether to play as either the character Alexios or his sister Kassandra.

Early on in the game, while the character is still on their home island of Kephallonia and the player is working their way through what serves as an extended tutorial section, they are tasked by their mentor Markos to undertake the 'An Eye for an Eye' quest and steal the Obsidian Eye, the eye of the Cyclops of Kephallonia, an obsidian prosthetic eye belonging to the head of the island's criminal gang. The theft is in retaliation for the Cyclops sending his men to harass Markos and Alexios/Kassandra in response to Markos not settling a debt; Markos plans to sell the eye to pay the money that he owes.

The individual is known as the Cyclops because he is missing his left eye. When the player arrives at the Lair of the Cyclops in Kleptous Bay, they find the Cyclops torturing the sea captain Barnabus because the latter happened to mention having encountered a 'one-eyed monster' on his travels, leading the Cyclops to think that he was insulting him. The Cyclops is very clear to both Barnabus and Alexios/Kassandra: he does not like to be referred to as the Cyclops. In response, Alexios/Kassandra inserts the eye into the backside of a nearby goat, which provokes the Cyclops into attacking, and the player must defeat and kill him. Subsequently retrieving the eye earns the player the 'Stink Eye' trophy, and the eye can then be either sold for 2750 drachmae or retained as part of the player's inventory.

This quest borrows liberally from both Greek mythology and Greek history. While the Cyclops is human, and nothing to do with the mythological Cyclopes Brontes the Thunderer, Steropes the Lightning Bringer, and Arges the Bright One that the player must face later in the game, there

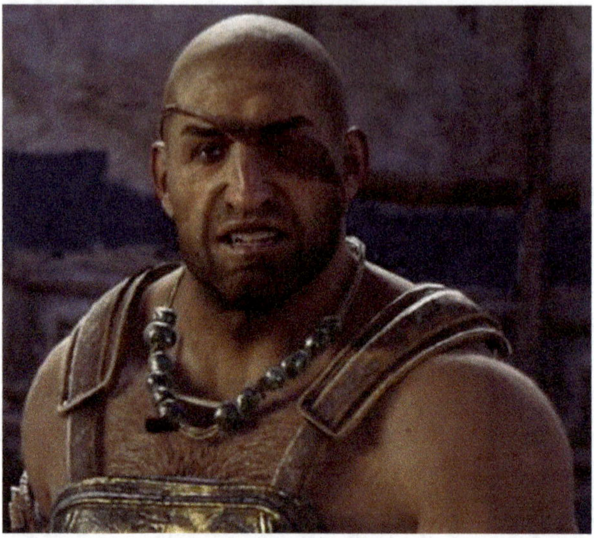

Figure 6.1 Still from *Assassin's Creed Odyssey*. Image courtesy of Ubisoft.

are several nods to the mythological creature Polyphemus, such as Barnabus' reference to encountering a one-eyed monster on a sea voyage, and the involvement of the goats.[1] Additionally, there are historical accounts of individuals who lost one of their eyes both being referred to by others as 'Cyclops', and disliking this practice, such as Philip II of Macedon (382–336 BCE) and Antigonus I (382–301 BCE).[2] However, as discussed earlier, the evidence for the existence of prosthetic eyes in classical antiquity is rather slim. Certainly, there are no definitive literary or documentary references, or even archaeological examples, of prosthetic eyes dating from the Classical period, which is when *Assassin's Creed Odyssey* is set.[3] But could an impaired individual like the Cyclops have utilised an obsidian prosthetic eye at this time? Certainly, obsidian was available in Classical Greece; a volcanic glass, it could be acquired from Milos, one of the islands in the Cyclades, and Gyali, one of the islands in the Dodecanese. The individual would have to be careful, however, as considering the sharpness of obsidian when broken, there would have been considerable risk involved in doing so.

[1] For the most famous ancient account of Polyphemus, see Hom. *Od.* 9.

[2] For discussion, see Draycott, 2018b.

[3] The earliest surviving prosthetic eye dates to the Mesolithic period, see Enoch, 2009.

In placing a visually impaired person at the centre of the narrative, *Assassin's Creed Odyssey* offers disability representation that is authentic and accurate to the historical period and setting (the game is set, after all, during the Peloponnesian Wars, and the debilitating Plague of Athens plays a significant role in the story and world-building), but it does fall back on the trope of the impaired individual as villain.[4] This is perhaps unsurprising; although Ubisoft employs a Greek historian and archaeologist, Dr. Stéphanie-Anne Ruatta, she is still reliant on existing historical and archaeological scholarship.[5]

To date, assistive technology of all kinds has been severely underrepresented in ancient historical scholarship, including (and especially) that which focuses specifically on impairment and disability.[6] This is somewhat surprising. Why have scholars of ancient impairment and disability paid so little attention to this area subject and not taken advantage of the information that the subject can provide for social history, cultural history, medical history, and the history of technology?[7] Examining the use of assistive technology in antiquity offers us an unprecedented glimpse into the lives of ancient people living with impairments and disabilities, and an opportunity to reconstruct certain otherwise unrecorded and hence unattested aspects of their lived experiences. And, considering what we know about ancient living conditions and standards, it is entirely possible that what we might today consider an overlooked minority was, in fact, a significant majority.[8]

Pieces of ancient assistive technology are objects, and as such they can be said to have object biographies or artefact biographies.[9] Depending upon the piece of ancient assistive technology in question, we can access some of these biographies, or parts of these biographies, in detail.[10] A piece of ancient assistive technology such as a prosthesis was designed, commissioned, manufactured, used, and eventually deposited, sometimes as

4 For explorations of the use of impairment and disability in popular culture, see Alaniz, 2014; Allen, 2013.

5 For an interview in which Dr Ruatta discusses the process, see Reinhard, 2019.

6 For an attempt to begin to address this oversight in relation to mobility impairments in the Roman Republic and Empire, see Graham, 2017.

7 For an attempt to undertake this sort of interdisciplinary enquiry in relation to the use of respirators in the nineteenth century; Jennifer Wallis' '"To be Eccentric or Fashionable": Respirators, Style, and Science in the Nineteenth Century' (unpublished article, via personal communication).

8 See Graham, 2013, p. 268, for her suggestion of 'a sliding scale of impairment'. See Pudsey, 2017, p. 24, for her observation that 'in all likelihood, hundreds of thousands, if not millions, of living people in the Roman world would have been experiencing disability'.

9 For discussion of these terms and their implications, see Gosden and Marshall, 1999.

10 See, for example, the detailed research that has been undertaken on the ancient Egyptian prosthetic toes: Finch, 2019.

a votive offering at the end of its life, or as part of its user's/wearer's burial, mummification, or cremation. Over the course of this study, I have attempted to flesh out this process using a combination of ancient literary, documentary, archaeological and bioarchaeological evidence, and a degree of impressionistic inference based on comparative material from other periods of history and the modern and contemporary world. I have shown that there is enough evidence for one particular type of assistive technology in particular – prostheses – to begin the process of understanding and interpreting them, their use, and their users. Using the data set of 107 literary references and 54 archaeological examples, it is possible both to identify broad trends and to drill down into the detail of individuals. There were many different types of prostheses, there was considerable variation – individualisation, in fact – in their form and their function, and both men and women used them, albeit in considerably different ways.

Objects are integral to human actions; they affect the human experience of the world, and an individual's lived experience. The human body plus material objects such as clothing, footwear, and accessories are all props in the performance of identity/identities, communicating both what the individual wishes to project, but also what their audience sees, whether the individual has factored that in to their communication or not. As such, it can be rewarding to consider ancient assistive technologies as a type of dress, although they are not generally included in studies on the subject of ancient dress.[11] One exception to this general rule can be found in Mireille Lee's *Body, Dress, and Identity in Ancient Greece*, which acknowledges certain types of assistive technology – prostheses and walking sticks – as worth considering:

> Handheld accessories might be considered less meaningful than other aspects of dress on account of the ease with which they may be removed by the user. On the other hand, the manipulation of such objects by the dressed individuals suggests that they might be especially charged. Their importance is underscored by the fact that they are frequently worn by those who are otherwise 'undressed'.[12]

Perhaps this inclusion is due to her decision to undertake a phenomenological approach to the study of dress:

> As an embodied social practice, dress must be considered in terms of its relationship with the body. Indeed, neither the body nor dress can be

[11] For a concise explanation as to why 'dress' is the best term to use, see Lee, 2015, p. 21.
[12] Lee, 2015, p. 171.

> understood in isolation; each derives its meaning from the other, dress is the medium through which the biological body becomes a social body.[13]

Ancient assistive technologies were not only an extension of the body but also an extension of the self. Although physically unimpaired individuals may well have used certain types of ancient assistive technology as accessories, such as hair pieces to supplement their own hair in the creation of elaborate hairstyles or staffs to indicate their political or religious offices, physically impaired individuals used them for different reasons, and under these circumstances they were not simply accessories. Consequently, ancient assistive technologies can be described as technologies of participation, since they rendered their users/wearers able to participate more fully in society. So Marcus Sergius Silus' iron hand enabled him to participate first in military activity as a soldier and later in political and religious activity as a praetor, Mindon's wooden leg enabled him to participate in agricultural activity as a farmer, and any number of Jewish women's golden, silver, bone, ivory, and wooden teeth enabled them to participate in social activities as viable candidates for marriage. Thus, the use of ancient assistive technologies was undoubtedly performative. While an ancient assistive technology such as a prosthesis concealed the impairment to a degree, with an extremity prosthesis covering the stump or a dental prosthesis covering the missing tooth or teeth, they could not do so in such a way as to conceal the impairment entirely.[14] What they could do, however, was redirect attention away from the impairment to the technology and, in doing so, reframe the interaction from a negative one to a positive one: a means of demonstrating wealth, status, good taste, ingenuity, etc.

In addition, the use of an ancient assistive technology altered its user's/wearer's relationship with their own body and with the physical environment that their body inhabited. We should consider the sensory experience of using a piece of ancient assistive technology, of being in sustained physical contact with organic and inorganic materials such as leather, wood, bone, ivory, hair, gems, and metal. While a user/wearer of an extremity prosthesis, a wig, or a hairpiece experienced the sensation of having something next to their body for a prolonged period of time, and the sweating, itching, and other less-than-pleasant physical sensations that resulted, a user of a cosmetic prosthesis such as a dental appliance or an eye

[13] Lee, 2015, p. 230.

[14] For a rare example of an ancient prosthesis said to be of such high quality that no one knew its user/wearer was impaired; see Suetonius' comments on the emperor Otho's wig at *Oth.* 12.

had to insert something into their body and experience the sensation of having something not just next to their body but inside their body for a prolonged period of time. Depending upon the type of ancient assistive technology used or worn, its user/wearer might be able to manipulate it to a greater or lesser extent. A wig or hairpiece could potentially be styled as desired, a prosthetic hand could be used to hold something in place, a staff could serve a variety of purposes ranging from a support to a tool to a weapon. Or a piece of ancient assistive technology might succeed in manipulating its user/wearer, causing them to make significant changes to their life in order to facilitate its presence. Someone using/wearing a prosthesis had to move in a different way to someone not wearing a prosthesis: their movements had to be slower, more considered, and more careful; if their prosthesis became separated from their body, it was a source not only of potential danger but also one of potential embarrassment.[15] Someone who used/wore a prosthesis for many years would see it come to affect the body itself. These effects included leaving visible marks on the surface of the body, ranging from chafing and blisters to build up of calluses to wear on the teeth that were used to help place it.[16] Yet they also left marks on the interior of the body that, while invisible to the user/wearer and their peers, still had a tangible effect upon their quality of life, such as stress fractures and alterations to bones.[17] It is clear that certain types of assistive technology – prostheses first and foremost among them – were viewed as an extension of the body, perhaps even part of the body, as indicated by the fact that they were included in their users' burials not as grave goods but attached to the body in death exactly as they had been in life, and excluded from restrictive sumptuary legislation.[18]

Yet not everyone was accepting of ancient assistive technologies, with anxieties regarding human enhancement dating back as far as the Archaic period.[19] But is 'enhancement' the best term to use in this context? A piece of ancient assistive technology, even a prosthesis, did not physically enhance its user: for example, ancient extremity prostheses did not enable their users to run, and ancient dental prostheses did not enable their users to chew. One key exception is the case of the wings designed by Daedalus

[15] For examples of ancient reactions to wigs coming loose ranging from amusement to disgust, see Hor. *Sat.* 1.8.47–50; Ov. *Ars am* 3.250; Avienus, *Fables* 11.7–12.

[16] See, for example, the wear on the teeth of the skeleton with the weaponised right-hand prosthesis caused by consistently using them to tighten the leather straps that secured the knife-hand to the wrist: Micarelli et al., 2018.

[17] See, for example, the stress fractures identified on the scapula of the skeleton with the impaired leg and interpreted as an indicator of crutch use: Belcastro and Mariotti, 2000.

[18] *Laws of the Twelve Tables* 10.8–9.

[19] Mayor, 2018.

for use by himself and his son Icarus to facilitate their escape from Crete.[20] While these are described as 'prosthetic', they were not prostheses in the sense that they were replacing or supplementing a missing or immobilised body part. Rather, they were augmentations. And, for Icarus at least, this attempt at augmenting one's physical body and overcoming its natural limitations proved fatal. While a user of ancient assistive technology could perhaps be described as a cyborg, they could certainly not be described as posthuman.

Finally, there are clear similarities between certain aspects of ancient assistive technology usage and contemporary assistive technology usage, and the process of exploring these can offer us insights into the relationship between humans and objects that has been ongoing throughout the whole of human history.

[20] Palaephatus, *On Unbelievable Things* 12.

References

Acton, Peter (2014) *Poiesis: Manufacturing in Classical Athens*. Oxford: Oxford University Press.

Adams, Ellen (2017) 'Fragmentation and the Body's Boundaries: Reassessing the Body in Parts', in Draycott, Jane and Graham, Emma-Jayne (eds.) *Bodies of Evidence: Anatomical Votives Past, Present and Future*. Abingdon: Routledge, pp. 193–213.

Adams, Ellen (2019) 'The Psychology of Prostheses: Substitution Strategies and Notions of Normality', in Draycott, Jane (ed.) *Prostheses in Antiquity*. London: Routledge, pp. 180–208.

Adams, Ellen (ed.) (2021a) *Disability Studies and the Classical Body: The Forgotten Other*. London: Routledge.

Adams, Ellen (2021b) 'Using, Creating and Showcasing Disability Supports and Services', in Adams, Ellen (ed.) *Disability Studies and the Classical Body: The Forgotten Other*. London: Routledge, pp. 89–91.

Africa, Thomas W. (1970) 'The One-Eyed Man Against Rome: An Exercise in Euhemerism', *Historia* 19.5, pp. 528–38.

Alaniz, José (2014) *Death, Disability, and the Super Hero: The Silver Age and Beyond*. Jackson: University Press of Mississippi.

Aldhouse-Green, Miranda (2004a) 'Crowning Glories: Languages of Hair in Later Prehistoric Europe', *Proceedings of the Prehistoric Society* 70, pp. 299–325.

Aldhouse-Green, Miranda (2004b) 'Chaining and Shaming: Images of Defeat, from Llyn Cerrig Bach to Sarmitzegetusa', *Oxford Journal of Archaeology* 23.3, pp. 319–40.

Allan, Kathryn (ed.) (2013) *Disability in Science Fiction: Representations of Technology as Cure*. New York: Palgrave Macmillan.

Allason-Jones, Lindsay (2005) *Women in Roman Britain*. York: Council of British Archaeology.

Allwood, Emma H. (2015) 'Is Disability Fashion's Forgotten Diversity Frontier?', *Dazed Digital*: https://bit.ly/1URhV7v (accessed January 2021).

Anagnostou-Laoutides, Eva (2015) 'Herodas' *Mimiamb* 7: Dancing Dogs and Barking Women', *Classical Quarterly* 65.1, pp. 153–66.

Anglesey, G. C. H. V. P. (1961) *One-leg: The Life and Letters of Henry William Paget, 1st Marquess of Anglesey*. London: Cape.

Antikas, Theodore G. and Wynn-Antikas, Laura K. (2015) 'New Finds from the Cremains in Tomb II at Vergina Point to Philip II and a Scythian Princess', *International Journal of Osteoarchaeology* 26.4, pp. 682–92.

Arena, Valentina (2012) *Libertas and the Practice of Politics in the Late Roman Republic*. Cambridge: Cambridge University Press.

Armstrong, Keith (2014) 'Possibly the First Wheeled Walking Aid (Revised)', available online at www.academia.edu/7448296/Possibly_the_first_wheeled_walking_aid_Revised_by_Keith_Armstrong (accessed August 2022).

Audollent, Auguste (1921) 'Les tombes des Martres-de-Veyre', *Man* 21, pp. 161–4.

Audollent, Auguste (1923) 'Les tombes gallo-romaines à inhumation des Martres-de-Veyre (Puy-de-Dôme)', *Mémoires présentés par divers savants à l'Académie des inscriptions et belles-lettres (Paris)* 13, pp. 275–328.

Aufderheide, Arthur C. and Rodriguez-Martin, Conrado (1998) *The Cambridge Encyclopedia of Human Paleopathology*. Cambridge: Cambridge University Press.

Bagnall, Roger S. and Cribiore, Raffaella (2006) *Women's Letters from Ancient Egypt, 300 BC–AD 800*. Ann Arbor, MI: University of Michigan Press.

Bailey, Jillian F., Henneberg, Maciej, Colson, Isabelle B., et al. (1999) 'Monkey Business in Pompeii – Unique Find of a Juvenile Barbary Macaque Skeleton in Pompeii Identified Using Osteology and Ancient DNA Techniques', *Molecular Biology and Evolution* 16.10, pp. 1410–14.

Baker, Patricia (2011) 'Collyrium Stamps: An Indicator of Regional Practices in Roman Gaul', *European Journal of Archaeology* 14.1–2, pp. 158–89.

Bartman, Elizabeth (1999) *Portraits of Livia: Imaging the Imperial Woman in Augustan Rome*. Cambridge: Cambridge University Press.

Bartman, Elizabeth (2001) 'Hair and the Artifice of Roman Female Adornment', *American Journal of Archaeology* 105.1, pp. 1–25.

Barton, Tamsyn (1994) *Ancient Astrology*. London: Routledge.

Barton, Tamsyn S. (2002) *Power and Knowledge: Astrology, Physiognomics, and Medicine under the Roman Empire*. Ann Arbor, MI: University of Michigan Press.

Bartsch, Shadi (2006) *The Mirror of the Self: Sexuality, Self-Knowledge, and the Gaze in the Early Roman Empire*. Chicago, IL: University of Chicago Press.

Baumgartner, R. (1982) 'Fußprothese aus einem Frühmittelalterlichen Grab aus Bonaduz', *Helvetia Archaeologica* 51, pp. 155–62.

Beagon, Mary (2002) 'Beyond Comparison: M. Sergius Silus, Fortunae Victor', in Clark, Gillian and Rajak, Tessa (eds.) *Philosophy and Power in the Graeco-Roman World. Essays in Honour of Miriam Griffin*. Oxford: Oxford University Press, pp. 111–32.

Beagon, Mary (2005) *The Elder Pliny on the Human Animal: Natural History Book 7*. Oxford: Clarendon Press.

Beard, Mary (2009) *The Roman Triumph*. Cambridge, MA: Harvard University Press.

Becker, Marshall J. (2014) 'Dentistry in Ancient Rome: Direct Evidence Based on Teeth from Excavations at the Temple of Castor and Pollux in the Roman Forum', *International Journal of Anthropology* 29.4, pp. 209–20.

Becker, Marshall J. and Turfa, Jean M. (2017) *The Etruscans and the History of Dentistry: The Golden Smile through the Ages*. London: Routledge.

Belcastro, Maria Giovanna and Mariotti, Valentina (2000) 'Morphological and Biomechanical Analysis of a Skeleton from Roman Imperial Necropolis of Casalecchio di Reno (Bologna, Italy, II–III c. A. D.). A Possible Case of Crutch Use', *Collegium Antropolegicum* 24.2, pp. 529–39.

Benhamou, Reed (1994) 'The Artificial Limb in Preindustrial France', *Technology and Culture* 35.4, pp. 835–45.

Biddiss, Elaine A. and Chau, Tom T. (2009) 'Upper Limb Prosthesis Use and Abandonment: A Survey of the Last 25 Years', *Prosthetics and Orthotics International* 31.3, pp. 236–57.

Binder, Michaela, Eitler, Josef, Deutschmann, Julia, et al. (2016) 'Prosthetics in Antiquity – An Early Medieval Wearer of a Foot Prosthesis (6th Century AD) from Hemmaberg/Austria', *International Journal of Paleopathology* 12, pp. 29–40.

Birley, Anthony R. (1992) 'A Case of Eye Disease (Lippitudo) on the Frontier in Britain', *Documenta Ophthalmologica* 81, pp. 111–19.

Black, E. W. (1986) 'Romano-British Burial Customs and Religious Beliefs in South East England', *Archaeological Journal* 143, pp. 201–39.

Blake, Sarah (2013) 'Now You See Them: Slaves and Other Objects as Elements of the Roman Master', *Helios* 39.2, pp. 193–211.

Bliquez, Lawrence J. (1983) 'Classical Prosthetics', *Archaeology* September/October, pp. 25–9.

Bliquez, Lawrence J. (1996) 'Prosthetics in Classical Antiquity: Greek, Etruscan, and Roman Prosthetics', in *ANRW* II 37.3, pp. 2640–76.

Bliquez, Lawrence J. (2014) *The Tools of Asclepius: Surgical Instruments in Greek and Roman Times*. Leiden: Brill.

Bradley, Keith (2005) 'The Roman Child in Sickness and in Health', in George, Michele (ed.) *The Roman Family in the Empire: Rome, Italy, and Beyond*. Oxford: Oxford University Press, pp. 67–92.

Bradley, Mark (2009) *Colour and Meaning in Ancient Rome*. Cambridge: Cambridge University Press.

Breckenridge, James D. (1981) 'Again the "Carmagnola"', *Gesta* 20.1, pp. 1–7.

Breitwieser, Rupert (ed.) (2012) *Behinderungen und Beeinträchtigungen/Disability and Impairment in Antiquity*. Oxford: Archaeopress.

Brown, Elspeth (2002) 'The Prosthetics of Management: Motion Study, Photography, and the Industrialized Body in World War 1 America', in Ott, Katherine, Serlin, David, and Mihm, Stephen (eds.) *Artificial Parts, Practical Lives: Modern Histories of Prosthetics*. New York: New York University Press, pp. 241–81.

Brozzi, Mario (1993) 'Strumento medico ricuperato in una tomba longobarda', *Forum Iulii* 17, pp. 35–8.

Brule, Pierre (2006) 'Bâtons et bâton du mâle, adulte, citoyen', in Bodiou, Lydie, Frère, Dominique, and Mehl, Véronique (eds.) *L'expression des corps: gestes, attitudes, regards dans l'iconographie antique*. Rennes: Presses universitaires de Rennes, pp. 75–83.

Buquet-Marcon, Cécile, Charlier, Philippe, and Samzun, Anaïck (2007) 'The Oldest Amputation on a Neolithic Human Skeleton in France', *Nature Precedings*, pp. 1–7.

Butler, Shane and Purves, Alex (2013) *Synaesthesia and the Ancient Senses*. London: Routledge.

Capasso, Luigi (1986) 'Etruria: Le Meraviglie dei Dentisti', *La Medicina nell'Antichità = Archeo Dossier (Novara)* 13, pp. 52–5.

Carbonelli, Giovanni (1908) 'Il "Brachiale Herniarium" nell'Alto Medio Evo', *Atti della Reale Accademia di Scienze e Lettere di Torino* 43, p. 261.

Carey, John (1973) *The Violent Effigy: A Study of Dickens' Imagination*. London: Faber.

Casson, Lionel (1994) *Travel in the Ancient World*. Baltimore, MD and London: Johns Hopkins University Press.

Cilliers, Louise and Retief, Francois P. (2013) 'Dream Healing in Asclepieia in the Mediterranean', in Oberhelman, Steven M. (ed.) *Dreams, Healing, and Medicine in Greece: From Antiquity to the Present*. Farnham: Ashgate, pp. 69–92.

Cohen, H. P. and Stern, N. (1973) 'References to Prosthetic Dentistry in the Talmud', *Bulletin of the History of Dentistry* 21.1, pp. 101–4.

Cokayne, Karen (2003) *Experiencing Old Age in Ancient Rome*. London: Routledge.

Collard, Franck and Samama, Evelyne (eds.) (2010) *Handicaps et sociétés dans l'histoire: L'estropié, l'aveugle et le paralytique de l'Antiquité aux temps modernes*. Paris: L'Harmattan.

Cootjans, Gerrit and Gourevitch, Danielle (1983) 'Les noms des dents en grec et en latin', *Revue de philologie, de littérature et d'histoire anciennes* 57, pp. 189–202.

Corbeill, Antony (1997) *Controlling Laughter: Political Humour in the Late Roman Republic*. Princeton, NJ: Princeton University Press.

Corbeill, Antony (2004) *Nature Embodied: Gesture in Ancient Rome*. Princeton, NJ: Princeton University Press.

Corson, Richard (1965) *Fashions in Hair: The First Five Thousand Years*. London: Peter Owen.

Couvret, Simone (1994) 'L'homme au bâton. Statique et statut dans la céramique attique', *Metis* 9–10, pp. 257–81.

Cox, J. Stevens (1977) 'The Construction of an Ancient Egyptian Wig (c. 1400 BC) in the British Museum', *Journal of Egyptian Archaeology* 63, pp. 67–70.

Craik, Elizabeth M. (2009) *The Hippocratic Treatise* On Glands*: Edited and Translated with Introduction and Commentary*. Leiden: Brill.

Craik, Elizabeth M. (2014) *The 'Hippocratic' Corpus: Content and Context*. London: Routledge.

Curle, James (1911) *A Roman Frontier Post and Its People: The Fort of New-stead in the Parish of Melrose*. Glasgow: James Maclehose and Sons.

Czarnetzki, Alfred, Uhlig, Christian, and Wolf, Rotraut (eds.) (1983) *Menschen des Frühen Mittelalters im Spiegel der Anthropologie und Medizin*. Stuttgart: Würtembergisches Landesmuseum.

Dalby, Andrew (2000) *Empire of Pleasures: Luxury and Indulgence in the Roman World*. London: Routledge.

Danelivicius, Zenonas (1967) 'SS Cosmas and Damian: The Patron Saints of Medicine in Art', *Journal of the American Medical Association* 201.13, pp. 145–9.

Darton, Y. (2010) 'Scapular Stress Fracture: A Palaeopathological Case Consistent with Crutch Use', *International Journal of Osteoarchaeology* 20.1, pp. 113–21.

Davis, Lennard (2002) 'Bodies of Difference: Politics, Disability, and Representation', in Snyder, Sharon L., Brueggemann, Brenda Jo, and Garland-Thomson, Rosemarie (eds.) *Disability Studies: Enabling the Humanities*. New York: The Modern Language Association of America, pp. 100–6.

Davis, Lennard (2013) *The End of Normal: Identity in a Biocultural Era*. Ann Arbor, MI: University of Michigan Press.

Dawson, Warren R. and Gray, Peter Hugh Ker (1968) *Catalogue of Egyptian Antiquities in the British Museum: 1. Mummies and Human Remains*. London: British Museum.

Dean-Jones, Lesley (2013) 'The Child Patient of the Hippocratics: Early Pediatrics?', in Grubbs, Judith E. and Parkin, Tim (eds.) *The Oxford Handbook of Childhood and Education in the Classical World*. Oxford: Oxford University Press, pp. 108–24.

Decker, Oliver (2016) *Commodified Bodies: Organ Transplantation and the Organ Trade*. London: Routledge.

Delbrueck, Richard (1914) *Carmagnola: (Porträt eines byzantinischen Kaisers)*. Rome: Loescher.

De Libero, L. (2002) 'Dem Schicksal trotzen. Behinderte Aristokraten in Rom', *Ancient History Bulletin* 16, pp. 87–96.

DeMarchi, Paola Marina (2006) 'Manufatti medici in contesti funerari: i cinti erniari.dalla diagnosi alla produzione', in Francovich, Riccardo and Valenti, Marco (eds.) *IV Congresso Nazionale di Archeologia Medievale. Pré-tirages (Scriptorium dell'Abbazia. Abbazia di San Galgano, Chiusdino – Siena, 26–30 settembre 2006)*, Florence: All'insegna del Giglio, pp. 440–6.

Derry, Douglas E. (1913) 'A Case of Hydrocephalus in an Egyptian of the Roman Period', *Journal of Anatomy and Physiology* 47.4, pp. 436–58.

Deubner, Ludwig (1907) *Kosmas und Damian: Texte und Einleitung*. Leipzig and Berlin: Scientia.

De Waele, Ferdinand J. (1927) *The Magic Staff or Rod in Graeco-Italian Antiquity*. The Hague: Erasmus.

Dillery, John (2005) 'Chresmologues and *Manteis*: Independent Diviners and the Problem of Authority', in Johnston, Sarah I. and Struck, Peter T. (eds.) *Mantikê: Studies in Ancient Divination*. Leiden: Brill, pp. 167–232.

Drachmann, Aage G. (1963) *The Mechanical Technology of the Greeks and Romans: A Study of the Literary Sources*. Copenhagen: Munksgaard, and Madison, WI: University of Wisconsin Press.

Draycott, Jane (2014) 'Who Is Performing What, and for Whom? The Dedication, Construction and Maintenance of a Healing Shrine in Roman Egypt', in Gemi-Iordanou, Effie, Gordon, Stephen, Matthew, Robert, McInnes, Ellen and Pettitt, Rhiannon (eds.) *Medicine, Healing, Performance: Interdisciplinary*

Approaches to Medicine and Material Culture. Oxford and Philadelphia, PA: Oxbow, pp. 42–54.

Draycott, Jane (2018a) 'Hair Loss as Facial Disfigurement in Ancient Rome?', in Skinner, Patricia and Cock, Emily (eds.) *Approaching Facial Difference: Past and Present*. London: Bloomsbury, pp. 65–83.

Draycott, Jane (2018b) 'Life as a Cyclops: Mythology and the Mockery of the Visually Impaired', in Kazantzidis, George and Tsoumpra, Natalia (eds.) *Morbid Laughter: Exploring the Comic Dimensions of Disease in Classical Antiquity*. Chicago, IL: Illinois Classical Studies, pp. 404–9.

Draycott, Jane (2019a) (ed.) *Prostheses in Antiquity*. London: Routledge.

Draycott, Jane (2019b) 'Introduction', in Draycott, Jane (ed.) *Prostheses in Antiquity*. London: Routledge, pp. 1–28.

Draycott, Jane (2019c) 'Prosthetic Hair in Ancient Rome', in Draycott, Jane (ed.) *Prostheses in Antiquity*. London: Routledge, pp. 71–96.

Draycott, Jane (2019d) *Roman Domestic Medical Practice in Central Italy from the Middle Republic to the Early Empire*. London: Routledge.

Draycott, Jane (2021) 'Prostheses in Classical Antiquity: A Taxonomy', in Adams, Ellen (ed.) *Disability Studies and the Classical Body: The Forgotten Other*. London: Routledge, pp. 93–116.

Draycott, Jane (in press a) 'Automata, Cyborgs, and Hybrids: Bodies and Machines in Antiquity', in Gerolemou, Maria and Kanzantzidis, George (eds.) *Iatromechanics*. Cambridge: Cambridge University Press.

Draycott, Jane (in press b) 'Staff or Stick? Cane or Crutch? Mobility Aids in Ancient Greece and Rome', in Bonati, Isabella (ed.) *Words of Medicine: Technical Terminology in Material and Textual Evidence from the Graeco-Roman World*. Berlin: De Gruyter.

Duffin, Jacalyn (2013) *Medical Saints: Cosmas and Damian in a Postmodern World*. Oxford: Oxford University Press.

Dunand, Françoise and Lichtenberg, Roger (1994) *Mummies: A Voyage through Eternity*. New York: Harry N. Abrams.

Dunand, Françoise, Heim, Jean-Louis, Henein, N. H., Barakat, H. N. and Castel, G. (1992) *Douch I: La nécropole. Exploration archéologique, Monographie des tombes 1 à 72: structures sociales, économiques, religieuses de l'Égypte romaine*. Cairo: Institut Français d'Archéologie Orientale du Caire.

Dupras, Tosha L., Williams, Lana J., Mayer, Marleen De, et al. (2010) 'Evidence of Amputation as Medical Treatment in Ancient Egypt', *International Journal of Osteoarchaeology* 20, pp. 405–23.

Edwards, Martha L. (2012) 'Philoctetes in Historical Context', in Gerber, David A. (ed.) *Disabled Veterans in History*. Ann Arbor, MI: University of Michigan Press, pp. 55–69.

Eitler, Josef and Binder, Michaela (2019) 'Evidence of a Late Antique Amputation in a Skeleton from Hemmaberg', in Draycott, Jane (ed.) *Prostheses in Antiquity*. London: Routledge, pp. 125–39.

Emery, Patrizia B. (1999) 'Old-Age Iconography in Archaic Greek Art', *Mediterranean Archaeology* 12, pp. 17–28.

Enoch, Jay M. (1996) 'Early Lens Use: Lenses found in Context with Their Original Objects', *Optometry and Vision Science* 73.11, pp. 707–15.

Enoch, Jay M. (1998) 'The Enigma of Early Lens Use', *Technology and Culture* 39.2, pp. 273–91.

Enoch, Jay M. (2007) 'Archeological Optics: The Very First Known Mirrors and Lenses', *Journal of Modern Optics* 54.9, pp. 1221–39.

Enoch, Jay M. (2009) 'A Mesolithic (Middle Stone Age!) Spanish Artificial Eye: Please Realize This Technology Is circa 7000 Years Old!', *Hindsight: Journal of Optometry History* 40.2, pp. 47–62.

Esser, A. (1959) Kannte die klassische Antike den Blindenhund?', *Monatsblätter für Augenheilkunde* 134, pp. 102–4.

Evans, Craig A. (2000) 'Parables in Early Judaism', in Longenecker, Richard N. (ed.) *The Challenge of Jesus' Parables*. Cambridge and Grand Rapids, MI: William B. Eerdmans Publishing Company, pp. 51–75.

Evans, R. J. (1999) 'Displaying Honourable Scars: A Roman Gimmick', *Acta Classica* 42.1, pp. 77–94.

Fabre, Georges (1981) *Libertus. Recherches sur les rapports patron-affranchi à la fin de la République Romaine*. Rome: École Française de Rome.

Figg, Laurann and Farrell-Beck, Jane (1993) 'Amputation in the Civil War: Physical and Social Dimensions', *Journal of the History of Medicine and the Allied Sciences* 48, pp. 454–75.

Finch, Jacky (2019) 'The Complex Aspects of Experimental Archaeology: The Design of Working Models of Two Ancient Egyptian Great Toe Prostheses', in Draycott, Jane (ed.) *Prostheses in Antiquity*. London, Routledge, pp. 29–48.

Fink-Bennett, D. M. and Benson, M. T. (1984) 'Unusual Exercise-Related Stress Fractures. Two Case Reports', *Clinical Nuclear Medicine* 9.8, pp. 430–4.

Fishman, Gerald A. (2003) 'When Your Eyes Have a Wet Nose: The Evolution of the Use of Guide Dogs and Establishing the Seeing Eye', *Survey of Ophthalmology* 48.4, pp. 452–8.

Fitzgerald, W. (2000) *Slavery and the Roman Literary Imagination*. Cambridge: Cambridge University Press.

Fletcher, Amy J. (1995) 'Ancient Egyptian Hair: A Study in Style, Form and Function'. 2 Vols. Manchester: University of Manchester, PhD thesis.

Fletcher, Joann (2005) 'The Decorated Body in Ancient Egypt: Hairstyles, Cosmetics and Tattoos', in Cleland, Liza, Harlow, Mary, and Llewellyn-Jones, Lloyd (eds.) *The Clothed Body in the Ancient World*. Oxford: Oxbow, pp. 3–13.

Fletcher, Joann (2016) 'The Egyptian Hair Pin: Practical, Sacred, Fatal', *Internet Archaeology* 42: http://dx.doi.org/10.11141/ia.42.6.5 (accessed January 2021).

Fletcher, Joann and Salamone, Filippo (2016) 'An Ancient Egyptian Wig: Construction and Reconstruction', *Internet Archaeology* 42: http://dx.doi.org/10.11141/ia.42.6.3 (accessed January 2021).

Fox, Alex (2020) 'Monkeys Found Buried in 2,000-Year-Old Egyptian Pet Cemetery', *Smithsonian Magazine*. www.smithsonianmag.com/smart-news/

monkeys-found-buried-2000-year-old-egyptian-pet-cemetery-180975667/ (accessed January 2021).

Fracchia, Carmen (2013) 'Spanish Depictions of the Miracle of the Black Leg', in Zimmerman, Kees, Fracchia, Carmen, de Jong, Jan, and Santing, Catrien (eds.) *One Leg in the Grave Revisited: The Miracle of the Transplantation of the Black Leg by the Saints Cosmas and Damian*. Groningen: Barkhuis, pp. 79–91.

Fredrick, David (ed.) (2002) *The Roman Gaze: Vision, Power and the Body*. Baltimore, MD and London: Johns Hopkins University Press.

Gale, Rowena, Gasson, Peter, Hepper, Nigel, and Killen, Geoffrey (2000) 'Wood', in Nicholson, Paul N. and Shaw, Ian (eds.) *Ancient Egyptian Materials and Technology*. Cambridge: Cambridge University Press, pp. 334–71.

Garland, Robert (1995, reissued 2010) *The Eye of the Beholder: Deformity and Disability in the Graeco-Roman World*. London: Bristol Classical Press.

Gatti Lo Guzzi, Laura (1978) *Il deposito votivo dall'Esquilino detto di Minerva Medica*. Studi e materiali di etruscologia e antichità italiche 17. Florence: Sanosoni.

Gerber, Douglas E. (1982) *Pindar's Olympian One: A Commentary*. Toronto, Buffalo, NY, and London: University of Toronto Press.

Gevaert, Bert and Laes, Christian (2013) 'What's in a Monster? Pliny the Elder, Teratology and Bodily Disability', in Laes, Christian, Goodey, Chris, and Rose, M. Lynn (eds.) *Disabilities in Roman Antiquity: Disparate Bodies* a Capite ad Calcem. Leiden: Brill, pp. 211–30.

Ghaly, Mohammed (2010) *Islam and Disability: Perspectives in Theory and Jurisprudence*. London: Routledge.

Giuliano, Antonio (1981) *Museo Nazionale Romano, Le sculture*. Rome: Museo Nazionale Romano.

Giuliano, Antonio (1985) *Museo Nazionale Romano, Le sculture*. Rome: Museo Nazionale Romano.

Glazebrook, Allison (2009) 'Cosmetics and Sôphrosunê: Ischomachos' Wife in Xenophon's Oikonomikos', *Classical World* 102.3, pp. 223–48.

Glinister, Fay (2000) 'Sacred Rubbish', in Bispham, Edward and Smith, C. (eds.) *Religion in Archaic and Republican Rome and Italy: Evidence and Experience*. Edinburgh: Edinburgh University Press, pp. 54–70.

Goggins, Sophie (2021) 'Displaying the Forgotten Other in Museums: Prostheses at National Museums Scotland', in Adams, Ellen (ed.) *Disability Studies and the Classical Body: The Forgotten Other*. London: Routledge, pp. 117–29.

Gosden, Chris and Marshall, Yvonne (1999) 'The Cultural Biography of Objects', *World Archaeology* 31.2, pp. 169–78.

Graham, Emma-Jayne (2013) 'Disparate Lives or Disparate Deaths? Post-Mortem Treatment of the Body and the Articulation of Difference', in Laes, Christian, Goodey, Chris F., and Rose, M. Lynn (eds.) *Disabilities in Roman Antiquity: Disparate Bodies:* A Capite ad Calcem. Leiden: Brill, pp. 249–74.

Graham, Emma-Jayne (2017) 'Mobility Impairment in the Sanctuaries of Early Roman Italy', in Laes, Christian (ed.) *Disability in Antiquity*. London: Routledge, pp. 248–66.

Greene, Elizabeth M. (2019) 'Metal Fittings on the Vindolanda Shoes: Footwear and Evidence for Podiatric Knowledge in the Roman World', in Pickup, Sadie and Waite, Sally (eds.) *Shoes, Slippers and Sandals: Feet and Footwear in Classical Antiquity*. London: Routledge, pp. 310–24.

Grmek, Mirko D. and Gourevitch, Danielle (1998) *Les maladies dans l'art antique*. Paris: Fayard.

Habinek, Thomas (2002) 'Ovid and Empire', in Hardie, Philip (ed.) *The Cambridge Companion to Ovid*. Cambridge: Cambridge University Press, pp. 46–61.

Hähn, Cathrin (2018) 'Mobility Limitations and Assistive Aids in the Merovingian Burial Record', Connelly, Erin and Künzel, Stefanie (eds.) *New Approaches to Disease, Disability and Medicine in Medieval Europe*. Oxford: Archaeopress, pp. 31–42.

Hallpike, Christopher R. (1969) 'Social Hair', *Man* 4.2, pp. 256–64.

Hamilton, David (2012) *A History of Organ Transplantation: Ancient Legends to Modern Practice*. Pittsburgh, PA: University of Pittsburgh Press.

Hasegawa, Guy R. (2012) *Mending Broken Soldiers: The Union and Confederate Programs to Supply Artificial Limbs*. Carbondale and Edwardsville, IL: Southern Illinois University Press.

Hayward, Lorna G. (1990) 'The Origin of the Raw Elephant Ivory used in Greece and the Aegean during the Late Bronze Age', *Antiquity* 64.242, pp. 103–9.

Henestrosa, C. (2018) 'Appearances Can Be Deceiving – Frida Kahlo's Construction of Identity: Disability, Ethnicity and Dress', in Wilcox, Claire and Henestrosa, C. (eds.) *Frida Kahlo: Making Herself Up*. London: V&A, pp. 66–82.

Hermes, Lisa (2002) 'Military Lower Extremity Amputee Rehabilitation', *Physical Medicine and Rehabilitation Clinics of North America* 13, pp. 45–66.

Hernigou, Philippe (2013) 'Ambroise Paré IV: The Early History of Artificial Limbs (from Robotic to Prostheses)', *International Orthopaedics* 37.6, pp. 1195–7.

Holleran, Claire (2012) *Shopping in Ancient Rome: The Retail Trade in the Late Republic and Principate*. Oxford: Oxford University Press.

Horn, Cornelia B. (2013) 'A Nexus of Disability in Ancient Greek Miracle Stories: A Comparison of Accounts of Blindness from the Asklepieion in Epidauros and the Shrine of Thecla in Seleucia', in Laes, Christian, Goodey, Chris F., and Rose, Martha Lynn (eds.) *Disabilities in Roman Antiquity: Disparate Bodies:* A Capite ad Calcem. Leiden: Brill, pp. 115–43.

Horstmanshoff, Manfred (2012) 'Disability and Rehabilitation in the Graeco-Roman World', in Breitwieser, Rupert (ed.) *Behinderungen und Beeinträchtigungen/ Disability and Impairment in Antiquity*. Oxford: Archaeopress, pp. 1–9.

Horstmanshoff, Manfred (2013) 'Klein gebrek geen bezwaar? Over de klompvoet in de oudheid', *Lampas* 46.1, pp. 203–21.

Hughes, Jessica (2008) 'Fragmentation as Metaphor in the Classical Healing Sanctuary', *Social History of Medicine* 21.2, pp. 217–36.

Hughes, Jessica (2017) *Votive Body Parts in Ancient Greek and Roman Religion*. Cambridge: Cambridge University Press.

Ioannidou, Christy Emilio (2015) 'Diving in Ancient Greece during the Late Archaic and Classical Period', *Archaeology and Science* 10, pp. 111–20.

Isaac, Benjamin (2004) *Racism in Antiquity*. Princeton, NJ: Princeton University Press.

Jackson, Ralph (2005) 'Holding on to Health? Bone Surgery and Instrumentation in the Roman Empire', in King, Helen (ed.) *Health in Antiquity*. London: Routledge, pp. 97–119.

James, Simon (2010) 'The Point of the Sword: What Roman-era Weapons Could Do to Bodies – and Why They Often Didn't', in Busch, Alexandra W. and Schalles, Hans-Joachim (eds.) *Waffen in Aktion. Akten der 16. Internationalen Roman Military Equipment Conference (ROMEC), Xantener Berichte 16*. Mainz: Von Zabern, pp. 41–54.

Johnson, Horton A. (2005) 'Fish Bile and Cautery: Trachoma Treatment in Art', *Journal of the Royal Society of Medicine* 98, pp. 30–2.

Jones, Alexander (2017) *A Portable Cosmos: Revealing the Antikythera Mechanism, Scientific Wonder of the Ancient World*. Oxford: Oxford University Press.

Joshel, Sandra R. (1992) *Work, Identity and Legal Status at Rome: A Study of the Occupational Inscriptions*. Norman, OK and London: University of Oklahoma Press.

Joshel, Sandra R. (1995) 'Female Desire and the Discourse of Empire: Tacitus's Messalina', *Signs* 21.1, pp. 50–82.

Kalligeropoulos, D. and Vasileiadou, S. (2008) 'The Homeric Automata and Their Implementation', in Paipetis, Stephanos A. (ed.) *Science and Technology in Homeric Epics*. London: Springer, pp. 77–84.

Kanz, Fabian and Grossschmidt, Karl (2009) 'Dying in the Arena: The Osseous Evidence from the Ephesian Gladiators', in Wilmot, Tony (ed.) *Roman Amphitheatres and Spectacula, a 21st-Century Perspective: Papers from an International Conference Held at Chester, 16th-18th February, 2007*. Oxford: British Archaeological Reports, pp. 211–20.

Kenna, Victor E. G. (1961) 'The Return of Orestes', *Journal of Hellenic Studies* 81, pp. 99–104.

Kinder, John M. (2015) *Paying with Their Bodies: American War and the Problem of the Disabled Veteran*. Chicago, IL and London: University of Chicago Press.

Kirkup, John (2007) *A History of Limb Amputation*. London: Springer.

Krierer, Karl R. (2004) *Antike Germanenbilder*. Vienna: Verlag der Österreichischen Akademie der Wissenschaften.

Krötzl, Christian, Mustakallio, Kateriina, and Kuuliala, Jenni (2015) *Infirmity in Antiquity and the Middle Ages: Social and Cultural Approaches to Health, Weakness and Care*. Farnham: Ashgate.

Kwass, Michael (2006) 'Big Hair: A Wig History of Consumption in Eighteenth Century France', *American Historical Review* 111.3, pp. 631–59.

Laes, Christian (2008) 'Learning from Silence: Disabled Children in Roman Antiquity', *Arctos* 42, pp. 85–122.

Laes, Christian (2011) 'How Does One Do the History of Disability in Antiquity? One Thousand Years of Case Studies', *Medicina nei Secoli* 23.3, pp. 915–46.

Laes, Christian (2013) 'Raising a Disabled Child', in Grubb, Judith E. and Parkin, Tim (eds.) *Oxford Handbook of Childhood and Education in the Classical World*. Oxford: Oxford University Press, pp. 125–44.

Laes, Christian (2014) *Beperkt? Gehandicapten in het Romeinse rijk*. Leuven: Davisfonds.

Laes, Christian (ed.) (2017) *Disability in Antiquity*. London: Routledge.

Laes, Christian (2018) *Disabilities and the Disabled in the Roman World: A Social and Cultural History*. Cambridge: Cambridge University Press.

Laes, Christian (2019) 'Power, Infirmity and "Disability": Five Case Stories on Byzantine Emperors and Their Impairments', *Byzantinoslavica* 77.1–2, pp. 211–29.

Laes, Christian (2020) '*Pedes habent et non ambulabunt*: Mobility Impairment in Merovingian Gaul', in Kuuliala, Jenni and Rantala, Jussi (eds.) *Travel, Pilgrimage and Social Interaction from Antiquity to the Middle Ages*. London: Routledge, pp. 183–204.

Laes, Christian, Goodey, Chris, and Rose, M. Lynn (eds.) (2013) *Disabilities in Roman Antiquity: Disparate Bodies* a Capite ad Calcem. Leiden: Brill.

Lanciani, Rodolfo (1898) *Ancient Rome in the Light of Recent Discoveries*. Boston, MA and New York: Houghton, Mifflin and Company.

Langmuir, Erika (2006) *Imagining Childhood*. New Haven, CT and London: Yale University Press.

Lapatin, Kenneth D. S. (2001) *Chryselephantine Statuary in the Ancient Mediterranean World*. Oxford: Oxford University Press.

Lawler, Lillian B. (1929) 'Two Portraits from Tertullian', *Classical Journal* 25.1, pp. 19–23.

Leary, Timothy J. (1996) *Martial Book XIV the Apophoreta*. London: Duckworth.

Lee, Mireille (2015) *Body, Dress and Identity in Ancient Greece*. Cambridge: Cambridge University Press.

Lehmhaus, Lennart (2019) '"An Amputee May Go Out with His Wooden Aid on Shabbat": Dynamics of Prosthetic Discourse in Talmudic Traditions', in Draycott, Jane (ed.) *Prostheses in Antiquity*. London: Routledge, pp. 97–124.

Leigh, Matthew (1995) 'Wounding and Popular Rhetoric at Rome', *Bulletin of the Institute of Classical Studies* 40.1, pp. 195–215.

Levine, Molly M. (1995) 'The Gendered Grammar of Mediterranean Hair', in Eilberg-Schwartz, Howard and Doniger, Wendy (eds.) *Off with Her Head! The Denial of Women's Identity in Myth, Religion and Culture*. Berkeley/Los Angeles, CA and London: University of California Press, pp. 76–130.

Li, Xiao, Wagner, Mayke, Wu, Xiaohong, et al. (2013) 'Archaeological and Palaeopathological Study on the Third/Second Century BC Grave from Turfan, China: Individual Health History and Regional Implications', *Quaternary International* 290–1, pp. 335–43.

LiDonnici, Lynn R. (1995) *The Epidaurian Miracle Inscriptions: Text, Translation and Commentary*. Atlanta, GA: Scholars Press.

Lilja, Saara (1965) *The Roman Elegists' Attitude to Women*. New York: Garland.

Loebl, W. Y. and Nunn, John F. (1997) 'Staffs as Walking Aids in Ancient Egypt and Palestine', *Journal of the Royal Society of Medicine* 90.8, pp. 450–4.

Lorimer, H. L. (1936) 'Gold and Ivory in Greek Mythology', in Bailey, C., Bowra, C. M., Barber, E.A., Denniston, J. D., and Page, D. L. (eds.) *Greek Poetry and Life: Essays Presented to Gilbert Murray on His Seventieth Birthday, January 2, 1936*. Oxford: Clarendon Press, pp. 14–33.

Majno, Guido (1975) *The Healing Hand: Man and Wound in the Ancient World*. Cambridge, MA: Harvard University Press.

Mann, Robert W., Thomas, Michael D., and Adams, Bradley J. (1998) 'Congenital Absence of the Ulna with Humeroradial Synostosis in a Prehistoric Skeleton from Moundville, Alabama', *International Journal of Osteoarchaeology* 8, pp. 295–9.

Matthews, Lydia (2019) 'Health and Hygiene', in Harlow, M. (ed.) *A Cultural History of Hair in Antiquity*. London: Bloomsbury, pp. 85–96.

Mayor, Adrienne (2018) *Gods and Robots: Myths, Machines and Ancient Dreams of Technology*. Princeton, NJ and Oxford: Princeton University Press.

Mays, Simon A. (1996) 'Healed Limb Amputations in Human Osteoarchaeology and their Causes: A Case Study from Ipswich, UK', *International Journal of Osteoarchaeology* 6, pp. 101–13.

Meadows, J. W. (1945) 'Pliny on the Smaragdus', *Classical Review* 59.2, pp. 50–1.

Meiggs, Russell (1982) *Trees and Timber in the Ancient Mediterranean World*. Oxford: Clarendon Press.

Merei, G. and Nemeskeri, J. (1958) 'Palaeopathologische Untersuchungen an ägyptischen Mumien aus der Römerzeit', *Virchows Archiv für pathologische Anatomie und Physiologie und für klinische Medizin* 331.5, pp. 569–72.

Micarelli, Ileana, Paine, Robert, Giostra, Caterina, et al. (2018) 'Survival to Amputation in Pre-antibiotic Era: A Case Study from a Longobard Necropolis (6th–8th Centuries AD)', *Journal of Anthropological Sciences* 96, pp. 1–16.

Michler, Markwart (1963) 'Die Klumpfusslehre der Hippokratiker: eine Untersuchung von De articulis, Cap. 62; mit Übersetzung des Textes und des galenischen Kommentars', *Sudhoffs Archiv für Geschichte der Medizin und der Naturwissenschaften Beihefte*, Heft 2. Wiesbaden: Steiner.

Milburn, Olivia (2017) 'Disability in Ancient China', in Laes, Christian (ed.) (2017) *Disability in Antiquity*. London: Routledge, pp. 106–8.

Minozzi, Simona, Fornaciari, Gino, Musco, Stefano, and Catalano, Paola (2007) 'A Gold Dental Prosthesis of Roman Imperial Age', *American Journal of Medicine* 120, e1–e2.

Minozzi, Simona, Lunardini, Agata, Catalano, Paola, Caramella, Davide, and Fornaciari Gino (2013) 'Dwarfism in Imperial Rome: A Case of Skeletal Evidence', *Journal of Clinical Research Bioethics* 4.3, pp. 1–5.

Mitchell, Alexandre G. (2013) 'Disparate Bodies in Ancient Artefacts: The Function of Caricature and Pathological Grotesques among Roman

Terracotta Figures', in Laes, Christian, Goodey, Chris F. and Rose, Martha Lynn (eds.) *Disabilities in Roman Antiquity: Disparate Bodies:* A Capite ad Calcem. Leiden: Brill, pp. 275–98.

Mitchell, Alexandre (2017) 'The Hellenistic Turn in Bodily Representations: Venting Anxiety in the Terracotta Figurines', in Laes, Christian (ed.) *Disability in Antiquity*. London: Routledge, pp. 182–96.

Moghadasi, Abdorezza N. (2014) 'Artificial Eye in Burnt City and Theoretical Understanding of How Vision Works', *Iranian Journal of Public Health* 43.11, pp. 1595–6.

Mulder, Tara (2017) 'Adult Breastfeeding in Ancient Rome', *Illinois Classical Studies* 42.1, pp. 227–43.

Murray, Craig D. (2005) 'The Social Meanings of Prosthesis Use', *Journal of Health Psychology* 10.3, pp. 425–41.

Murray, Craig D. and Fox, Jezz (2002) 'Body Image and Prosthesis Satisfaction in the Lower Limb Amputee', *Disability and Rehabilitation* 24.17, pp. 925–31.

Nelson, Max (2002) 'A Note on the ὄλισβος', *Glotta* 76, pp. 75–82.

Neumann, Boaz (2010) 'Being Prosthetic in the First World War and Weimar Germany', *Body & Society* 16.3, pp. 93–126.

Nirenberg, Sheila and Pandarinath, Chethan (2012) 'Retinal Prosthetic Strategy with the Capacity to Restore Normal Vision', *Proceedings of the National Academy of Sciences of the United States of America* 109.37, pp. 15012–17.

Noel, Anne-Sophie (2019) '"Prosthetic Imagination" in Greek Literature', in Draycott, Jane (ed.) *Prostheses in Antiquity*. London: Routledge, pp. 159–79.

Nriagu, Jerome O. (1983) 'Occupational Exposure to Lead in Ancient Times', *The Science of the Total Environment* 31, pp. 105–16.

Nutting, Herbert C. (1922) 'Oculus Effodere', *Classical Philology* 17.4, pp. 313–18.

Oberhelman, Steven M. (2014) 'Anatomical Votive Reliefs as Evidence of Specialization at Healing Sanctuaries in the Ancient Mediterranean', *Athens Journal of Health* 1.1, pp 47–62.

O'Connor, Erin (2000) *Raw Material: Producing Pathology in Victorian Culture*. Durham, NC: Duke University Press.

Olson, Kelly (2009) 'Cosmetics in Roman Antiquity: Substance, Remedy, Poison', *Classical World* 102.3, pp. 209–310.

Olson, Kelly (2012) *Dress and the Roman Woman: Self-Representation and Society*. Abingdon: Routledge.

Orizaga, Rhiannon Y. (2013) 'Roman Cosmetics Revisited: Facial Modification and Identity', in Della Casa, Philippe and Witt, Constanze (eds.) *Tattoos and Body Modifications in Antiquity: Proceedings of the Sessions at the EAA Annual Meetings in the Hague and Oslo, Zurich Studies in Archaeology* 9, pp. 115–20.

O'Sullivan, Timothy (2011) *Walking in Roman Culture*. Cambridge: Cambridge University Press.

Ott, Katherine, Serlin, David, and Mihm, Stephen (eds.) (2002) *Artificial Parts, Practical Lives: Modern Histories of Prosthetics*. New York: New York University Press.

Paipetis, Stephanos A. (2010) *The Unknown Technology in Homer*. London: Springer.

Paley, Frederick A. (1868) *The Odes of Pindar*. Cambridge: Deighton, Bell and Co.

Papaioannou, Sophia (2006) 'The Poetology of Hairstyling and the Excitement of Hair Loss in Ovid "Amores" 1,14', *Quaderni urbinati di cultura classica* 83.2, pp. 45–69.

Parkin, Tim G. (2003) *Old Age in the Roman World: A Cultural and Social History*. Baltimore, MD: Johns Hopkins University Press.

Paule, Maxwell T. (2017) *Canidia: Rome's First Witch*. London: Bloomsbury.

Pazzini, Adalberto (1935) 'Il significato degli "ex voto" ed il concetto della divinita guaratrice', Atti della Accademia Nazionale dei Lincei, Classe di Scienze Morali, Storiche e Filologiche 6, pp. 42–79. Reprinted in Pazzini, Adalberto (1941) *La Medicina Primitiva*. Milan and Rome: Editoriale Arte e Storia, pp. 105–31.

Petrie, William F. (1927) *Objects of Daily Use*. London: British School of Archaeology in Egypt.

Petsalis-Diomidis, Alexia (2006) 'Amphiaraos Present: Images and Healing Pilgrimage in Classical Greece', in Maniura, Robert and Shepherd, Rupert (eds.) *Presence: The Inheritance of the Prototype within Images and Other Objects*. Aldershot: Ashgate, pp. 205–29.

Pezzin, Lillian. E., Dillingham, Timothy. R., MacKenzie, Ellen J., Ephraim, Patti and Rossbach, Paddy (2004) 'Use and Satisfaction with Prosthetic Limb Devices and Related Services', *Archives of Physical Medicine and Rehabilitation* 85.5, pp. 723–9.

Phillips, Oliver (2002) 'The Witches' Thessaly', in Mirecki, Paul A. and Meyer, Marvin W. (eds.) *Magic and Ritual in the Ancient World*. Leiden: Brill, pp. 378–85.

Pinheiro, Marília F. (2006) 'Utopia and Utopias: A Study on a Literary Genre in Antiquity', in Byrne, Shannon N. (ed.) *Authors, Authority and Interpretation in the Ancient Novel: Essays in Honour of Gareth F. Schmeling*. Ancient Narrative Supplementum 5: Barkhuis, pp. 147–71.

Plantzos, Dimitris (1997) 'Crystals and Lenses in the Graeco-Roman World', *American Journal of Archaeology* 101.3, pp. 451–64.

Porter, Chloe, Walter, Katie L., and Healy, Margaret (2017) *Prosthesis in Medieval and Early Modern Culture*. London: Routledge.

Prag, A. J. N. W. (1990) 'Reconstructing King Philip II of Macedon: The "Nice" Version', *American Journal of Archaeology* 94.2, pp. 237–47.

Pudsey, April (2017) 'Disability and *infirmitas* in the Ancient World: Demographic and Biological Facts in the longue durée', in Laes, Christian (ed.) *Disability in Antiquity*. London: Routledge, pp. 22–34.

Pullin, Graham (2009) *Design Meets Disability*. Cambridge, MA and London: The MIT Press.

Raditsa, Leo (1985) 'The Appearance of Women and Contact: Tertullian's De Habitu Feminarum', *Athenaeum* 63, pp. 297–326.

Raevskij, D. S. (1982–3) 'The Scythian Genealogical Legend', *Anthropology & Archaeology of Eurasia* 21, pp. 33–66 and pp. 80–122.

Redfern, Rebecca (2010) 'A Regional Examination of Surgery and Fracture Treatment in Iron Age and Roman Britain', *International Journal of Osteoarchaeology* 20, pp. 443–71.

Reinhard, Andrew (2019) 'Consulting for Ubisoft on Assassin's Creed: Odyssey', *Archaeogaming* 19/ 04/2019, available online at https://archaeogaming.com/2019/04/19/consulting-for-ubisoft-on-assassins-creed-odyssey/ (accessed January 2021).

Remensnyder, John P., Bigelow, Mary E., and Goldwyn, Robert M. (1979) 'Justinian II and Carmagnola: A Byzantine Rhinoplasty?', *Plastic and Reconstructive Surgery* 63.1, pp. 19–25.

Richlin, Amy (1992) *The Garden of Priapus: Sexuality and Aggression in Roman Humor*. New York and Oxford: Oxford University Press.

Richlin, Amy (1995) 'Making up a Woman: The Face of Roman Gender', in Doniger, Wendy and Eiberg Schwartz, Howard (eds.) *Off with Her Head!: The Denial of Women's Identity in Myth, Religion and Culture*. Berkeley, CA: University of California Press, pp. 185–213.

Rigonos, Alice S. (1994) 'The Wounding of Philip II of Macedon: Fact and Fiction', *Journal of Hellenic Studies* 114, pp. 103–19.

Roberts, Charlotte and Manchester, Keith (2010) *The Archaeology of Disease*. Stroud: History Press.

Roberts, Charlotte A., Knusel, Christopher J. and Race, Lynne (2004) 'A Foot Deformity from a Romano-British Cemetery at Gloucester, England, and the Current Evidence for *Talipes* in Palaeopathology', *International Journal of Osteoarchaeology* 14, pp. 389–403.

Roby, Courtney (2016) *Technical Ekphrasis in Greek and Roman Science and Literature: The Written Machine between Alexandria and Rome*. Cambridge: Cambridge University Press.

Rodríguez-Álvarez, Emilio (2018) 'The Archaeology of Sponges: Middle Range Theory and Divers in Ancient Greece', available online: www.researchgate.net/profile/Emilio_Rodriguez-Alvarez/publication/282337666_The_Archaeology_of_Sponges_Middle_Range_Theory_and_Divers_in_Ancient_Greece/links/5c75304a92851c6950425fb5/The-Archaeology-of-Sponges-Middle-Range-Theory-and-Divers-in-Ancient-Greece.pdf (accessed January 2021).

Roeschlein, R. A. and Domholdt, E. (1989) 'Factors Related to Successful Upper Extremity Prosthetic Use', *Prosthetics and Orthotics International* 13.1, pp. 14–18.

Rose, Martha Lynn (2003, reissued 2013) *The Staff of Oedipus: Transforming Disability in Ancient Greece*. Ann Arbor, MI: University of Michigan Press.

Rosenfeld, Amnon, Dvorachek, Michael, and Rotstein, Ilan (2000) 'Bronze Single Crown-like Prosthetic Restorations of Teeth from the Late Roman Period', *Journal of Archaeological Science* 27.7, pp. 641–4.

Rossignani, Maria P., Sannazaro, Marco and Legrottaglie, Giuseppina (2005) *La Signora del sarcofago: una sepoltura di rango nella necropoli dell'Università cattolica: ricerche archeologiche nei cortili dell'Università Cattolica*. Milan: Vita e pensiero.

Ryan, Stephen, Oaten, Megan, Stevenson, Richard J., and Case, Trevor I. (2012) 'Facial Disfigurement Is Treated Like an Infectious Disease', *Evolution and Human Behaviour* 33, pp. 639–46.

Rynearson, Nicholas (2003) 'Constructing and Deconstructing the Body in the Cult of Asklepios', *Stanford Journal of Archaeology* 2. www.semanticscholar.org/paper/CONSTRUCTING-AND-DECONSTRUCTING-THE-BODY-IN-THE-OF-Rynearson/ffb5d4ea334b53d8487e6743c7a828666e111509 (accessed August 2022).

Salazar, Christine (2000) *The Treatment of War Wounds in Graeco-Roman Antiquity*. Leiden: Brill.

Sansoni, Stefania, Wodehouse, A., and Buis, Arjun (2014) 'The Aesthetics of Prosthetic Design: From Theory to Practice', *International Design Conference – Design 2014*, pp. 975–84. www.designsociety.org/publication/35242/THE+AESTHETICS+OF+PROSTHETIC+DESIGN%3A+FROM+THEORY+TO+PRACTICE.

Santing, Catrien G. (2013) 'Cosmas and Damian as Representatives of a Diverse Medical Profession and Its Functions', in Zimmerman, Kees, Fracchia, Carmen, de Jong, Jan, and Santing, Catrien (eds.) *One Leg in the Grave Revisited: The Miracle of the Transplantation of the Black Leg by the Saints Cosmas and Damian*. Groningen: Barkhuis, pp. 127–36.

Sauer, Eberhard (1996) 'An Inscription from Northern Italy, The Roman Temple Complex in Bath and Minerva as a Healing Goddess in Gallo-Roman Religion', *Oxford Journal of Archaeology* 15.1, pp. 63–93.

Schultze, Clemence (2011) 'Encyclopaedic Exemplarity in Pliny the Elder', in Gibson, Roy and Morello, Ruth (eds.) *Pliny the Elder: Themes and Contexts*. Leiden: Brill, pp. 167–86.

Selinger, Reinhard (2012) 'Selbstrepräsentationen von Behinderung im Alten Ägypten: Körperprothesen an Mumien und Grabstatuen von Minderwüchsigen', in Breitwieser, Rupert (ed.) *Behinderungen und Beeinträchtigungen*. Oxford: Archaeopress, pp. 25–35.

Sensi, Luigi (1980–1) 'Ornatus e status sociale delle donne romane', *Annali della Faculta di Lettere e Filosofia Perugia-Sezione Studi Classici* NS 4, pp. 55–102.

Shanmugarajah, Kumaran, Gaind, Safina, Clarke, Alex, and Butler, Peter E. M. (2012) 'The Role of Disgust Emotions in the Observer Response to Facial Disfigurement', *Body Image* 9.4, pp. 455–61.

Sines, George and Sakellerakis, Yannis A. (1987) 'Lenses in Antiquity', *American Journal of Archaeology* 91.2, pp. 191–6.

Skinner, Patricia (2014) 'The Gendered Nose and Its Lack: Medieval Nose-cutting and Its Modern Manifestations', *Journal of Women's History* 26.1, pp. 45–67.

Smith, Susan (2016) '"Limbitless Solutions": The Prosthetic Arm, Iron Man and the Science Fiction of Technoscience', *Science Fiction and Medical Humanities* 42, pp. 259–64.

Smith, Marquard and Morra, Joanne (2006) *The Prosthetic Impulse: From a Posthuman Present to a Biocultural Future*. Cambridge, MA: MIT Press.

Sneed, Debby (2020) 'The Architecture of Access: Ramps at Ancient Greek Healing Sanctuaries', *Antiquity* 94.376, pp. 1015–29.

Snowden, Frank M. (1970) *Blacks in Antiquity: Ethiopians in Greco-Roman Experience*. London: Belknapp.

Snowden, Frank M. (1991) *Before Colour Prejudice: The Ancient View of Blacks.* Cambridge, MA: Harvard University Press.

Southwell-Wright, William (2013) 'Past Perspectives: What Can Archaeology Offer Disability Studies?', in Wappett, Matthew and Arndt, Katrina (eds.) *Emerging Perspectives on Disability Studies.* London: Springer, pp. 67–97.

Squire, Michael (ed.) (2016) *Sight and the Ancient Senses.* London: Routledge.

St Clair, Archer (2003) *Carving as Craft: Palatine East and the Greco-Roman Bone and Ivory Carving Tradition.* Baltimore, MD: Johns Hopkins University Press.

Stuckert, Caroline M. and Kricun, Morrie E. (2011) 'A Case of Bilateral Forefoot Amputation from the Romano-British Cemetery of Lankhills, Winchester, UK', *International Journal of Paleopathology* 1, pp. 111–16.

Sudhoff, K. (1917) 'Der Stelzfuss aus Capua', *Mitteilungen zur Geschichte der Medizin und der Naturwissenschaften* 16, pp. 217–93.

Sumler, Alan (2010) 'A Catalogue of Shoes: Puns in Herodas *Mime 7*', *Classical World* 103.4, pp. 465–75.

Swain, Simon (ed.) (2007) *Seeing the Face, Seeing the Soul: Polemon's Physiognomy from Classical Antiquity to Medieval Islam.* Oxford: Oxford University Press.

Talbert, Richard A. (2017) *Roman Portable Sundials: The Empire in Your Hand.* Oxford: Oxford University Press.

Taub, Liba (2017) *Science Writing in Greco-Roman Antiquity.* Cambridge: Cambridge University Press.

Thompson, Frederick H. (2003) *The Archaeology of Slavery.* London: Duckworth.

Thurston, Alan J. (2007) 'Paré and Prosthetics: The Early History of Artificial Limbs', *ANZ Journal of Surgery* 77.12, pp. 1114–19.

Tilley, Lorna (2012) 'The Bioarchaeology of Care', *The SAA Archaeological Record* 12.3, pp. 39–41.

Tilley, Lorna (2015) *Theory and Practice in the Bioarchaeology of Care.* London: Springer.

Tilley, Lorna and Schrenk, Alecia (2016) *New Directions in the Bioarchaeology of Care.* London: Springer.

Toner, Jerry (2015) 'Barbers, Barbershops and Searching for Roman Popular Culture', *Papers of the British School at Rome* 83, pp. 91–109.

Toynbee, Jocelyn M. C. (1973, reissued 2013) *Animals in Roman Life and Art.* Barnsley: Pen and Sword.

Trentin, Lisa (2011) 'Deformity in the Roman Imperial Court', *Greece and Rome* 58.2, pp. 195–208.

Trentin, Lisa (2013) 'Exploring Visual Impairment in Ancient Rome', in Laes, Christian, Goodey, Chris F. and Rose, M. Lynn (eds.) *Disabilities in Roman Antiquity: Disparate Bodies:* A Capite ad Calcem. Leiden: Brill, pp. 89–114.

Trentin, Lisa (2017) 'The "Other Romans": Deformed Bodies in the Visual Arts of Rome', in Laes, Christian (ed.) *Disabilities in Antiquity.* London: Routledge, pp. 233–47.

Trinquier, Jean (2002) 'Les vertus magiques et hygiéniques du vert dans l'antiquité', in Villard, Laurence (ed.) *Couleurs et vision dans l'antiquité classique.* Rouen: Publications de l'Université de Rouen, pp. 97–128.

Turfa, Jean M. and Becker, Marshall J. (2019) 'A Very Distinctive Smile', in Draycott, Jane (ed.) *Prostheses in Antiquity*. London: Routledge, pp. 49–70.

Upson-Saia, Kristi (2011) 'Resurrecting Deformity: Augustine on Wounded and Scarred Bodies in the Heavenly Realm', in Schumm, Darla and Stoltzfus, Michael (eds.) *Disability in Judaism, Christianity, and Islam: Sacred Texts, Historical Traditions and Social Analysis*. New York: Palgrave Macmillan, pp. 93–122.

Vainshtein, Olga (2012) '"I Have a Suitcase Just Full of Legs Because I Need Options for Different Clothing": Accessorizing Bodyscapes', *Fashion Theory* 16.2, pp. 139–70.

Van Dam, R. (1993) *Saints and Their Miracles in Late Antique Gaul*. Princeton, NJ: Princeton University Press.

Van Lommel, Kornell (2015) 'Heroes and Outcasts: Ambiguous Attitudes towards Impaired and Disfigured Roman Veterans', *Classical World* 109.1, pp. 91–117.

van Schaik, Katherine (2019) 'Living Prostheses', in Draycott, Jane (ed.) *Prostheses in Antiquity*. London: Routledge, pp. 140–58.

van Straten, Folkert T. (1981) 'Gifts for the Gods', in Versnel, Hendrick S. (ed.) *Faith, Hope, and Worship: Aspects of Religious Mentality in the Ancient World*. Leiden: Brill, pp. 65–151.

Vespa, M. and Zucker, A. (2020) 'Imiter ou communiquer? L'intention du singe dans la littérature gréco-romaine', *Metis* 18, pp. 233–50.

von Brun, W. (1926) 'Der Stelzfuss von Capua und die antiken Prothesen', *Archiv für Geschichte der Medizin* 18, pp. 351–60, table xiii.

Voultsiadou, Eleni (2007) 'Sponges: An Historical Survey of their Knowledge in Greek Antiquity', *Journal of the Marine Biological Association of the UK*, 87, pp. 1757–63.

Walter, Katie L. (2016) 'Fragments for a Medieval Theory of Prosthesis', *Textual Practice* 30.7, pp. 1345–63.

Warne, Vanessa (2008) 'Artificial Leg', *Victorian Review* 34.1, pp. 29–33.

Warne, Vanessa (2009) '"To Invest a Cripple with Peculiar Interest": Artificial Legs and Upper-Class Amputees at Mid-Century', *Victorian Review* 35.2, pp. 83–100.

Watkins, Calvert (2002) 'Pindar's Rigveda', *Journal of the American Oriental Society* 122.2, p. 432.

Weaver, David S., Perry, George H., Macchiarelli, Roberto, and Bondioli, Luca (2000) 'A Surgical Amputation in 2nd Century Rome', *The Lancet* 356, p. 686.

Wierschowski, Lothar (1995) 'Kriegsdienstverweigerung im römischen Reich', *Ancient Society* 26, pp. 205–39.

Wikander, Örjan (2008) 'Gadgets and Scientific Instruments', in Oleson, John P. (ed.) *The Oxford Handbook of Engineering and Technology in the Classical World*. Oxford: Oxford University Press, pp. 785–99.

Wild, John-Peter (1993) 'A Hairmoss Cap from Vindolanda', in Jaacks, G. and Tidow, K. (eds.) *Archäologische Textilfunde – Archaeological Textiles: Textilsymposium Neumünster 4.-7.5.1993 (NESAT V), Neumuenster 1994*. Neumünster: Textilmuseum Neumünster, pp. 61–68.

Wills, David (1995) *Prosthesis*. Stanford, CA: Stanford University Press.

Wilson, Andrew I. (2008) 'Machines in Greek and Roman Technology', in Oleson, John P. (ed.) *The Oxford Handbook of Engineering and Technology in the Classical World*. Oxford: Oxford University Press, pp. 337–66.

Wirthe, Henning (2010) *Die linke Hand: Wahrnehmung und Bewertung in der griechischen und römischen Antike*. Stuttgart: Franz Steiner Verlag.

Withey, Alun (2016) *Technology, Self-Fashioning and Politeness in Eighteenth Century Britain: Refined Bodies*. London: Palgrave Macmillan.

Wondergem, Marloes, Lieben, George, Brouman, Shirley, van den Brekel, Michiel W. F., and Lohouis, Peter J. F. M. (2016) 'Patients' Satisfaction with Facial Prostheses', *British Journal of Oral and Maxillofacial Surgery* 54.4, pp. 394–9.

Wood, H. (1883) 'Roman Urns Found Near Rainham Creek, on the Medway', *Archaeologica Cantiana* 15, pp. 108–10.

Wrenhaven, Kelly L. (2011) 'Greek Representations of the Slave Body: A Conflict of Ideas?', in Alston, Richard, Hall, Edith, and Proffitt, Laura (eds.) *Reading Ancient Slavery*. London: Bristol Classical Press, pp. 97–120.

Wyke, Maria (2002) *The Roman Mistress: Ancient and Modern Representations*. Oxford: Oxford University Press.

Zetzel, James E. G. (1996) 'Poetic Baldness and Its Cure', *Materiali e discussioni per l'analisi dei testi classici* 36, pp. 73–100.

Zimmerman, Kees (1998) *One Leg in the Grave: The Miracle of the Transplantation of the Black Leg by the Saints Cosmas and Damian*. Bunge: Elsevier.

Zimmerman, Kees, Fracchia, Carmen, de Jong, Jan, and Santing, Catrien (eds.) (2013) *One Leg in the Grave Revisited: The Miracle of the Transplantation of the Black Leg by the Saints Cosmas and Damian*. Groningen: Barkhuis.

Ziskowski, Angela (2012) 'Clubfeet and Kypselids: Contextualising Corinthian Padded Dancers in the Archaic Period', *Annual of the British School at Athens* 107, pp. 211–32.

Index Locorum

Ancient Documentary Sources
CIL III 2117, 148
CIL V 7044, 148
CIL VI 9402 = *Inscr. Grut.* 645, 89, 125
CIL VI 9403 = *ILS* 7713, 125–6
CIL VI 95, 148
CIL VI 2911, 148
CIL VI 6939, 148
CIL VI 7655, 149
CIL VI 7885, 149
CIL VI 9202, 148
CIL VI 9222, 148
CIL VI 9375, 149
CIL VI 9397, 149
CIL VI 9528, 149
CIL VI 33423, 149
CIL VI 37374, 149
CIL VI 37793, 149
CIL XI 1305 = *ILS* 3135, 4, 106
CIL XIV Suppl. P. 662 n. 14, 149
Epidaurian iamata A9 (*IG*[2] I, 121–122.9), 4, 43, 87
Epidaurian iamata A19 (*IG* IV[2], 1.19), 4, 43, 106
Epidaurian iamata B17, 158
Epidaurian iamata B18, 158
Epidaurian iamata C14, 158
Epidaurian iamata C21, 158
P.Giss. 20 = *W.Chr.* 94 = *P.Giss. Apoll.* 11, 7, 125–6

Ancient Literary Sources
Ach. Tat. 5.17, 8.5, 111
Ael. *NA* 7.21, 162
Ael. *VH* 1.26, 32
  2.26, 32
  4.17, 32
Agnellus of Ravenna, *Agnelli Liber Pontificalis Ecclesiae Ravennatis* c.137, MGH SSRLI 367, 93
Amm. Marc. 15.3, 57
  17.10, 35
  22.21, 32
  29.5.22, 56
  29.31, 56
Andocides, *On the Mysteries* 62, 158
Apollod. *Bibl.* 2.1–3, 7
App. *B Civ.* 2.76.318, 81
App. *Hann.* 8.118, 56
Apul. *Met.* 2.8, 106, 116
  2.30, 73–4
  9.12, 111
  11.8, 32
Arist. *Aves.* 1378–9, 61
Arist. *Eccl.* 1094, 61
Arist. *Pax* 1209–64, 147
Arist. *Ran.* 294, 61
Arist. *Sph.* 31, 136
Arist. *Cat.* 10.13a, 42–3
Arist. *De an.* 2.1, 472 B, 90
Arist. *Eth. Nic.* 1162b4, 166
Arist. *Gen. an.* 5.783b, 105
Arist. *Hist. an.* 585b, 133
  586a, 133
Arist. *Metaph.* 5.27.4, 43, 106
Arist. *Oec.*, 142
Arist. *Part. An.* 2.16.659a9, 146
Arist. *Pol.* 1254b25–7, 166
  1.4.3–4, 142
  8.21, 142
Arist. *[Pr.]* 32.3, 32.5, 145
Arist. *Rhet.* 1367a32–3, 9, 166
Arist. *On Marvellous Things Heard* 58/834b, 89
Arist. *On the Pythagoreans* Fr. 191(1), 32
Arist. *Thesm.* 258, 32, 112
Arr. *Anab.* 4.7.3–4, 56, 83
Arr. *Ind.* 6.9, 121
Artem. *On.* 1.18, 111
  1.22, 111
  1.30, 111
  4.30, 166
Ath. 6.248f (Satyrus, *Life of Philip* fr. 3, *FHG*3.161, fr. 24), 87
  8.338a, 133
  10.415a-b, 32
  12.524d, 86

August. *Ep.* 34 (*Epistle* 133), 82
Avienus, *Fables* 11.7–12, 32, 117, 174

Babylonian Talmud Chagiga 3a, 32
Babylonian Talmud, Nedarim 66a–b, 32, 98
  66b, 36, 147
Babylonian Talmud, Shabbat 65a, 98, 151
Babylonian Talmud, Yebamot 102b–103a, 32
Babylonian Talmud Yoma 78b, 32

Caelius Aurelianus, *Chronic Diseases* 1.12, 3.131, 109
Caes. *BCiv.* 3.53.4, 35, 81
Caes. *BGall.* 7.4, 82
Caes. *BHisp.* 12, 56
Calp. *Ecl.* 1.7, 144
Cass. Dio. 11 Zonaras 8.15, 83
  54.9.8–9, 40
  57.17, 158
  60.2.3, 158
  67.7.4, 122
  80.2, 32, 117
Cato, *Agr.* 135, 65
Celsus, *Med.* 1.4.1, 109
  3.18.8, 109
  3.20.4, 109
  3.23.7, 109
  4.2.6, 109
  4.2.9, 109
  4.11.8, 109
  5.26.1, 47
  6.1.1, 105
  6.12, 9, 32, 79, 96, 147
  6.14, 77
  6.2.2, 109
  6.6.8 E, 109
  6.6.15, 109
  6.7.1 D, 109
  6.7.4, 109
  6.7.8 B, 109
  7.7.8 B, 77
  7.7.15 D, 109
  7.33.1, 47
  9.1, 77
  12.1, 79
Cic. *Leg.* 2.24.60, 96
Cic. *Off.* 1.38, 46
  3.11, 55
Cic. *Phil.* 8.15, 46
  8.16, 49
Cic. *Pis.* 19, 83
Cic. *Tusc.* 2.52, 85
Claud. *Cons. Hon.* 4.446–7, 121
Clement of Alexandria, *The Instructor* 3.63.1–2, 114
Cyprian, *Letters* 77.3, 111

Dem. 27.9, 147
  54.20, 158
Dig. 9.2.5.3, 84
  39.4.16.7, 121, 150
Din. 1.36, 158
Dio Chrys. *Or.* 8.28, 32, 59, 88, 141, 150
Diod. Sic. 1.11.3, 53–4
  1.78.3, 81
  1.78.4–5, 35, 81–2
  2.58.4, 43
  3.52, 32
  4.64.3–4, 68
  23.16, 83
  33.7.6–7, 110
  33.14.3, 55, 82
Diog. Laert. 5.9, 84
  9.59, 85
  11, 32
Dion. Hal. *Ant. Rom.* 5.23.2–25, 35, 81
Diosc. 5.94, 145

Epiph. *Adv. haeres.* 64.70.5–17 (*Apocryphon of Ezekiel* fr. 1), 159
Eugentius, *Mythologies* 2.15, 7
Eur. *Hec.* 65–7, 157
  261, 157
  281, 157
Eur. *Phoen.* 1546, 160
  1548–9, 157
Eutr. 1.383, 121

Flor. 2.13.50, 81
  2.30, 86
  2.30.25, 121
Frontin. *Str.* 3.15.4, 56
  4.7.32, 81
  4.17, 54

Gal. *Comp. Loc.* 1.2, 102
Gal. *Hipp. Art.* 18A.667–83K, 48
Gal. *Ind.* 4–5, 10, 138
Gal. *MM* 14.8, 105, 108
Gal. *Nat. Fac.* 3.13.192, 48
Gal. *Subf. Emp.* 6.54, 90
Gal. *Aff. Dig.* 4 5.17–18 K, 84, 86
Greek Anthology
  9.11 (Philippus or Isodorus), 158–9
  9.12 (Leonidas of Alexandria), 159
  9.13 (Plato the Younger), 159
  9.13B (Antiphilus of Byzantium), 159
  9.233 (Erycius), 32, 35, 61, 144

11.68 (Lucilius), 32, 35, 116
11.307, 142
11.310 (Lucilius), 32, 35, 115, 116
11.408 (Lucilius), 97
11.374 (Macedonius), 32, 35, 115, 146
6.254 (Myrinus), 32, 123
Gregory of Tours, *VM* 3.9, 5, 25, 32, 66, 130
4.41, 5, 25, 32, 66, 67

Hermesianax, *Fragments (Leontion)* 2.4, 35, 84
Herod. 6, 135
6.57–73, 135, 152
6.87–8, 152
7, 135
7.56–64, 135, 152
Hdt. 3.146.3, 158
4.71.2, 139
4.8–10, 79
9.36–7, 29, 32, 61, 129, 146
9.37, 8, 57
9.38, 8, 57
Herodian, *History of the Empire* 4.7.3, 32
Hes. *Op.* 51, 68
Hippoc. *Art.* 33.9–10, 9, 32, 79, 96, 147
53, 68, 132, 142
58, 68, 71, 127, 132
62, 133,
68–9, 46,
Hippoc. *Carn.* 14, 105
Hippoc. *Gland.* 4, 105
Hippoc. *Mochl.* 20, 68
21, 68
23, 68, 132
24, 68
32, 133
Hippoc. *Morb. sacr.* 3, 133
Hippoc. *Mul.* 1.11, 9
Hippoc. *Nat. mul.* 1.11, 9
Hippoc. *Nat. puer.* 9, 105
Hom. *Il.* 18.410–18, 142, 154–9
Hom. *Od.* 9, 170
Hor. *Epod.* 5, 74
Sat. 1.8.47–50, 32, 35, 74, 97, 115, 116, 117, 174
Hyg. *Fab.* 83, 7, 8, 32

Jacob de Voragine, *Legenda Aurea/The Golden Legend* 2.143.4, 1
Joseph. *AJ* 14.10, 86
Joseph. *BJ* 1.9, 86
5.455, 56
Joseph. *Vit.* 47, 32
177, 54
Juv. 5, 111
6, 117
6.120–2, 32, 35
12.81, 111
13.164–65, 121

Laws of the Twelve Tables 10.8–9, 32, 96, 147, 174
Lev Rabbah 4.5, 159
Livy 24.42, 158
34.52.12, 111
45.44, 111
Livy, *Epit.* 95, 56
Lucan *Pharsalia* 3.603–26, 50–1
6.213–16, 35, 81
6.413–587, 74
Luc. *Alex.* 40, 32
Luc. *De Merc. cond.* 5, 162
Luc. *De Salt* 54, 32
Luc. *Dial. meret.* 8, 112
11.4, 32, 117
39.11, 116
Luc. *Dial. mort.* 416, 32
Luc. *Imag.* 5, 107–8
Luc. *Ind.* 6, 32, 61, 146, 151, 157
Luc. *Pod.* 54–7, 68
Luc. *Rhet.* 24, 32, 35, 98, 115
Luc. *Somn.* 6–13, 142
Luc. *Tox.* 10, 35
62, 35
Luc. *Ver. hist.* 1.22, 32, 152
1.25, 32, 88
Luke 5.17–26, 158
22.50–1, 4
Lycoph. *Alex.* 72–80, 145
149, 7
Lys. 4.9, 158
24.7, 167
24.11, 163
24.12, 163

Macrob. *Sat.* 1.26, 157
2.7, 109
7.10, 105
Mart. 1.72, 32, 35, 97–8, 115, 149
2.29.9–10, 100
2.34, 98
2.41, 115
2.74, 111
2.82, 86
3.38, 32
3.51, 98
3.54, 98
3.85, 83–4
3.90, 98
4.38, 98
4.58, 98
5.37.8, 121
5.43, 32, 35, 98, 115

Mart. 1.72 (cont.)
 5.49, 105
 5.49.12–13, 113
 5.68, 121
 5.84, 98
 6.12, 32
 7.18, 98
 7.58, 98
 8.33.22, 100
 9.38, 32, 35, 98, 115, 116
 9.4, 98
 9.78, 98
 10.25, 98
 10.100, 32, 61, 146
 11.19, 98
 12.23, 32, 35, 98, 115, 116
 12.25, 87
 12.45, 32, 35
 12.82, 105
 12.84, 32
 14.26, 121, 150
 14.46, 32
 14.56, 35, 115
Mark 1.1–12, 158
Matthew 9.1–8, 158
Mekilta on Exodus 15:1, 159
Mishnah Shabbat 6.5, 32
 6.8, 32

Non. 1, *Hermotimus* 86, 111
Nonnus, *Dion.* 2.427–35, 35, 50
 15.24–30, 32
 22.196–202, 35, 50
 47.587–93, 89

Ov. *Am.* 1.14., 106, 115–16, 121
Ov. *Ars am* 2.4.37–44, 122
 3.135–58, 116
 3.159–68, 121
 3.163–8, 113, 121
 3.242–50, 106, 116, 121
 3.244–7, 117
 3.249–50, 117, 174
Ov. *Her.* 6.83–94, 74
Ov. Met. 6.405, 7, 32
 6.613–18, 84
 14.654–660, 32

Palaephatus, *On Unbelievable Things* 12, 9, 175
Palestinian Talmud, Shabbat 6.5, 88, 89, 99, 151
Palestinian Talmud, tractate Nedarim 9. 41c, 36, 147
Palestinian Talmud/Yerushalmi Nedarim 9.8 (41c), 32, 89, 98
Paul, 1 *Corinthians* 11.4–8, 112
Paul of Aegina, *Medical Compendium* 6.40.3, 47
 84, 48
Paus. 5.13.4–6, 32
Pers. 6.46–7, 122
Petron. *Sat.* 67, 85
 110, 32, 111, 117, 122, 132
Philo, *That the Worse Is Wont to Attack the Better* 48, 85
Philostr. *Ep.* 22, 32, 115
Philostr. *Imag.* 1.30.7–11, 8, 32
Philostr. *VA* 6.11.18–19, 154
Philostr. *VS* 2.1.588, 164–5
Pind. *Ol.* 1.37, 8, 32
Plaut. *Amph.* 1.1.306, 111
Plaut. *Aul.* 53, 86
 188–9, 35, 86
Plaut. *Cur.* 392–400, 87
Plaut. *Mil.* 1388–9, 84
 1430, 87
Plaut. *Pers.* 797, 86
Plaut. *Rud.* 5.2.16, 111
Plaut. *Trin.* 463–5, 86
Plin. *Ep.* 6.2.2, 100
 7.27, 111
 18.9–10, 167
Plin. *HN* 7.11.50, 133
 7.29, 32, 35, 51, 59, 147, 157
 7.37.124, 79
 8.7, 149
 28.6.24, 32
 33.40, 145
 33.78, 147
 34.59, 45
 34.95, 65, 140
 35.40.147–8, 149
 37.66–7, 90
[Plut.] *Cons. Ad Apoll.* 22, 85
Plut. *Mor.* 18d, 133
 647f–648a, 144
 652f, 108
Plut. *Mor. De frat. amor.* 3.1, 8, 9, 29, 32, 146
 761 C, 57
Plut. *Mor. De Is. et Os.* 4, 110
Plut. *Mor. Lives of the Ten Orators: Antiphon* 849B–D, 85
Plut. *Mor. On Exile* 606B, 83
Plut. *Vit. Caes.* 45.1, 81
Plut. *Vit. Cam.*, 35
Plut. *Vit. Eum.* 14.3, 158
Plut. *Vit. Flam.* 13.6, 111
Plut. *Vit. Galb.* 13.4, 106
Plut. *Vit. Lys.* 9, 55
Plut. *Vit. Num.*, 32

Plut. *Vit. Per.* 27, 158
Plut. *Vit. Pomp.* 71.4, 81
Plut. *Vit. Popl.* 16.4–7, 81
Plut. *Vit. Sert.* 4.2, 35, 81
Polyb. 1.81, 56
3.78, 32, 143
30.18, 111
Porph. *Pyth.* 28, 32
Procop. 3.3.9, 55
3.8.4–55, 83
Prudent. 2.145–8, 160

Quint. 297, 167
297.4, 167
297.13, 167
358, 54
362, 54
372, 54–5
Quint. *Inst.* 8.3.75, 46, 49
8.5.2, 57
Quintus Curtius *History of Alexander* 3.16, 56
Quint. Smyrn. 3.479, 157
5.446–7, 157

Sall. *Hist.* 1.88, 81
Scribonius Largus, *Compositiones medicamentorum* 161, 134
Sen. *Controv.* 10.2, 85
Sen. *Ep.* 27.5–8, 163–4
95.20–1, 106, 108
124.22, 121
Sen. *Ira* 3.26.3, 121
5.17.1, 82
5.18.1–2, 82
5.20.1–2, 82
5.9.2, 90
7.3–4, 82–3
Sen. *QNat.* 1.3.9, 91
1.6.5–6, 91
Sen. *Thy.* 145, 7
Serv. 8.564, 111
Sext. Emp. *Math.* 255–256, 32
Soph. *OC* 867, 157
Phil. 743–50, 45
Stat. *Silv.* 3.3.89, 147
Stat. *Theb.* 94–7, 32, 59, 141
Strabo, *Geog.* 2.30, 49
12.759, 86
16.31, 86
Suet. *Aug.* 24.1, 57
83, 42
91, 158
Suet. *Calig.* 11.1, 34, 117
27, 86
47, 122
Suet. *Claud.* 5, 54, 58
Suet. *Dom.* 18.1, 106
18.2, 106
Suet. *Galb.* 9, 54, 106
21.1
Suet. *Iul.* 45.1–2, 106
51.1, 106
68.4, 35, 81
Suet. *Ner.* 26.1, 32, 117
31, 149
Suet. *Oth.* 12, 32, 113
Suet. *Tib.* 61.6, 42

Tac. *Agr.* 39, 122
Tac. *Germ.* 3.84, 86
19, 112
38, 121
Talmud Sanhedrin 91a–b, 159
Talmud Yerushalmi Shabbat 8:8, 8c, 32
Tertullian, *On the Apparel of Women* 2.7.1–2, 113–14
Theophanes the Confessor *Chronicle* 6187, 92
Chronographia, 32
Theophr. *Hist.* pl. 1.3.2, 131, 146
5.7.7, 68, 131, 146
9.5.2, 144
Tib. 1.4–63–4, 8, 32
Tosefta Shabbat 5:1–2, 32
Tosephta, *Parah.* 3.8, 86
Tractate Nedarim 9; 41c, 89

Val. Max. 1.7, 158
2.8, 158
3.4, 84–5
6.3, 57
6.6, 166
9 External 8, 55, 83
Varro, *Rust.* 1.17, 166
Verg. *G.* 3.7, 9, 32
Vitr. *De arch.* 5.9.5, 90
7.5.8, 90

Xen. *Cyr.* 1.3.2, 32, 112
8.2.5, 134
Xen. *Hell.* 2.1.31, 55
Xen. *Mem.* 1.54, 49
3.10.9, 147
Xen. *Oec.* 6.2, 142
10.2–3, 7, 102–3

Index

amputation, 7, 12, 14, 17, 38, 40, 42, 52, 58, 65, 66, 71, 76, 124, 151
  arm, 49, 59
  as mutilation, 57
  as punishment, 53, 82
  as torture, 55
  bioarchaeological evidence for, 42, 44, 49, 65
  cause of, 45
  fingers, 57
  foot, 8, 49, 57, 61, 129
  hand, 54
  leg, 12, 19, 25, 45, 49, 61, 144
  result of military action, 14, 50
  surgical techniques for, 43, 45, 47, 48
Anglesey Leg, 14, *See also* Marquess of Anglesey
animal assistance, 152, 159, 163, *See also* living protheses
Asklepios, 4, 7, 87, 106
assisitive technology
  canes, crutches, staffs, and sticks, 157
assistive technology, 11, 16, 25, 28, 38, 42, 45, 69, 125, 127, 130, 132, 134, 142, 146, 153, 154, 156
  automata, 122, 154, 166
  canes, crutches, staffs, and sticks, 38, 42, 59, 63, 67, 68, 69, 71, 130, 132, 134, 137, 152
  corrective footwear, 130, 133, 134
  lenses, 91
  litter or sedan chair, 158
  staff as eyes, 68, 160
  walking frames, 38, 42
  wheeled conveyances, 31, 69, 152

baldness, 4, 43, 105, 106, 108, 113, 115, *See also* hair loss
  views on, 106, 108
blindness, 4, 43, 77, 157, 158, 161, 166, 168
  guide dog, 161, *See also* living prostheses

Cairo Toe, 37, 63, 127, 146, 168
Capua Limb, 25, 37, 63, 67, 91, 137, 139, 147, 150
caregiving, 156, *See also* living protheses
children, 31, 41, 69, 85, 105, 124, 157
cosmesis, 11, 76
cosmetics, 36, 102, 115, 142
  alkanet, 102, 103
  kommotikon, 102
  kosmetikon, 102
  white lead, 98, 102, 103

deafness, 10, 168
dentistry, 94
  Etruscan, 94, 96, 142
dentures, 47, 98, 100, 143
dildo, 135, 152, *See also* phallus
disability, 11, 20, 22, 27, 28, 39, 42, 92, 129, 156, 163, 164, 171
disease, 9, 44, 47, 49, 58
  alopecia, 108
  gangrene, 19, 46
  gout, 108, 134
  hydrocephalus, 69, 133
  of the eye, 77, *See also* eye ailments
  ringworm, 109
  tuberculosis, 25, 66

epilepsy, 109
exhibits
  Glasgow School of Art
    'Prosthetic Greaves', 16
  National Museum of Scotland
    Technology by Design, 21
  V & A Museum
    Alexander McQueen Savage Beauty, 20
    Frida Kahlo Making Herself Up, 18
eye ailments
  cataract, 77, 87
  ophthalmia, 109
  trachoma, 77
eyepatch, 87

fractured bones, 67, 69, 132, 139, 149, 174

greaves, 16, 139
Greville Chester Toe, 63, 127, 168

hair, 31, 35, 73, 74, 75, 76, 87, 91, 97, 104, 173
  modification
    dying, 110, 115
    plucking grey/white, 109, 110
  natural loss
    illness, 117
  replacement. *See* wigs
  sacrifice, 110
    pars pro toto, 110, 111
    votive, 106
  shaving
    as punishment/mutilation, 111
    medical treatment, 109
    religious ritual, 110
  styling, 115, 119
hair loss, 4, 104, 106, 116, 122, 144
  natural, 104, 105
    age, 105, 106
    illness, 107, 109
  women
    moral judgement, 106, 108
hairpiece. *See* wigs
healing sanctuary, 4, 5, 43, 106
Hemmaberg Limb, 37, 137, 147

insanity, 109

Julius Caesar, 56, 81, 82, 86

Kahlo, Frida, 19

law, 100
  Chinese, 25
  Egyptian, 81
  Hindu, 53
  Roman, 96, 166
    Twelve Tables, 96, 147
living prostheses, 38, 154, 156, 159, *See also* caregiving
  animals
    ape/monkey, 162
    dog, 168
    donkeys/mules, 163
    horse, 163
  children, 157
  slaves, 157, 166
luxuria, 151, 153

manufacturers, 27, 125
  armourer, 139
  carpenter, 27, 126, 130, 136
  cutler, 137
  eborarius, 137, 149
  faber ocularíarius, 125
  goldsmith, 137, 143, 147
  kōloplastēs, 126
  leather-worker, 27, 130
  metal-worker, 27
  nagra, 126
  shoemaker, 135
  silversmith, 137
  wig-maker, 112, 114, 121
Marquess of Anglesey, 12, 15
medical treatises
  Archigenes, 47
  Celsus, 46, 77, 96, 98, 109, 147
  Galen, 48, 105, 108, 137
  Heliodorus, 47
  Hippocrates, 45, 47, 48, 68, 96, 98, 104, 127, 130, 131, 147, 154
  Paul of Aegina, 159
miraculous healing, 4, 5, 25, 43, 66, 106, 158
missing
  body part, 9, 10, 30, 175
  ear, 75
  eye, 4, 11, 76, 87, 169
  foot, 65
  limb, 11, 65
  nose, 11, 75, 76
  shoulder, 8
  teeth, 96, 99, 173
mobility, 29, 66, 68, 71, 92, 129, 130, 132, 133, 139, 150, 158, 162
mutilation, 35, 43, 56, 82, 83, 84, 111
  castration, 84
  facial, 35, 82, 92, 93
  punishment, 25, 56
  self, 9, 57, 84, 85
  torture, 82

occupational hazards, 144

phallus, 135, 152, *See* dildo
Povegliano Veronese Hand, 37
prostheses, 5, 6, 7, 8, 9, 11, 12, 13, 15, 18, 25, 27, 28, 29, 30, 37, 42, 45, 58, 59, 65, 66, 67, 71, 122, 136, 139, 141, 142, 146, 151, 152, 157, 172, 174
  body part
    eye, 61, 88, 89, 90, 91
    facial, 35, 74, 100, 137
    foot, 31, 65
    hair, 31, 104, 112, 123
    hand, 10, 31, 51, 61
    leg, 12, 23, 31, 63, 65
    nose, 92, 137
    shoulder, 8, 10

prostheses (cont.)
teeth, 31, 149, 173
thigh, 10
toe, 31, 61, 128
grave goods, 25
makers of, 124, 127, 135, *See also* manufacturers
material
bronze, 63, 65, 147
diamond, 61, 89
gold, 10, 61, 137
iron, 10, 147
ivory/horn, 8, 10, 61, 137, 149
leather, 65, 147
malachite, 61, 89
silver, 137
wax, 74
wood, 61, 63, 65, 137, 146, 147

tooth extraction, 77, 79, *See also* dentistry
transplantation, 1, 2
Turfan Limb, 25, 26, 63
type of amputation
surgical techniques for, 44

votive, 106, 108, 123, 172
anatomical, 5
manufacture of, 126, *See also* manufacturers

wigs, 5, 10, 30, 38, 112, 113, 115, 116, 117, 120, 121, 122, 123, 142, 143, 150, 166, 173
'captive hair', 121, 150
'Indian hair', 121, 150
archaeological evidence for, 117, 119, 120, 123
human hair, 119, 166
linen, 119, 120, 150
plant fibres, 120, 150
witches, 73, 74, 97
wood, 5, 8, 10, 21, 61, 63, 65, 68, 98, 130, 136, 146, 147, 173
ash, 21
bay, 68, 131, 146
citrus, 149
elm, 146
fig, 151
holly, 146
imported, 146, 147
Judas-tree, 146
mallow, 131, 146
olive, 61, 131, 146

For EU product safety concerns, contact us at Calle de José Abascal, 56–1°,
28003 Madrid, Spain or eugpsr@cambridge.org.

www.ingramcontent.com/pod-product-compliance
Lightning Source LLC
LaVergne TN
LVHW010335220926
848484LV00004BB/905

* 9 7 8 1 0 0 9 1 6 8 3 9 7 *